Health Freaks

Health Freaks

America's Diet Champions and the
Specter of Chronic Illness

· ·

TRAVIS A. WEISSE

The University of North Carolina Press Chapel Hill

© 2024 Travis A. Weisse
All rights reserved
Set in Charis by Westchester Publishing Services
Manufactured in the United States of America

Complete Library of Congress Cataloging-in-Publication Data for this title is
available at https://lccn.loc.gov/2024021609.

ISBN 978-1-4696-8299-0 (cloth: alk. paper)
ISBN 978-1-4696-8300-3 (pbk.: alk. paper)
ISBN 978-1-4696-8301-0 (epub)
ISBN 978-1-4696-8302-7 (pdf)

Cover art created by PaintedDreams/stock.adobe.com using AI.

For Kathleen

Contents

Illustration

Health Freaks

Introduction

The Mise en Place

. . . .

I grew up in the 1990s, the only child of a pair of certifiable health freaks. My parents live for the singular, relentless pursuit of dietary perfection. Since the late 1970s, they have experimented with many different diet programs, but their underlying goal has always been the same: to eat as healthily as humanly possible. As you can imagine, dear reader, this upbringing cultivated in me—a scrawny towheaded know-it-all kid bedecked with a bowl cut and white knee socks—an unusual relationship with food to say the least. My dad, renowned as the family "food police," trained me to be especially defensive against the most commonplace of American foods. I was on guard during every meal in the school cafeteria, on edge every time a plate circulated at friends' or extended family's houses, and suspicious of every restaurant. I was a dietary anomaly in every social group I moved through for never having even sampled cow's milk, cheese, beef, bacon, hotdogs, or ham. It was not just animal products either: my lunchbox virtually never saw a brand name. I keenly remember salivating over the occasional piece of fruit leather. The foods I toted along with me were a dubious blend of boring and bizarre. And I could never seem to persuade my friends to accept peeled broccoli stems in exchange for illicit chips or cookies.

Like the households of many "health enthusiasts" (my mom's preferred term), we were not gourmets. My parents are both capable, inventive cooks, but they have always been skeptical of if not outright averse to cooking oil, sugar, and salt, which precluded most of the flavors of any mainstream cuisine. In those halcyon days, we were among the few reliable customers of our local Denver Vitamin Cottage, which has since become a large chain of health food stores that goes by Natural Grocers. There were never lines at the checkout when my parents started shopping there in 1986, wielding reusable yarn bags years before the wellness-obsessed hipsters and the rest of the preppy Whole Foods crowd would invade with their canvas totes. Colorado had its share of granolas, of course, but we did not live in hippie Boulder or a ski-bum mountain town. In our suburban stiffness, we would not have fit in with them anyhow. Of the hippies, my parents would say, "We find them uncomfortable"—although virtually everything we ate we owed to their trailblazing.

Not belonging to any health-oriented communities and not being "cookbook people," my parents invented a cooking style of their own through trial and error. They cobbled together a rotating cast of weekly recipes built to mimic dishes they liked at restaurants or expensive prepared foods from the store, albeit heavily modified to suit their dietary idiosyncrasies. In the end, the dishes they created scarcely resembled the originals because we could not eat a meal with fewer than ten vegetables in it and another dozen or so assorted spices and herbs. Our kitchen stores never wanted for such health food store treasures as carob, couscous, Edensoy soy milk, Rice Dream rice milk, millet, pitas, rice cakes, Bragg's Liquid Aminos, and Tofu Pups. These staples were supplemented by a relatively large backyard garden where we grew zucchini, strawberries, tomatoes, carrots, raspberries, pumpkins, corn, and sunflowers. Even today, the food my parents eat is not for the faint of heart (which is not to say it is not good!) because everything, from salads and hot cereal to smoothies and pies, is jam-packed with nutrient-boosting ingredients and thoroughly spiced (did I mention they eschew salt?). Still, it was not unheard of for members of my extended family to escape dinner at our house and get fast food on the way home. Oh, how I envied them!

Though my parents had always seemed so firm in their dietary choices when I was growing up, such certainty betrays the varied paths they took on their lifestyle journey. Remarkably, my parents' health quests began separately. For my dad, a turning point was his sophomore year in high school. As a kid, he and his friend would put a cardboard plug in the change return chute of a vending machine, collect the trapped coins, and reinsert them into the machine to gorge on stolen candy. He was a self-proclaimed addict, eating so much he would make himself sick. Then, he stumbled on an episode of the TV drama *Marcus Welby, M.D.* in which the title character treats a young male patient complaining of stomach aches. When the patient was diagnosed with diabetes, my dad saw in the character's fate a dire warning for his own health. He stopped eating sweets cold turkey at age fourteen. When my parents met several years later, he was still entirely sugar-free; he stiffly refused birthday cakes, holiday pies, soda, and even gum, politesse be damned. Through the end of his adolescence, my dad tried to eat healthily based on his limited understanding of nutrition, but that mostly meant that he binged on protein. He wolfed steak and eggs for breakfast, chugged a gallon or more of milk a day, and demolished Big Macs. Though he claims to have heard that red meat was unhealthy on the news, he did not yet understand the reasoning or the environmental politics; he kept eating it.

Shortly after meeting my dad, yet for unrelated reasons, my mom renounced dairy from her own diet. Like many a young couple living in the shadow of the Rocky Mountains, my parents were drawn inexorably to the outdoors. But whenever they hiked, my mom wheezed uncontrollably, at times unable to catch her breath. When she had a full panel of allergy tests done, asthma was eventually diagnosed. Adamant that she did not want to rely on an inhaler, my mom started perusing the natural healing section at the bookstore. Who could say what drew her to Bernard Jensen's page-turner *Tissue Cleansing Through Bowel Management*, but his theory that ingesting cow's milk triggered systemic inflammation, which in turn caused the body to produce excessive mucus, was all the explanation my mom needed.[1] When quitting dairy relieved her asthma, she says, it encouraged them to ask, "What else can we fix?"

Beyond allergy relief, Jensen claimed, based on comparative anatomical studies with animals, that the human colon was not, evolutionarily speaking, "supposed" to digest meat. Human colons, he argued, more closely resembled the colons of frugivores than carnivores. Eating meat we were ill-suited to process, he reasoned, gradually polluted the colon, resulting in a cascade of chronic ailments. After reading Jensen's theories, my parents grew all the more hesitant about meat eating, and both promptly scheduled colonics—a heterodox procedure that flushes and "detoxifies" the colon with gallons of purified water. Things only ramped up from there. Through the 1980s and 1990s they experimented with lots of other dietary models: the Pritikin Program, the McDougall Program, The Zone. "We melded into who we are today," my mom says.

Though they had toyed with vegetarianism for several years, they did not commit to a fully vegan diet until 1984 when my mom watched the 1978 cult horror mockumentary *Faces of Death*.[2] She had been given it by her father. The VHS cover art boasted grimly that the content had been "Banned in 46 Countries" for its gory footage of death and mutilation, both human and animal. In the film, the main character, a pathologist called Dr. Francis B. Gross, warns viewers that the carnage they are about to see is real: disturbing shots of bloated human corpses and cycling accidents interspersed with grisly images of sheep hanging from meat hooks and a particularly vivid scene where a monkey is beaten to death with a hammer, its head carved open, and its brain devoured. As a mondo movie, some of the scenes *were* genuine—reproduced from unaired newsreels deemed too disturbing for public broadcast—but much of the film (including the monkey brain scene) was staged. Appalled and scarred, my mom declared then that she would no longer eat meat of any kind. Not even having seen the film, my dad agreed.

Shortly after having made their dietary tryst though, my parents were invited to a family friend's house for a birthday party. Unbeknownst to them, their friend's new father-in-law was an executive at Monfort Beef, who had generously catered the birthday party with his own prime cut steaks. Facing tremendous social pressure to enjoy such an expensive treat, my parents capitulated. "We didn't tell them beforehand that we weren't going to eat it," my mom recalled. "It was just assumed that everyone would love to have a $100 steak. So we choked it down, and that was the last time we had beef." Despite the risk of his own social ostracization, my dad has claimed beef was "easy to give up" because he "never believed this macho thing that beef is good for men to grow muscle and all this bullshit."

It should be said, however, that my parents' obsession with perfecting their bodily health is also steeped in decades of familial trauma. My mom is still haunted by images of her grandfather smoking out of the stoma in his throat, of her alcoholic uncle wasting away, of the traumatic death of her younger brother awaiting a heart transplant. While having her hips replaced, my maternal grandmother developed liver cirrhosis from taking too much Tylenol. We have had relatives follow everything their doctor advised yet die anyway. In some cases, medical care itself precipitated these declines: overfilled prescriptions, false diagnoses, and premature releases from hospitals. Witnessing other friends and family members suffer and die from preventable conditions only inflamed my parents' shared passion to take their health into their own hands. My mom's attitude toward all this can be bleak and unforgiving: "If you didn't put any effort into your health, then you got zip. I don't care how much money you have, you've got nothing. I watched lots of people ready to retire, who did all the right things except for their health, then their kids get all the retirement and they get nothing. And that's sad."

Despite believing firmly in science, my parents resent the health care system for its cost, its emotional vacuity, its arrogance in the face of its own limits, and most of all its conspicuous neglect of preventive health measures. "You have to care about your own health," my mom cautions, "because doctors can't see you long enough to care about you." Negative personal experiences and decades of alternative health media have also sown in my parents a certain reluctance toward using technocratic interventions like chemotherapy, pharmaceuticals, and radiation (even dental X-rays), but they do not shy away from vaccines. Still, by rigorously policing the inputs to their bodies, my parents strive to avoid the fates of so many of their friends and family. They seek nothing short of extinguishing all future risk of their developing cancer, heart failure, diabetes, and all the modern world's other killers. They do not just want to coast into the fabled longevity "blue zone," they want to be capable and strong as centenarians.[3] Their chief goal, in my mom's words, is "to have the longest 'health span' [they] can possibly have." If they could stay active and independent, they would do anything to live forever.

In the past few years, the world has evolved to better reflect my parents' long-held dietary convictions. The things we ate that were once rare and deeply unpopular are seeing a surging market today. People are cutting back on beef and experimenting with faux meats, nut milks, ancient grains, and heirloom vegetables. My parents' latest kick is the Whole Foods Plant Based diet. Many of their heroes post slick informational videos on YouTube, which my parents eagerly devour. They have become dedicated subscribers of Michael Greger, Joel Fuhrman, Joel Kahn, Rhonda Patrick, Mic the Vegan, and a myriad of others.

Still, a gradual transformation driven, as theirs has been, by years of inklings and tinkering has its downsides. It's "easy to get sucked into [nutritional] reductionism," my dad admits. "We were in that spot." He does not think there is anything wrong with being nutritionally obsessed though. "Some people might classify us with that 'orthorexia' label," he says, referring to the hypothesized medical condition characterized by an excessive pursuit of healthy food; "I dismiss it because I don't think there's anything wrong with it—it's not like we're doing something harmful. We're trying to make things better. It makes no sense that that's a bad thing." For all their eccentricities, their lifestyle works for them. They do not take any regular medications, they are active, and mostly they are pain-free. When doctors analyze my parents' blood, they are usually shocked at the results. Doctors have even paraded my parents before their office staff and publicly praised them. My mom beams as she says, a bit too self-satisfied, "It feels like the reward for all of the striving."

What's in a Diet?

When I first became interested in studying diet and nutrition as a historian of medicine, I quickly realized that most critical analyses of American dieting culture (whether in the academic or popular press) confined their attention exclusively to yo-yo or crash dieting for weight loss. The story behind America's population-wide shame spiral regarding our collective waistlines is well-known by this point. It began in earnest when clinical measurements of human body weight were first published by physicians in standardized indexes. Statistically normalized standards were drawn around the data to indicate which bodies were acceptable, "normal," or "healthy," and which were evidently not.[4]

As these medical concepts were exported into American homes through commodities such as the bathroom scale or as standardized clothing sizes, they encouraged people (especially women) to understand and position themselves relative to fixed, discrete, numerical standards.[5] To contort themselves into the appropriate shape, Americans purchased all manner of products and media, and adopted a wide range of new personal habits. In some ways, the new pressure to "reduce"—as dieting to lose weight was once known—was reminiscent of Victorian-era corseting albeit modified to accommodate new scientific instruments and rationales. But the twentieth-century cults of youth and thinness were also massively amplified by the new manufacturers of bodily idealizations: the rising tide of women's magazines in the 1880s and 1890s, the advent of department stores, and in the 1910s, Hollywood. Together, these institutions sculpted a new conspicuous consumption model targeting middle- and upper-class urban white women that in the ensuing decades would slowly spread to everyone else. This legacy continues apace today with massive psychosocial pressure on the internet and social media to cultivate a particular bodily aesthetic (one that still typically holds thinness in high regard). Many Americans have since discovered for themselves that the race for weight loss simply cannot be won; no matter the efforts made and prices paid, the fat body stubbornly resists dietary reform.

Nothing of my experiences or what I knew of my parents' journey made sense in this weight-loss–centered model of the diet world, nor did the many other rich features of diet culture. While diets have been not-so-subtly restructuring our self-image, they have grown into engines of the global economy. As kingmakers for the latest and greatest superfoods, from quinoa to acai berries, diets help create billion dollar markets for obscure products, reshaping and even upending local economies and threatening indigenous communities in the process.[6] Popular dietary advice appears in nearly every tabloid, magazine, and newspaper; it accompanies nearly every alternative medical practice and wellness technique; and it is intimately entwined with every sport (professional or amateur) and all the ultrapopular fitness cults, from yoga to CrossFit. Political radicals from the right propagate dietary myths just as eagerly as the left. Diets pepper our food supply with alluring buzzwords and ominous acronyms, they guilt us into choking down foods we may dislike because they have been deemed good for us, and they compel us to consume things that scarcely resemble food (for example, activated charcoal, protein powder, and cotton balls). As more Americans abide by an ever-widening array of dietary restrictions, once-humdrum events like potlucks, barbecues, and shared meals at holidays have devolved into a Gordian knot of social accommodation.

The diet cultures featured in this book held ideals of health, longevity, disease prevention, and bodily restoration at their center. Scholars of fatness and disability have demonstrated repeatedly that health, fitness, and longevity are not value-neutral concepts, and the programs featured here certainly did not promote a "health at every size" or disability-inclusive mentality. The weight loss and fitness industries have clearly shaped much of our global thinking about fatness, food, health, sex appeal, the able body, and embodiment (for better or worse), and my aim is not to overturn these well-established arguments. Instead, I hope to broaden the narrative by presenting a different branch in the history of American dieting, one that was more self-consciously animated by dissatisfaction with the health care system. Rather than focus on the drive toward the ideal body per se, this book will examine how certain popular diets attracted and treated patients struggling with (or trying desperately to avoid) chronic ailments such as heart disease and cancer. In taking this perspective, I hope to fundamentally reorient our historical conception of dieting culture(s) by articulating the public role that diets played in shaping the twentieth-century American health environment. Changes in the disease landscape over the course of the twentieth century transformed health care and patient expectations thereof, fueling the transformation of popular diets into a new kind of vernacular or alternative medicine, one that inspired the droves of loyal followers I have lovingly termed "health freaks" to take their health into their own hands.

American Health Freaks

Although I recognize that labeling anyone—let alone my own parents—a health freak could seem a bit harsh, following the lead of food historians Warren Belasco and Harvey Levenstein I intend the phrase to invoke the freak scene of the 1960s and 1970s, which coincided with the era when my parents (and many of the patients in this book) were first "turning on" to alternative healing cultures.[7] Members of the freak scene—often conflated with hippies—were social and political radicals; they embodied a passionate devotion to a subculture that was not widely understood or accepted by the mainstream. This revolutionary "freak" serves as a useful archetype for the many dietary enthusiasts featured in this book. I find the term "health freak" especially fitting to use in this context because it seems to have originated from that era whereas comparable (yet more clearly ableist) phrases such as "neat freak" or "clean freak" only arose in the middle to late 1980s.[8] By contrast, health freak has usually been used only playfully to denote someone who exerts uncommon levels of restraint over their lifestyle to promote a greater sense of personal embodied health.

To understand and appreciate the full breadth of motivations driving the dieters in this book, it is imperative to think expansively about embodied health and well-being. Dieters from different cultures, who participated in different programs with different medical histories, conceptualized the intangible essence of health and longevity in innumerable ways. Some understood their health as an extension of a complex political or religious cosmology whereas others merely sought relief from daily symptoms of chronic disease. These sometimes overlapping, sometimes mutually exclusive logics predict the contemporary formulation of "wellness," which rhetoric scholar Colleen Derkatch describes as "the optimization of an individual's daily life across multiple domains (physical, psychological, social, and spiritual), emphasizing function over dysfunction, agency over passivity, and overall well-being over mere bodily health."[9] Instead of understanding health as just one among many different factors motivating dietary pursuits, following Derkatch I view health as a wide lens through which myriad other social concerns can be made legible. By centering dieters' concerns with the health care system, this book seeks to highlight the degree to which these consumer-patients' social attitudes and cultural experiences undergirded their idiosyncratic conceptions of bodily health.

Chronic Dissatisfaction

Though the American dieting tradition long predates the mid-twentieth century, the generation of "diet gurus" who emerged after World War II marked a fundamental shift in how dieting was understood and enacted.[10] While dieting for one's health was not a novel concept per se, it changed significantly in shape and character alongside the increased epidemiological significance of chronic disease in the American health landscape. As the scientific health care system grew in efficiency, fewer people succumbed to infections (especially during childhood) and average life spans increased. After wonder drugs such as penicillin and public vaccinations mostly brought to heel the contagious epidemics that had ravaged earlier generations, their relative absence buoyed the number and severity of complex chronic degenerative conditions—heart disease, cancer, adult-onset diabetes, osteoporosis, rheumatoid arthritis—which filled the vacuum of morbidity and mortality.

Although chronic diseases were not new when they became the nation's leading killers in the 1950s, in the decades prior they had still been primarily understood as natural sequelae of aging rather than as illnesses unto themselves. As these bodily states became more overtly medicalized, public expectations remained high that laboratory science would continue to produce miracles that could quash chronic ailments as easily as infectious ones.[11] Emboldened by their two-front victory in World War II—made possible in large part by scientific advances—Americans began conceptualizing good health and a longer life as not only technologically possible but necessary: a core human right. Yet rather than advocate for broad preventive measures (whether austere behavioral changes or costly social or environmental modifications) to reduce the total population risk of all chronic diseases at once, twentieth-century biomedicine instead largely conceptualized and treated chronic conditions as it had infectious ones: siloed conditions that would prove amenable to targeted pharmaceutical and technoscientific intervention at the level of the individual patient. Though we often speak casually of chronic disease as a naturalized umbrella category of illness, in practice the approach of the United States to each disease exists in its own sphere, equipped with its own medical specialty, fundraising associations, patient advocacy groups, and research apparatus.[12] The separation of efforts meant these diseases were made to compete against others for scarce resources.

In a system prioritizing research and treatment over primary prevention and care, chronic conditions became most visible in moments of acute crisis (heart attacks, strokes, seizures, etc.). Once a disease had progressed to this point, the standard treatment protocol called for advanced technoscientific interventions such as intensive drug therapies, radical surgeries, and burdensome self-management regimes. Heart disease required stents, bypass surgery, and statins; cancer required chemotherapy and radiation; diabetes called for insulin and potentially dialysis. There was rarely a cure waiting on the other side of all this new medical care, just more treatments as the inevitable complications arose.[13] As institutional medicine adapted to the new epidemiological reality, aspects of daily life once excluded from scientific medicine (diet, exercise, and other lifestyle choices) were (re)introduced as risk factors requiring vigilant minimization in a sprawling new medical surveillance system. But rather than promote healthy lifestyles, biomedicine prioritized early detection. Physicians assessed risk with powerful diagnostic technologies (cytological, immunological, radiological) through which diseases became more defined by measurable laboratory markers than by patients' self-reported experiences.[14]

Though nutrition scientists were beginning to uncover some of the dietary underpinnings of the major chronic diseases in the 1930s and 1940s, the scientific community remained relatively hesitant to popularize or act on these connections until the preponderance of evidence became clearer. There were early suggestions by pioneering researchers such as physiologist Ancel Keys that nutrition was a potential risk factor in the network of causes underpinning degenerative diseases like heart disease, but his studies were controversial and roundly criticized.[15] Even after the controversial release of the 1978 McGovern Report, the first government document explicitly tying diet to chronic disease, some scientists voiced discomfort because they felt the evidence was still too weak.[16] Meanwhile, Americans struggled to maintain healthy eating habits against the deluge of processed goods in the national food ecosystem. For average Americans, scientific nutrition ignored the practical and cultural elements of eating that were so central to everyday life, offering only abstract quantitative tools like calorie counting that, like fad diets, facilitated a neoliberal perspective on food choice, reflecting a uniquely American understanding of patienthood and citizenship vis-à-vis market efficiency.[17]

As it became more obvious in the 1960s and 1970s that medical science was not exactly coming to the rescue (at least within the life spans of the patients then staring down death), new patient anxieties emerged concerning this new class of conditions that it could no longer be assumed physicians had the power to vanquish. The rising regime of risk management and self-surveillance in medicine gave people with severe chronic conditions the impression that medical institutions were needlessly calloused toward the lived experience of being sick or condemned to die. Disappointed, disillusioned, and scared, millions of Americans ventured into the open market for types of care they deemed more appropriate to the gravity of their conditions.

To counter the relative quiet of public health authorities, diet gurus and other twentieth-century health radicals became some of the first public figures in the United States to loudly condemn orthodox medicine and the increasingly artificial food environment as the twin engines behind America's growing incidence of chronic disease. Alongside their criticisms, diet gurus offered accessible alternatives to medicine complete with the patient-centered approach Americans craved.

Living to Diet, Dieting to Live

This book examines a critical slice of the transformation of diets into lifestyles, identities, and complementary healing systems by scrutinizing the lives and careers of the experts behind four important dietary movements, whose work predicted and defined our contemporary diet and wellness culture: Alvenia Fulton (1907–1999), Michio Kushi (1926–2014), Nathan Pritikin (1915–1985), and Robert C. Atkins (1930–2003). These diet gurus pioneered diets that were the most successful of their kind between the late 1950s and the early 2000s, and each of these gurus seeded a movement that continues to dominate the dietary landscape today. Alvenia Fulton was a key founder of the contemporary Black vegan movement; Michio Kushi's legions of macrobiotic followers supplied critical infrastructure to the natural health food movement; Nathan Pritikin was a direct inspiration for the Whole Foods, Plant-Based diet; and Robert Atkins's diet revolution pioneered much of the science and cultural appeal of the ongoing low-carbohydrate craze, evident in popular programs such as the protein-heavy Paleolithic and fat-laden ketogenic diets. Each of the diet programs featured here claimed to heal the body through the selective application of lifestyle changes, and they were led by gurus who earned substantial followings by embodying a hope for radical cultural reform and bodily restoration through targeted individual behavior modifications. To that end, this book focuses primarily on diets that fit the criteria of intentional, value-driven movements that were shaped by the gurus' own lives, including their personal experiences with eating and with chronic illness.

Each body chapter is narrowly focused on a particular diet movement, but between the four main chapters are nestled three *entremets* chapters meant to elucidate the larger arc of the conflict between organized medicine, health heterodoxy, and the food system. I chose the term "entremets," which derives from classic French cookery and translates fittingly to "between servings," ironically. Though the concept of a small bite between meals is decidedly diet unfriendly, the elite gourmandism the term evokes is meant to clash against the rejection of haute cuisine that American fad diets represent. Reclaiming the nomenclature of fine dining for these decidedly "unfine" dietary practices is a call for respect—to appreciate diet gurus for their earnest artistry, if nothing else.

The gurus featured in this book were exquisitely well-positioned to address American patients' widespread dissatisfaction with hegemonic medicine and corporate food; they were keenly sensitive to the politics of eating, healing, and living, and they erected thriving microcultures catering to these overlapping sentiments. Each guru carefully straddled the line between science and humanity; each presented earnest critiques of the medical system but, cleverly, also cloaked their health claims in the language, notations, and prestige of science. Their programs spoke the language of calories, macronutrients, vitamins, and physiological processes as confidently and fluidly as credentialed experts. Sandwiched between personal, relatable anecdotes about food choice or illness, some gurus presented themselves as doctors, others cited medical literature, and still others conducted their own clinical trials. Yet in the same breath where they explained probiotics or polyphenols, the guru might wax poetic on cleansing and detoxing, yin and yang, or vital energies. However cherry-picked or distorted their medical evidence may have been, the diet gurus in this book nevertheless sought to make such information legible and accessible to their audiences while speaking to the cultural experience of eating and the lived reality of being sick.

Diet gurus found an opening because, as a scientific field, nutrition is among the most difficult and complex. Just accounting for all the millions of different biochemical, cultural, environmental, and anatomical variables simultaneously *in vivo* (even in laboratory mice) is a daunting task, let alone finding meaningful signals in all that noise and communicating that information simply to the general public. Making socially aware and livable guidelines based on imprecise knowledge—especially for a public as large and diverse as that of the United States—is nigh impossible. Yet the public need for safe diet guidelines that simultaneously account for cultural variability, cost, and disease prevention is too urgent to wait for clear scientific consensus (as if the current regulations meet such criteria anyway). Still, diet gurus—who have never been beholden to broad consensus in the same way as scientists or policy makers—have historically been able to exercise greater flexibility in their approach. Not needing to reach or represent all Americans or the scientific community as a whole, gurus have had the freedom to target specific groups with more pertinent information tailored to their interests and needs. Regardless of the veracity of the gurus' dietary claims, learning to eat from diet gurus clearly empowered dieters to learn about and thus take agency over their own health.

The preference among certain classes of patients for heterodox care is often explained away by critics as the result of delusion, helplessness, or misinformation.[18] As a result, most of the public health efforts to dissuade patients from adopting alternative health epistemologies and practices assume that patients who veer toward unproven therapies are simply too ignorant of science to discern between legitimate and illegitimate claims. Yet because of patients' epistemic fluidity, the battle between science and pseudoscience for patients' hearts and minds has seldom been won in the arena of hard evidence. What largely drove the patients in this book toward pseudoscientific practices was an alignment of healing practices with other kinds of closely held social values. To attract and maintain populations of devoted followers, gurus donned an eclectic mantle of expertise drawn from such disparate sources as Eastern religious philosophy, African herbalism, Indigenous foodways, and, of course, Washington, DC, Beltway medical and nutrition science. They then mobilized their experience in these various domains to deliver a kind of personalized medicine tailored to a particular audience.[19] Gurus' careful and savvy messaging concerning difficult issues of race, gender, age, sexuality, class, and taste, as well as their careful positioning relative to national and international politics, was far more persuasive to their followers than were their narrow physiological claims about the functions of proteins or carbohydrates in the body—the substance of most scientific critiques leveled against them.

Unbound by the institutional or ethical guardrails of medicine, popular diets can be understood as producing invaluable heuristics for members of the public who lack the literacy, privilege, time, or interest to dissect medical literature on their own. They are, by necessity, imperfect, market-oriented solutions. Though the diets in this book located the blame for chronic disease incidence in unequal American social structures, they nevertheless laid the responsibility to recover from or resist those social forces squarely on the shoulders of the individual patient-consumer. There is clearly an ideological contradiction in the core premise here, but to spread their ideas in capitalist America, diet gurus (who were largely forbidden from practicing medicine outright) had little recourse but to find audiences in the marketplace. Unable to directly influence the institutional levers they blamed for Americans' health problems, diet gurus worked from the bottom up, empowering private citizens to use their consumptive choices to resist the system as best they could to create health-forward lives on their own.

Because they were at risk of being prosecuted, alternative healing movements and cultures, including mass-market diets, have had to be protective over their privacy and suspicious of interlopers. Heterodox healers have always been at a legal disadvantage as well. Unlike the legally circumscribed and standardized educational and professional paths taken by orthodox medical experts, diet gurus' professional trajectories have not always been so straightforward. Although some gurus were trained alternative healers, others were physicians, and others had no formal training at all. This power imbalance between regular and heterodox healing has affected the stories we are able to tell—as cultural pariahs, alternative healing groups' records have not been preserved as rigorously as have the records of the medical establishment. Where heterodox organizations' records have been preserved, the documents have been collected selectively and haphazardly—often by the very physicians who most antagonized them.[20] This has skewed the documentary record itself, allowing unfair presumptions about sectarian healers to proliferate unchallenged.[21]

By spotlighting the heretofore unexamined diversity of diet gurus and their followers, and the overlooked medical subtext of the nation's premier diets, this book seeks to expunge several persistent myths about American dieting culture as a whole: that twentieth-century dieting was predominantly a pastime for affluent, white women; that diets were primarily undertaken for weight loss; and that those who followed these programs were either ignorant of medical science or hopelessly gullible, or both. Beyond foregrounding the medical dimensions of these diet programs, each chapter also offers a biographical glimpse at the bizarre, sometimes fantastic origins of a different diet, its leaders, major disciples, and electrified devotees. I reconstruct the overarching narrative of each diet program by tracing its social networks—especially their intersections with popular culture, diverse patient groups, and major social movements—and by comparing and contrasting its political exigencies, transformations, and adaptations. Together, these case studies upend the traditional historical conception of who has dieted and why.

This book is framed so as to *critically appreciate* the perspective and politics of the members of alternative healing and eating cultures, but it should not be understood as advocating such practices. It is not meant as an attack against nutrition science, the food industry, the medical establishment, or their champions. There is clearly much to criticize about the modern

American diet industry and much to legitimately fear about health fraud and certain heterodox healing practices. For example, it is clear that food environments replicate and reinforce structural inequalities; yet, as agents of neoliberalism, diets insist on constant self-policing and vigilance, unfairly tasking the system's victims with ameliorating its failures. Moreover, some of the practices espoused by the protagonists of this book lacked conventional medical merit and may have actually been harmful. In this book, I am not attempting to defend dieting culture(s) from any of these or other legitimate claims to social or physical harm. Rather, I seek to put their actions and beliefs into relief against the backdrop of American health care to better illuminate the heterodox healing community's firm conviction that the medical orthodoxy has made major mistakes, oversights, and misguided choices that have endangered the health and well-being of millions of Americans.

To fully appreciate the gurus' and their patients' stories and perspectives requires reckoning with the fact that many patients and gurus were earnest in their beliefs and pursuits of alternative health measures. Shared belief structures provided a common bond that transformed otherwise humdrum diet programs into full-fledged healing communities. This is not a new idea; the esteemed physician William Mayo already understood this dynamic well in 1932. In a letter to the former president of the American Medical Association, Morris Fishbein—a rabid anti-quackery figure in his own right—Mayo claimed, "The dishonest quack is easy to handle. As a matter of fact, he soon discredits himself, but the honest advocate of foolish medical theories is more difficult. The more he is opposed, the more strongly he is convinced that he is right and the more disciples he is able to gather around him."[22] Less cynically (and less self-interestedly), diet gurus—who were persecuted by the medical establishment as quacks—offered what they truly believed to be humane alternatives to regular medicine, and their patients loved them for it. Patients from around the world chose diet gurus' care—in full knowledge of its consequences and legitimacy—over that offered by conventional physicians. By taking health radicals' attitudes seriously, I show that what they sought as they ventured into the dark, quasi-medical forest is worthy of our attention.

1 A Farewell to Chitterlings

Dr. Alvenia Moody Fulton, Soul Food, and the
Advent of Black Veganism

· ·

It is a paradox to be sure—the astounding aspect of an American black
flinging away his barbecue bone for a celery stalk. On the other hand,
many blacks in this land of meat and honey had never been accus-
tomed to meat on their daily menus—at least not until they had
attained that ultra-refined hotshot status that made them card-carrying
members of the middle class. Therefore it has followed in the peculiar
pattern of the classical absurdity, that some American blacks who can
now afford filet have elected instead to dine on raw carrots and
cabbage juice.

—*Ebony* Magazine, 1974

Soon after a young Dick Gregory (1932–2017) caught the attention of Hugh
Hefner in 1961, he became the first Black comic to break the color barrier
when he performed at the Chicago Playboy Club.[1] His incisive wit onstage
forced white audiences to encounter—many for the first time—the structural advantages afforded by their race. In one of his best-known jokes,
Gregory recounted sitting down at a restaurant in the Jim Crow South and
being told by the server, "We don't serve colored people here," to which
Gregory replied, "That's all right, I don't eat colored people. Just bring me
a whole fried chicken."[2] In 1965 Gregory was listed in *Time* magazine as one
of the four major Black male comedians in America.[3] Yet just as his stand-
up career finally began to bloom, by 1966 Gregory turned away from comedy to assist the Black freedom struggle. After first hosting a controversial
march in Chicago and running two failed write-in campaigns for political
office, he abandoned conventional activist tactics for his own idiosyncratic
methods: leveraging his body and his fame to address problems of a personal, national, and global scope. In addition to becoming an outspoken
vegan and health activist, Gregory staged dozens of fasting protests (sometimes coupled with long-distance runs) to bring attention to a panoply of
political issues.

While Gregory has been widely (and rightly) credited as an influential figure in shaping the Black American diet, he did not develop his dietary program or his philosophy of strategic food refusal in isolation. He learned everything he espoused from a self-proclaimed expert in fasting for both health and weight loss, a Chicago-based naturopath named Alvenia Moody Fulton. Fulton empowered Gregory to deploy his body as his chief political tool, and under her careful instruction he became a civil rights icon for whom nutrition, fasting, and prayer were a panacea for the world's problems. Although Fulton was the pioneering advocate of therapeutic fasting and corrective nutrition in Black America, her radical and eclectic health philosophy has escaped historical attention because her ideas have typically been read through the lens of Dick Gregory's career in health activism and other Black food reform efforts that ran through the 1960s and 1970s.

This chapter brings Fulton to the fore, following the contours of her life from the early roots of her nutritional philosophy to the foundation of her health food store and her civil rights engagement with Dick Gregory. Her career ran parallel to several major transformations for Black Americans: unprecedented northern migration, integration, and urbanization; the meteoric rise in chronic disease burden complicated by medical inequality; burgeoning pride in Black cultural heritage and identity exemplified by the "soul" trend in music, dance, and food; and the heated inter- and intraracial politics of the Black freedom struggle. During this time of public upheaval, Fulton unironically sold healthy vegetarian staples, weight loss plans, supplements, and nature cures—practices that had been historically associated with white health promoters and heterodox healers—as a novel solution for many of the crises facing Black America.

As a diet guru, Fulton performed critical cultural labor by translating ideas from the overwhelmingly white alternative medical community—and subsequently the natural health food movement—for an urban Black audience. She reformulated ideas from each tradition in line with her own understanding of Black history and Black health and the needs of her community—a community entrenched in a battle for the recognition of its civil rights. Fulton drew on her own experience with illness and dietary cure to create a replacement for soul food, which was increasingly being blamed for the high rates of heart disease among Black men. Although by the 1970s Fulton was only one voice in a crowd of soul food critics, she offered a unique perspective that carefully threaded the needle between demands for a Black identity based in authentic cultural heritage and civil rights era health goals.

Dr. Alvenia Moody Fulton

The self-styled "Queen of Nutrition" was born Alvenia Moody on May 17, 1906 in Pulaski, Tennessee. Her family owned a 156-acre farm—a rarity in Gilded Age America—and was almost entirely self-sufficient.[4] The Moody family produced all their own fruits in a private orchard from which they preserved their own jam; they grew vegetables in a large garden; they milled their own grain; they slaughtered and cured meat from their own livestock; they milked their own cows, churned their own butter, and even fermented and stored barrels of sauerkraut.[5] Fulton's family also relied heavily on non-traditional medicine, emphasizing treatments derived from plants that could be foraged from the nearby woods or streams or cultivated locally. Fulton's mother was a trained healer and midwife in the vernacular healing traditions handed down from her enslaved ancestors, having been apprenticed by her own mother, Fulton's grandmother. Fulton described her mother's herbalism in her book *Radiant Health through Nutrition*: "I vividly remember the roots, barks, herbs, leaves, sulphur, molasses, onions, kerosene, olive oil and Black Draught. We had vinegar baths and sulphur rubs, those were the medicines used and the medical practices followed."[6]

Both the heritage cuisines and vernacular healing traditions that African Americans developed relied extensively on the complex ethnobotanical legacy of slavery. Those who were enslaved—having been captured from throughout the African continent—employed and shared a wide variety of African healing practices, even cultivating traditional African herbs. Historian Sharla Fett describes how enslaved people imported seeds and grasses to the Americas, planting the licorice seeds that hung from traditional necklaces they wore and the dried wild grasses that slavers strew across the deck of ships through the Middle Passage.[7] Enslaved people adopted, borrowed, or traded knowledge of local plants and healing secrets with Indigenous cultures throughout the American continents and the Caribbean, and they imbibed elements of European healing traditions, including orthodox medicine. The Atlantic exchange in healing knowledge yielded a staggering and eclectic *materia medica* made even more impressive by the breadth of functions that any given herb or root could serve. These vernacular herbal practices are still widely (if secretly) used today, owing to the painful legacy of medical discrimination, experimentation, and abuse at the hands of mainly white orthodox physicians.[8]

Though Fulton wrote that herbalism was a powerful formative force in her development as a nutritionist and healer, it did not take root until relatively late in life. As a young adult, Fulton attempted careers as a practical nurse, rural school teacher, and midwife before enrolling at Tennessee State Normal College and settling on a career as a preacher.[9] Her mother—along with every man on both sides of her family—had been a leader in the Baptist or African Methodist Episcopal (AME) churches. Not only was Fulton the first woman to enroll and graduate from Greater Payne Theological Seminary in Birmingham, Alabama, she was the first woman to preach at several major churches in Kentucky, Alabama, Tennessee, Ohio, and Kansas. Along the way, she met and took the name of her husband, Reverend O. M. Fulton.[10]

By the early 1950s, Fulton had moved from the South to start a new life in Chicago. It is not clear what motivated this shift, but her move (perhaps inadvertently) aligned with the path taken by millions of other Black migrants during the Second Great Migration. Beginning in the 1910s and lasting through the 1970s, northern cities like Chicago became major destinations for African Americans migrating from the South. During the first Great Migration (1910s–1930s), rural Southern African Americans—who primarily found employment as servants for white kitchens or in unskilled manufacturing jobs in Chicago's meatpacking houses—began splitting single flats into as many as six separate kitchenettes to combat the dearth of affordable living spaces in Chicago.[11] When Fulton founded her natural health food business there in 1957, Chicago was still undergoing massive demographic shifts as a result of the Second Great Migration (1940–1970), when hundreds of thousands of Black Americans resettled from the urban South into the already crowded urban North. Although World War II and the New Deal promised thousands of skilled manufacturing jobs in the North, the cities failed to provide new housing to accommodate the newest wave of migrants, and existing Black neighborhoods "virtually burst at the seams."[12] Historian Jessica Harris argues that quickly thereafter, when affluent whites abandoned the city for the suburbs, new Black migrants were "relegated to living in inner-city neighborhoods that were slumping into deterioration."[13]

Unsurprisingly, the health of these overfull urban Black communities lagged behind their white neighbors, and before her natural health awakening, Fulton's health was no exception. For thirty years, Fulton was in and out of doctors' offices, suffering from a wide array of ailments for which she tried all manner of orthodox therapies and patent medicines. In 1954, her health took a sudden turn for the worse. She writes about undergoing two major hospitalizations: one for bleeding duodenal ulcers and another shortly thereafter for complications from uterine fibroid tumors. Her nurses even instructed her to stop working as her condition worsened, and she was put on a strict diet without fresh or whole fruits and vegetables—only cooked or strained foods and dairy. In both cases, she felt orthodox medical treatments were failing her and prayed for recovery.

It was during these personal brushes with serious illness that Fulton was first alerted to the relationship between diet and disease. Rather than continue what she perceived to be useless orthodox medical procedures, she decided to pursue radical, nonchemical treatment options and began attending public lectures on natural healing and health foods in Chicago. Sociologist Laura J. Miller explains that health lecturers were common and widely popular from the late nineteenth century through the early 1960s and often toured through such major cities as Chicago. The circuit regularly featured speakers on diverse subjects, including self-improvement, natural foods, and herbal medicine.[14] Fulton attended lectures from a wide range of speakers, including the most influential health proselytizers of the era: Paul Bragg, Gayelord Hauser, and Martin Pretorius.[15]

From the lectures she attended, Fulton found relief from illness; in recovery, she found inspiration. She developed her health program, with its signature emphasis on vegetarianism and restorative health through juicing and fasting, from the same procedures that healed her. From one lecture she attended during her bout with ulcers, Fulton learned of an unpublished study that had been running for the previous four years being conducted by a Stanford University doctor, Garnett Cheney. Cheney was testing "vitamin U therapy" on inmates with peptic ulcers at San Quentin Prison near San Francisco. The regular doses of raw cabbage juice—apparently rich in "vitamin U"—reportedly had positive results, and many of the inmates recovered without incident.[16] Fulton's ulcer, though intestinal rather than gastric, vanished after a cabbage juice regime as well.[17] Likewise, while she was hospitalized for fibroid complications she came upon another health lecturer, Max O. Garten, who advertised therapeutic fasting as a revolutionary new cure for tumors. As with her ulcer, Fulton sought Garten's advice, experimented with his therapy, and promptly found relief. In praise of her experience with Garten, Fulton wrote, "Fasting had brought me closer to God and to a better life."[18] After her complete recovery, she turned away from her life in ministry to teach her community about the powers of nutrition, plant foods, and healing herbs.

Fultonia Health Food and Fasting Center

In 1955, Fulton opened the Pioneer Natural Health Institute out of her home at 65th Street and Eberhardt Avenue in the West Englewood neighborhood of Chicago. The institute began as a small reading group and prayer circle for Fulton's friends to whom she would provide a variety of healing services and products. Fulton was by no means the first African American to combine religious faith and healing. Black spiritual leaders have, throughout American history, had a dually powerful and intimate role in Black communities, and this power has often extended to organizing or offering medical services. Soon after its opening, the institute had so many customers that her small home was overwhelmed. As she told a reporter from the *Chicago Daily Defender*, "I was pushed out of my house into a store on a shoestring, and found that there was not another business of this kind in the black community."[19] She initially imagined her store as a combined natural health food store and vegetarian restaurant with a predominantly Black clientele—the first of its kind in the country.

When her first brick-and-mortar store opened in 1957, she christened it the Fultonia Health Food and Fasting Center. It was a nondescript building located in the middle of the shopping district on the 500 block of East 63rd Street near "two taverns, a candy store, two cleaners, a bakery, a barber shop, a print shop, a restaurant, and a storm window shop."[20] All that was visible from the street—aside from a plain white sign with thick black letters hanging over the entrance—was a window display showcasing a menagerie of "chloro caps, herbolax, extraction of garlic, passion flower, living beauty cream and vitamin E jars selling for $4.75."[21] Those enthusiastic health-seekers who opened Fultonia's door were greeted by a unique olfactory assault: a peculiar interplay between the funk of dried African herbs, the tang of barbecued soy "chicken," and the earthy sweetness of freshly blended carrot juice. Guests encountered the "glamorous tropical decor of rippling fountains, mock palm trees and thatched roof" that Fulton carefully designed to encourage both weight loss and relaxation.[22]

Fulton's business remained relatively inconspicuous, attending mostly to the needs of her local community, until 1966 when she sent an "unsolicited container of funny-looking salad" to Dick Gregory's office during his write-in campaign to unseat the controversial Richard J. Daley as mayor of Chicago.[23] Gregory initially feared the salads to be a Trojan horse, assuming Daley had laced them with arsenic to poison him.[24] When he learned they were intended as a promotional device for Fulton's dietary lifestyle program, Gregory and his wife Lillian visited Fulton at her store, where they had their first consultation.

As a former high school track star turned 270-pound chain-smoking alcoholic, Gregory was a stranger to health-seeking behavior. In 1964, he felt that, as a pacifist in the mold of Martin Luther King Jr. and Mohandas Gandhi, he needed to abstain from violence against humans and animals, so he went vegetarian. At this point, Gregory continued to smoke and drink heavily. When he first visited Fultonia, Gregory only sought advice on safe fasting techniques, not wholesale dietary change. Fulton obliged. As a teaching experiment, she even joined Gregory for his first fast—in protest of the Vietnam War—which was scheduled to last the forty days between Thanksgiving and New Year's Day.[25]

Fulton's signature fast was tailored to each client; Gregory's began with a series of fifteen enemas using Fulton's special colon-cleansing formula, moved to a raw fruit and vegetable juice diet, and eventually transitioned to nothing but distilled water with honey and lemon, and an occasional seaweed pill.[26] After concluding this initial fast, Gregory swore off cigarettes and alcohol, and converted his ethical vegetarianism and political fasting regimens to a sleek, totalizing yet health-oriented diet philosophy that verged on fruitarianism.[27] Armed with his new diet and fasting regimen, Gregory swiftly lost two-thirds of his body weight—descending to a skeletal ninety-seven pounds—but he felt more energetic and enthusiastic than ever.[28] Though politics remained at the forefront of his dietary activism, Gregory's partnership with Fulton—and his entire conception of what it meant to be healthy—was built on the promise of being physically vigorous enough to perform and survive the extreme acts of protest he had in mind.

Fulton's program became the basis of all of Gregory's fasting protests, hunger strikes, and awareness campaigns. Over the next several decades, he fasted dozens of times to bring attention to a wide array of political issues. In 1973, he vowed to fast until all American prisoners of the Vietnam War had been released; in 1976, he fasted to bring attention to hunger in the United States; in 1979, he spent four months fasting in Iran hoping to persuade the Ayatollah Khomeini to release the hostages from the American embassy. He fasted for an astonishing 167 days in 1984 to bring attention to world hunger. At other times he fasted in support of women's rights, in opposition to apartheid in South Africa, and against police brutality in the United States.[29] Between each fast, Gregory gained much of his weight back only to lose it all again dramatically during the next fasting protest, embodying what literary scholar Doris Witt has described as "the grotesque trope of the expanding and contracting Black man."[30] During this period, Fulton and Gregory also collaborated several times, taking trips to teach Black college students and other civil rights activists how to fast as an act of protest.

As Gregory's dietary feats gained notoriety, Fulton leveraged his publicity to recruit more celebrities to her cause, earning her the title "Dietitian to the Stars." Denizens of West Englewood must have watched in amazement as celebrities and foreign nationals disappeared into Fultonia week after week alongside the more familiar young couples and "food stamp survivors."[31] Among these pilgrims, savvy onlookers may have recognized actors (Ossie Davis, Ruby Dee, Gloria Swanson, Billie Dee Williams, Ben Vereen, Michael Caine, and Cicely Tyson), athletes (Jesse Owens, Jim Kelly, Gale Sayers, Bill Walton, Ernie Banks, and Muhammad Ali), comedians (Redd Foxx, Dick Gregory, George Kirby, and Godfrey Cambridge), public personalities (Oprah Winfrey, Sheila Goldsmith, Diane Weathers, and Freda Payne), and musicians (Roberta Flack, Della Reese, Mahalia Jackson, Ramsey Lewis, Stevie Wonder, Stan Getz, John Lennon, Johnny Nash, Lola Falana, Taj Mahal, and all members of Earth, Wind, and Fire, and the James Brown band).[32] Her small store also reportedly received visitors from around the world, including such places as Peru, India, Jamaica, the Bahamas, New Guinea, Barbados, and Australia.[33]

Fultonia had something for everyone and every budget, from local families seeking a wholesome meal to celebrities looking to splurge on mystical secrets. In 1968, Dick Gregory broke his fast in protest of the Vietnam War to dine at Fultonia on a meal of soy "chicken" salad, brown rice, a fresh salad, carrot juice, and wheat bread that cost just $2.25.[34] For her other wealthy clients, Fulton prepared "secret formula diet juices for $125 a shot."[35] If the client could afford it, Fulton would even package her special concoctions and dietary products in dry ice and ship them anywhere in the United States through O'Hare Airport, as she was reported to have done on several occasions for the James Brown band.[36]

In many respects, Fulton's business model closely resembled others under the umbrella of American health heterodoxy, and her entrepreneurship was evidently successful. By 1972, she claimed to have sold her $120 thirty-day fasting program to over 10,000 people.[37] To attract such a large following, Fulton had to maintain a relatively high media profile beyond her exposure through Dick Gregory. Her nutritional practice and philosophy were featured on their own terms several times throughout the 1970s in *Ebony* magazine, which, by its publisher's estimate in 1962, circulated to 56 percent of all Black Americans.[38] Fulton also ran a nutritional advice column for the *Chicago Defender*, one of the nation's premier Black newspapers, and three weekly syndicated radio shows where she offered nutritional advice to callers from across the country.[39] She made several appearances on local and national television.[40] She authored five books.[41] And she even lectured abroad, on as many as five separate occasions, in such places as "Africa, Europe, and the Far East."[42] She won several awards for her work as a local, feminist community leader as well, and she was regularly featured in the *Chicago Metro News*, the self-proclaimed "largest black oriented weekly in the [Chicago] metropolitan area."[43] In 1977, Fulton opened a fasting institute in Union Pier, Michigan, the first step in making her brand into a chain, with unrealized plans to expand to Mexico.[44]

Underneath the pretense of her identity as a celebrity guru, Fulton's grounded approach to nutrition was best displayed in her community-oriented work: her radio shows, activism, local interviews, and her column for the *Chicago Defender*, "Eating for Health . . . and Strength." In these media, her advice was situational and flexible rather than rigid and ideological. Though she gave advice on how to prepare wholesome vegetarian meals and wrote polemics on the dangers of the industrial food system, Fulton spent much of her time answering everyday community questions regarding proper nutrition, including such difficult subjects as how to feed a family on a budget, handle picky eaters, or take care of elderly parents.

The tone of Fulton's writing oscillated between that of a nutritionist armed with scientific knowledge and that of a prophet replete with divine wisdom. Her written work blended those traditions central to her own development as a healer: the herbalism passed down through generations of women in her family, the traditions of preaching and ministering to the sick in the Black church, and the received wisdom of white drugless healers. At times, her writing was debonair and filled with charming colloquialisms that struck a grandmotherly chord; at other times, she could be blunt or even scolding. A 1974 profile of Fulton in *Ebony* magazine captured this ambivalence in her persona well: "Trying to confront Alvenia Fulton with any objections whatsoever is a little like standing in front of an herbal wizard, part Earth-Mother, part witch-doctor, and wondering why the battle is lost. She stares down reservations with deep honey-colored eyes and thrusts out her high-energy vitamin cocktail along with a fearsome array of diagrams depicting ruined, rotten colons. . . . Then suddenly her face brightens with promise of the famous Fultonia solution that wards off such misery."[45]

Drawing from her earlier career in the Black church, Fulton thoroughly blended her nutritional ideology with her religiosity. She explicitly located justification for fasting in the Bible, highlighting the theme—common in scriptural parables—of self-denial leading to personal strength and reward. Her unshakeable faith was reflected in the text of her books and dietary manuals where Fulton unflinchingly hybridized religious and scientific verbiage. Because her clientele sought spiritual care but also trusted the basic tenets of Western medicine, she wrote each book like a sermon peppered subtly with citations of contemporary medical literature. Interwoven between the dipoles of science and religion were heterodox remedies and personal anecdotes of ill health, triumph, weight reduction, and redemption. Fulton saw health not as an isolated biomedical pursuit, but as an embodied endeavor suffused with religious meaning.

As a preacher, Fulton learned how to reach out to and capture the imagination of a community—a talent she eagerly applied to her nutritional endeavors. Through her local advice columns and other community outreach, Fulton kept her finger on the pulse of Black communities' everyday anxieties about health. Hearing community members' frustrations with their health revealed overlaps with her own experience of chronic illness and disillusionment with scientific medicine. In these community narratives, Fulton recognized the signs of nutritional dysfunction throughout the country, especially in Black neighborhoods, and marshaled her resources to intervene where regular medicine would not.

Racial (Hyper)Tension and Heart Disease

While the rates of many acute and chronic diseases—including pneumonia, influenza, tuberculosis, and syphilis—remained much higher among African Americans than whites during 1960s and 1970s, the major cause of death in Black communities during the 1960s was the same as for the nation as a whole: coronary heart disease (CHD).[46] In 1960, the *Chicago Daily Defender* newspaper reported that 58 percent of all deaths in Black and white Chicago that year were caused by heart disease.[47] Data from the National Center for Health Statistics show that, in the 1960s and 1970s, the rate of CHD in men of all races far outstripped that in women, with the highest rate of mortality from heart attacks in white men.[48] Curiously, in the late 1950s the Black press began reporting that Black communities suffered higher rates of hypertensive disease than whites, though these reports correlated with lower overall mortality from CHD.

Because hypertension was widely considered to be a risk factor for CHD, high hypertension rates among Blacks posed a difficult medical puzzle. A 1962 article in *Ebony* commented that this discrepancy was "the great enigma of the American Negro's heart disease problem."[49] Physicians as far back as the antebellum period had been aware of differences in blood pressure along racial lines, and the first reference to African Americans' consistently higher rates of hypertension as a disease state was published in the 1930s. In the 1950s, the Framingham Heart Study—though there were no African Americans in its first cohort—concluded erroneously that Black rates of heart disease were comparable to whites.[50] Only with the publication of data in 1960 from the first cohort studies to examine Black heart disease risk, the Charleston and Evans County Georgia Heart Studies, was it established that Black mortality was, in fact, lower than for whites, despite high hypertensive morbidity.[51]

After US heart disease incidence peaked in the mid-1960s, data from the National Center for Health Statistics demonstrated that there was a steady decline in CHD mortality across all demographic groups.[52] But because heart disease mortality declined faster for white patients than for Black patients, Black men became the nation's leading victims of heart attacks in the early 1980s.[53] These statistics may not offer the entire story, however, because much Black heart disease went unrecorded during the 1960s and 1970s owing to hospital discrimination and unequal access to care.[54] There were even myths spread among white doctors—from the 1950s to the mid-1980s—that Blacks suffered very little to no heart disease at all, even while it was the leading cause of death.[55] This systematic weakness in the recognition of CHD incidence among African Americans signals the need to pay increased attention to anecdotal and cultural impressions of historical disease burden.

As it became clear that the higher morbidity rates among African Americans were tied to structural racism, medical discrimination and unequal access to care became central issues for civil rights groups.[56] In the late 1960s, the recognition of the invisible hypertensive crisis spurred multiple efforts by civil rights groups to address disparities in health care. The Black Panther Party, for example, devoted significant political energies to mobilizing against health disparities and attempted to build an independent medical infrastructure to test for sickle cell disease, bolster childhood nutrition, and combat medical discrimination and unequal treatment.[57] As part of their free health clinic mission, the Black Panther Party began conducting free blood pressure screenings in major cities, including Chicago, with the hope of motivating Black men in particular to seek treatment.[58]

Fulton, too, saw high rates of hypertension as part of a larger systemic prejudice against Black men. Just as Black men were disproportionately inducted into the Vietnam War, institutionalized with mental illness, and incarcerated by the criminal justice system, Fulton argued that Black men were conspicuously absent in their social roles because of unequal medical outcomes that resulted from poor nutrition.[59] One of Fulton's major goals was, therefore, to reduce the amount of disease among Black men, ensuring longer, healthier, and more productive lives.[60] In a 1976 editorial published in a community circular, Fulton wrote provocatively,

> Black men are too scarce and too valuable to continue dying so young from preventable diseases, resulting from diet deficiencies, such as heart attacks, high blood pressure, gout, diabetes and strokes. There is no longer any doubt that the rapid increase in cancer of the colon (the big gut) among black men in the last ten years is exaggerated by faulty diet. Feeding your husband from quick food outlets, stuffing his [face] with food filled [with] chemical coloring and sweetening, may give you more leisure for social invitations. It may also introduce you to a lonely young widowhood.[61]

Fulton had watched as housing segregation and a lack of high-paying jobs conspired against Black migrants whose health also suffered as waves of cheap, processed foods flooded low-income neighborhoods.[62] From her perspective, the path to escaping the harsh realities of Black medical care in the civil rights era was through the stomach.

Fulton's recognition of dietary influences on heart health aligned with developments in the medical community. In 1953, just before Fulton began attending health lectures, physiologist Ancel Keys published the first scientific evidence connecting diet and heart disease. And while the diet-heart hypothesis remained controversial among scientists until the early 1980s, by the late 1950s, a significant portion of the white public began adopting heart-healthy diets following the publication of Keys's low-fat cookbook *Eat Well and Stay Well*.[63] Similar attention to heart disease was delayed among African Americans, but by at least 1968 the *Defender* and other Black press outlets had begun to recommend the American Heart Association's modest dietary changes to the "coronary prone."[64] Yet early dietary recommendations like Keys's Eurocentric Mediterranean diet held little cultural appeal for Black audiences. Fulton recognized that to encourage Black Americans to choose healthier food, she would need to confront a powerful countervailing trend: the rise of soul food.

Soul Food and the Civil Rights Movement

Though the term "soul food" only gained its modern currency in the 1960s, the cuisine itself descended from the much older tradition of Southern "homestyle" or "down-home" cooking that had predominated among Southern Blacks since slavery.[65] In the South, this cooking style is virtually synonymous with comfort food and is well-known for its golden cornbread; savory, slow-cooked pork; crispy fried chicken; and hearty, flavorful stews of okra and black-eyed peas. Alongside bold seasoning, soul food also implies a flair for improvisation and resourcefulness stemming from a history of making do with inadequate provisions.

The Southern-style fare first made its way north with the movement of working-class families during the first Great Migration but enjoyed limited popularity beyond this narrow segment. Down-home cooking—though expensive to maintain—was important to the first generation of Southern transplants because it provided the smells and tastes of home in an otherwise harsh and unfamiliar environment.[66] However, until the 1960s most middle-class Blacks in the urban North disdained Southern cuisine as "backwards" and distanced themselves from those who consumed it because the newcomers "did not conform to [native Black] Chicagoans' carefully cultivated standards of respectability."[67] It was only as urban Southern migrants joined the middle class in northern cities during the Second Great Migration that the cultural importance of Southern cooking—now rebranded as soul food—surged. The explosion of soul-inspired restaurants was encapsulated eloquently by poet Amiri Baraka: "There are hundreds of tiny restaurants, food shops, rib joints, shrimp shacks, chicken shacks, 'rotisseries' . . . that serve 'soul food'—say, a breakfast of grits, eggs, sausage, pancakes and Alaga syrup—and even tiny booths where it's at least possible to get a good piece of barbecue, hot enough to make you whistle, or a chicken wing on a piece of greasy bread."[68]

As a Southern migrant herself, Fulton was no stranger to soul food, but neither was she a fan. Although Fulton's neighborhood was not home to Chicago's most iconic soul food restaurants—Gladys', Soul Eatery, and Pearl's Place—her 63rd Street shopping district nevertheless abounded with bars and restaurants catering to these tastes.[69] In her published reflections, Fulton attributed many of her early health problems to overeating the foods that predominated in Southern cooking, such as the home-grown meat and dairy products on her father's farm.[70] It was clear to Fulton early on, therefore, that the growing chronic disease rates in struggling Black communities were underscored by the rising popularity of soul food. From her perspective, soul food left much to be desired nutritionally: it was high in fat, cholesterol, salt, and refined carbohydrates. In her weekly column for the *Defender*, Fulton proudly quoted a Black physician as having said, "Eating hog guts and fat pork is like drinking pure lard. I know of no blankety-blankety surer way to destory [sic] your arteries, damage your heart and invite diabetes than living on such a blankety-blankety diet."[71] For its heavy reliance on greasy and processed foods, soul food was anathema to the preservation and empowerment of Black bodies.

That soul food was inherently unhealthy was not lost on Black diners, but it was not enough to curb their appetite. According to culinary historian Adrian Miller, "As early as the 1920s, Black doctors had exhorted readers to change their down home cooking diet."[72] For some Black Americans, sociologist Janet Shim argues that, along with cigarettes and alcohol, eating soul food may have blunted the harms of racism.[73] Critical race scholar Amie Breeze-Harper extends this argument suggesting that "Black people may eat unhealthier foods because they don't have what they need to properly heal from racialized trauma, as well as other legacies of racialized colonialism."[74] Undoubtedly for some, the evocative history implied by soul food—and its irresistible taste—were compelling despite the health implications. Yet soul food's political weight made it especially difficult to extricate from peoples' lives compared with other unhealthy food choices. Historian Frederick Douglass Opie asserts, "In northern cities, politically rejecting soul food meant rejecting part of one's African diasporic urban identity."[75] To understand soul food's centrality to Black politics and identity—and thereby to appreciate the scale of the barriers Fulton faced in introducing natural health foods—it is instructive to reexamine soul food's origins by interrogating its historicity.

From its inception in the mid-1960s, soul food intentionally harkened back to the cuisine of enslaved people at a historical moment when Black Americans were attempting, largely for the first time, to celebrate Black culture openly. In music, dance, and food, soul was the rejection of the perception among whites of Blacks' otherness, inferiority, and lack of cultural contributions. During the Black Power movement, soul food became an edible manifestation of the spiritual continuity between contemporary Black Americans and the suffering of their disenfranchised ancestors. Because it spoke to a near universal experience of Blackness, it quickly provided a site of cultural unity and exchange for Black Americans across class and geographical boundaries. The cuisine emphasized thriftiness because of what thriftiness implied about the resilience and creativity of Black Americans, yet the soul restaurant scene was quickly populated by upscale restaurants attracting a more affluent Black clientele.

Though the phrase "soul food" was intended to recall an authentic slave diet, historians of Black foodways have shown that soul food's purchase on historical accuracy has always been tenuous. First, scholars of Southern foodways point to a great diversity of Southern regional cuisines developed during slavery that were omitted from the definition of soul food: the seafood and corn chowders of the Chesapeake Bay; the mélanges of seafood and rice characteristic of the Carolina Lowcountry; and the spicy meat, vegetable, and rice stews of the Gulf South's Creole cuisine.[76] Second, the narrative that cultural nationalists used to delineate soul food as its own cuisine in the early 1960s hinged on the fact that enslaved people had inferior food provisions (and cooking equipment) compared with plantation owners, supplemented with the meager spoils of privately tended gardens and forest foraging. Soul food self-consciously drew upon this history of racial disparity, rejecting white Southern cuisine as the heir to opulent plantation feasts, with their uncritical celebration of expensive ingredients and reliance on elite (and impractical) cooking techniques. The rebranded subsistence-cum-radical Black cuisine, by contrast, favored ingredients that were cheap and plentiful—neck bones, pig's feet, organ meats, dandelion, collard, and turnip greens—and made liberal use of hog fat, spices, and herbs to fry and season them to perfection. Yet, in 1966 when Stokely Carmichael, as leader of the Student Nonviolent Coordinating Committee, outlined the basis of soul food in an influential position paper, he "focused on the most hard-core poverty foods of . . . Black Belt Mississippi," which, "cemented soul food with Blackness, pork, and poverty in the public imagination."[77]

Soul food paralleled the broader Southern cuisine more than cultural nationalists were prepared to admit. It so closely resembled white Southern cuisine in method, ingredients, and flavor because both culinary traditions were coproduced through the intimate violence of domestic slavery.[78] Enslaved women, who were responsible for meal preparation on plantations, were well-educated in every element of elite technical cooking and thus played a central role in defining white Southern cookery.[79]

Unsurprisingly, they also transferred these skills to after-hours meal preparation in slave quarters.[80] The boundary between Black and white Southern cuisines was therefore more political than substantive. According to Black chefs, it was not the ingredient list, but the soul—an intangible mix of "black spirituality and experiential wisdom"—behind the food that elevated homestyle cooking into another cuisine entirely.[81]

Where soul food had unimpeachable political importance was in the restaurants themselves, which served as critical loci for activist organizing. Black-owned restaurants had historically provided a safe space where Black diners were guaranteed welcome amid an otherwise hostile and segregated restaurant culture. In the 1950s and 1960s, when the rising political inclinations of African Americans collided with a lack of friendly public meeting spaces, activists flooded Black-owned institutions: churches, salons, and soul food restaurants. As historian Fred Opie argues, quoting Martin Luther King Jr., Southern soul food restaurants became places "where people went to eat, meet, rest, plan and strategize."[82]

The Soul Food Rebellion

While Fulton respected the political power of the soul food diet with its connections to Black tradition and ancestry, she also recognized that soul food damaged Black bodies. In that way, soul food undermined the social mission it was intended to fulfill. Rather than replace soul food and risk undercutting the cultural authority it held, she recognized that by simply reframing its cultural narrative and the way its ingredients were mobilized to create dishes, she could intervene in the worst dietary habits in her community: "While [healthy food] may be nutritionally sound, to the Black person's palate it is often tasteless. There is much in the traditional Southern diet that, without the abuse of salt and animal fats, could be more nutritious and tasteful to the black appetite than the most well-planned hospital diet or the store-bought, highly processed foods that black people have been programmed to think of as symbols of middle-class successfulness."[83]

By advocating changing the signature cooking styles of soul food, and thus altering the flavor and nostalgia of classic dishes, Fulton risked alienating those she intended to convert. So to avoid appearing drab and flavorless—or worse, culturally aloof—Fulton shifted the emphasis behind consuming a heritage diet. Instead of simply "healthifying" the existing soul food regimen, Fulton rediscovered and celebrated healthier—if forgotten—elements of the Southern diet, creating a more "natural" cuisine that Gregory playfully referred to as "soil food."[84] In one of her weekly columns, she wrote, "[Enslaved peoples'] diets contained certain nutrient values or more of us would have perished. Food was grown without . . . chemical fertilizers. . . . Our ancient diet was rich as well in greens, which in turn are rich [in] minerals. Our flour was unbleached and our corn bread was made from whole grains unbleached. The lowly dandelion, used as a spring tonic, is rich in vitamin A. They are just as good today. Eat them when they are young and tender before the flowers form."[85] Whereas soul food posited a slave diet structured around fried meats, Fulton imagined one centered around whole grains and wild foraged roots, herbs, and weeds, echoing her early apprenticeship with African American vernacular healing. Along these lines, Fulton and Gregory cowrote a 1974 cookbook, *Dick Gregory's Natural Diet for Folks Who Eat*, which evicted fried meat, exchanged overcooked vegetables for fresh raw ones, and disposed of the traditional grease jar in favor of safflower oil—when frying was necessary at all. Fulton said what she served was not really "sure 'nuff" soul food, but it "sure [was] good for the soul."[86]

Despite the cultural pressures favoring soul food, Fulton was not alone in staging a dietary revolution in Black America. As the mainstream civil rights coalition began to fracture, cultural pride in soul food started chafing against some of the more radical visions for the future of Black America. Some critics worried that soul food was an inadequate wellspring for African American identity, let alone cultural pride, because it recalled (fondly) centuries of white oppression. But the critique that animated most of the resistance to soul food was its inherent unhealthiness—especially the unhealthiness of the narrow scope of "authentic" Southern foods that made it into Carmichael's influential definition of the cuisine. Opie categorizes both factions as "food rebels," emphasizing their collective efforts to reform African American diets in the late-1960s and 1970s.[87]

Perhaps the most vocal critic of soul food was Elijah Muhammad, the charismatic leader of the Black separatist group the Nation of Islam, who argued that soul food celebrated the fact that slaveholders denied enslaved people access to quality foods.[88] For over a decade Muhammad ran a self-authored column in the Nation's weekly newspaper, *Muhammad Speaks*, entitled "How to Eat to Live," and he published two books of the same title in 1967 and 1973, respectively.[89] In place of a standard (African) American diet, Muhammad advocated a strict dietary regimen that blended elements of scriptural *halal*—the Islamic code of pure eating outlined in the Quran—and a roughly pescatarian diet. Muhammad further admonished his read-

ers to avoid processed foods—especially those from white food manufacturers and distributors. According to Muhammad, processed foods had not
only been drained of their purity but many were also being poisoned by
"white devils" to further the project of racial oppression and genocide.[90] To
circumvent the ubiquity of both soul food and processed foods, Muhammad operated a chain of Nation-owned farms, distributors, grocers, farm-
to-table restaurants, and delis—famed for their bean pie slinging street
hawkers.[91] Despite the Nation's extremism and militancy, Muhammad's
nutritional philosophy nevertheless enjoyed broad circulation among non-
Muslim African Americans via *Muhammad Speaks*, which was popular for
its news coverage of the Black diaspora.[92]

The Nation of Islam was not alone in advocating a diet untouched by
white hands. Rastafarian immigrants from the Caribbean, for instance,
imported their own (vegan) diet *ital*, which emphasized growing and
eating food as closely to nature as possible and resisting processing.[93]
Afro-Caribbean immigrant chefs like Tonde Lumumba imported these
foods and dietary principles into radical urban neighborhoods in the
1970s and 1980s.[94] The importation of Afro-Caribbean fare mirrored the
push in the mid-to-late-1970s to broaden Black heritage cooking beyond
soul food by introducing soulful cooking styles from throughout the African diaspora. After the publication of cookbooks like Vertamae Grosve-
nor's *Vibration Cooking* and Helen Mendes' *African Heritage Cookbook*,
West African dishes never before tasted in the United States—spicy with
thick curry-like peanut sauces and cassava—began to grace African
American dinner tables.[95] For these cultural nationalists, new international flavor profiles and ingredients provided a richer, more global understanding of Blackness, and the clearest glimpse yet of a past untouched
by white conquest.[96]

Other responses to the nutritional vacancy of soul food were less radical. In 1974, Ben Ami Ben-Israel, the founder of the controversial African
Hebrew Israelites—who believed that Black Americans were the true heirs
of Israel—opened his Chicago restaurant, Original Vegetarian Soul.[97] Ben-
Israel hoped to improve the diet of African Americans, not by shifting the
culture, but by swapping out pork (forbidden by Jewish custom anyway) and
other meaty mains for lighter—yet equally fried—fare like barbecued tofu
"catfish." Original Vegetarian Soul was a harbinger of the many vegetarian
"soulless" restaurants to come as a wave of Black chefs up and down the
Eastern Seaboard found an audience of young Black college students eager
to eschew eating animals.[98]

While other food rebels were certainly aware of the medical implications of a soul food regimen and mobilized health claims in the advertisements for their corrective diets, Fulton was the only practicing healer among them, which gave her a distinct perspective. Although Black Hebrews, Rastas, and Black Muslims each promoted eating well as a mechanism to undo the harm done to Black bodies through racial oppression, their diets were still subservient to larger politico-religious ideologies. Fulton's restorative nutrition program, by contrast, was coextensive with her ideology.[99]

Fulton's White Healing Practices

Tracing the source of Fulton's dietary philosophy reveals a complicated network of alternative holistic health practices. This network, which I have collapsed under the banner of the white alternative health movement, encompasses naturopathy, the natural health food movement, and other diet-based, holistic alternatives to orthodox medicine and mainstream nutrition science. What holds the white alternative health movement together is similar to what sociologist Laura Miller argues coheres in the natural health food movement: defiance of "jurisdictional claims of professional physicians, dieticians, and pharmaceutical companies [enacted] by asserting an equivalent, if not superior, right to advise people on health issues and to develop health aids."[100] Despite their differences, alternative healers have been classified together since the nineteenth century, when healers outside the scope of scientific medicine were variedly called "heterodox," "sectarians," or outright "quacks." Grouping these practices together diminished their differences from one another and eroded their political power. Yet the number of people and practices that were lumped together under the umbrella of heterodox healing was dramatically expanded in the twentieth century with the American Medical Association's push in 1961 against the ill-defined specter of "food faddism" or "nutritional quackery" (see entremets II).

There had been robust attempts to unite health and food reform at least as early as the mid-nineteenth century, though most resulted in informal allegiances such as the health lecture circuit, which fostered an open exchange of ideas among a wide variety of different practitioners. Much of Fulton's practice, from brown rice and soy cutlets to juice fasting and enemas, can be traced directly to the lectures she attended from the radical luminaries of white Protestant alternative health. For example, one article reported that Fultonia sold "colorful cans of coconut meal, graham crackers, brown sugar, yeast and wheat germ," among which the signature products of two major health icons stand out: Sylvester Graham and Gayelord Hauser.[101] Graham, an American Presbyterian minister and popular nineteenth century vegetarian health promoter, located the root of illness in sin and excessive stimulation—including alcohol and spices. Hauser, a German immigrant, was a leading figure in the early days of the American natural foods movement and was best known for advocating five "super foods": wheat germ, brewer's yeast, skim milk, blackstrap molasses, and yogurt.

The health lectures Fulton attended only partially describe her immersion in white medical heterodoxy; she also completed degree programs, served in professional organizations, and delivered lectures of her own. When Fulton fell ill in 1954, fasting guru and health lecturer Max O. Garten advised Fulton to pursue a formal education in nutrition and naturopathy. She briefly studied at the little-known American Institute of Science in 1958, earning a certificate as a Biochemical Therapist and Nutritional Counselor.[102] She then trained with naturopath Otis J. Briggs at the Lincoln College of Naturopathic Physicians and Surgeons in Indianapolis where she became, by her own assessment, the first African American to receive an ND degree.[103] Eventually, Fulton secured a PhD in nutrition from Donsbach University in 1980 at the age of seventy-three. In interviews, she explained that her doctoral degree in nutrition was part of a one-year study at home program; her dissertation was titled "Rejuvenation through Fasting."[104]

It is important to note that because alternative medicine was excluded from the state licensing and accreditation laws that governed regular medicine, practitioners like naturopaths had to establish their own internal standards of education and care. When those standards could not be agreed upon, factions split; thus, alternative medicine was plagued with potentially dubious educational opportunities like home study, correspondence courses, and outright diploma mills.[105] After the founder of naturopathy, Benedict Lust, died in 1945, the vision of a unified American Naturopathic Association splintered into at least six separate factions.[106] Consequently, the late-1950s—when Fulton earned her degree—was a time of chaos and decline for organized naturopathy in the United States. Similar cases could be made for her other programs as well. The degrees Fulton earned were not medically recognized, nor were the institutions formally accredited. Donsbach University, for example, was a correspondence school founded by Kurt Donsbach in Huntington Beach, California, in the late 1970s. Donsbach, who had been the president of the National Health Federation from 1975–89, was a high priority target of the American Medical Association and Food and

Drug Association's joint anti-quackery task force (see entremets II); he was reportedly making over a million dollars a year in fraudulent medical consultations alone.[107] Notably, Donsbach's correspondence-based PhD program (which cost around $1,000) used the *Dr. Atkins Diet Revolution* as a textbook (see chapter 4).[108] After receiving her degree, Fulton became a Registered Holistic Health Practitioner with the International Academy of Nutritional Consultants (IANC), an organization that had also been founded by Donsbach in 1979. The IANC, later renamed the American Association for Nutritional Consultants, was publicly accused of fraud by the anti-quackery activist Ben Goldacre after he successfully registered his dead cat, Hettie, as a nutritionist.[109]

When considered through the lens of orthodox medical standards, it is admittedly difficult to assess the formal education Fulton received in alternative medicine. However, although anti-quackery activists have decried schools like Donsbach University as frauds or diploma mills, it is clear that Fulton fully understood the legitimacy of the degrees that bore her name. Rather than deploying her degrees to unfairly exalt herself or to pass as an orthodox medical practitioner, Fulton proudly displayed her diplomas and certificates on the wall of her store to flout regular, credentialed medicine. She justified mocking the establishment on the basis that medical degrees conferred upon their recipients authority over the whole human body, despite the well-known dearth of nutritional education in medical schools. In a 1977 interview with a community paper, Fulton argued, "We have more hospitals, more doctors, more health cults, more great medical societies than all the other nations of the world put together, yet we continue to be the least well-fed of any of the so-called developed nations. My answer to this is that if the physicians of today will not become nutritionists, then the nutritionists must become doctors."[110] For Fulton, displaying credentials was not about securing the power of the medical establishment for herself— it was a brazen challenge to the legitimacy of certification as an unbiased assessment of one's healing capacity.

After health lectures waned in popularity in the 1960s, Fulton remained active in professional organizations for alternative healers and natural foods promoters. Attending alternative health conferences provided her with a social network and access to new trends in alternative treatments and practices, which she drew on continuously to update her offerings.[111] Fulton also earned notable recognition from this community. She became a member of the Holistic Doctor's Convention, she served as the secretary of the Natural Doctor's Convention, and she was elected as a fellow in the Society for Nutrition and Preventive Medicine.[112] She even caught the eye of the largest alternative medical organization in the country, the National Health Federation (NHF), presenting several times at their infamous National Congresses on Medical Monopoly (NCMM) (see entremets II). At the 1980 conference, she gave the keynote lecture where the NHF board members honored her message by serving vegetarian entrees cooked in spring water. After her address, she received their Pioneer of American Preventative Medicine award.[113]

In many ways, Fulton's alternative medical career was indistinguishable from any other white practitioner. She spread many of the same ideas about healing and diet, expressed the same concerns about agricultural chemicals and food processing, sold the same health products, earned the same certifications, and attended the same conferences as the disciples of white alternative medicine. Her philosophy of health reduced the full complexity of human disease to a singular nutritional cause and cure, just as theirs did. Accordingly, Fulton faced many of the same difficulties that white holistic practitioners faced in establishing credibility.

There is a tension, however, in Fulton's adoption and propagation of the products and tactics of white heterodox healing in that the health programs espoused and embodied by many natural food and health lecturers emerged in tandem with white supremacist or eugenic ideologies. Such popular icons of American health culture as John Harvey Kellogg, Bernarr Macfadden, and Adelle Davis were avid proponents of eugenics and mandated fasting, fitness, vegetarianism, and health foods as euthenic approaches to secure the future of the white race.[114] Although not every white health reformer framed their techniques in these terms, the ways in which the most prominent early American health reformers framed issues of personal health, physical fitness, and proper nutrition as markers of good citizenship—an idea that is itself classed, raced, and gendered—held a powerful defining influence over much of the public dialogue around health and nutrition in America through the twentieth century.[115]

The degree to which bigoted attitudes toward race remained in the health food movement through the late 1950s is unclear, especially regarding the content of popular lectures. Because public spaces were still often segregated—even if less rigidly—in northern cities, Fulton's mere presence at these lectures as a Black woman is notable. Fulton readily admitted that none of her Southside Chicago neighbors had encountered these white health lecturers or their ideas.[116] By at least the mid-1960s, with the rising counterculture, the explicitly ascetic and moralizing temperance philosophy that underpinned white heterodox healing at the beginning of the twentieth century was receding. Regardless, many of the alternative health and diet practices Fulton employed held racially coded meanings in select middle-class white communities. Fulton, however, was not a naive consumer of the information being sold at the lectures she attended.

Situating Fulton's life and work in the context of Black America reveals that rather than uncritically relaying white-coded health ideas to the public, she mobilized these attitudes, techniques, and products in an explicitly antiracist framework. Following Gregory's activist lead, Fulton directed her restorative diet program toward assisting the Black freedom struggle and alleviating the undue health burden on African Americans. She not only recommended her diet and fasting routine for physical ailments from malaise and low sex drive to gout and diabetes, she thought nutrition could ameliorate social ailments in Black communities like drug addiction and violence as well.[117] These concerns found their greatest expression in the work of Fulton's protégé, Dick Gregory, who not only became the public face of Fulton's ideology but the *de facto* public leader of Black veganism more generally for several decades.

Dick Gregory, Formula 4X, and Contemporary Black Veganism

As a male celebrity, activist, and aspiring politician, Dick Gregory's activities more easily and more frequently made appearances in the national news than did Fulton's. As the standard bearer for Fulton's ideology, however, Gregory's career trajectory as a health activist demonstrates more clearly the shape and extent of her legacy. As recommended by Fulton, Dick Gregory consumed only soy milk and fruit juice during his political fasts, but soon he began adding in a supplement he called Formula 4X. Formula 4X was a proprietary trail-mix-like blend of kelp, dried fruit, seeds, and nuts. Interestingly, Gregory initially credited Fulton with helping him invent the product, but this claim gradually disappeared in his later works, where he claims to have acted alone.[118] Although Gregory and Fulton initially designed the supplement to help people cope with and break from periods of extended fasting, soon after its development Gregory began imagining ways he could use 4X to create a dietary regimen that would advance his many social justice commitments. Gregory envisioned the product as having as many as five distinct uses, each gleaned from his own experience: to wean off fasts, to lose weight, to boost athletic performance, to eliminate poverty, and to conquer addiction.

Formula 4X was the supplement Gregory took to fuel his ultramarathon runs during fasting protests. When his athleticism began to spark public curiosity in the mid-1970s, Gregory began selectively granting elite athletes access to his 4X formula. One of its earliest successes was in helping champion runner E. Gordon Brooks break the world record speed for running from New York City to Los Angeles.[119] Gregory ran alongside Brooks on the return journey from LA to New York while fasting to bring attention to world hunger. Seeing Gregory accomplish such an amazing feat inspired other athletes to inquire about his secret, so he decided to license his formula out on a limited basis but with great success. In an interview, Gregory boasted that "[a] 4X regimen changed the Muhammad Ali who danced for 15 rounds against Jimmy Young to the Muhammad Ali who quickly conquered Richard Dunn in Munich, Germany."[120] Ali admitted as much in an interview after the Dunn fight, skyrocketing the demand for Gregory's supplement. Ali also credited 4X with helping him defeat Ken Norton for the third time in 1976, in one of the most disputed boxing matches in history. Gregory got several other major sales boosts: when he sold his formula to the Pittsburgh Pirates before they won the World Series; when he claimed 4X boosted the performance of world-class sprinter Houston McTear; when 4X healed the legendary Red Sox pitcher Bill "Spaceman" Lee's shoulder after a pitching injury; and when 4X helped Randy Jackson, the youngest of the Jackson brothers, recover after a near fatal car crash. Beyond proving Formula 4X's power to increase athletic performance, Gregory said he recruited celebrity athletes to destigmatize the formula so it was not perceived as a "poverty food."[121]

Gregory soon set his sights higher. In line with his civil rights philosophy to eradicate violence and to uplift Black people everywhere, he became interested in solving world hunger, one of the most visible blights on people of color. Beginning in November 1984, the first international media reports of an already two-year famine in Ethiopia emerged. Over the next several months, the world watched in horror as nearly 400,000 Ethiopians, many of them children, starved to death in one of the worst famines the modern world had ever seen. Not only was the country experiencing a severe drought, it was also undergoing a violent rebellion. During this period of turmoil, an additional 150,000 people were killed by fighting. Political leaders in Ethiopia cut off access and denied aid to areas with rebellious insurgents, exacerbating the political crisis and leaving many famine victims stranded. Countries from all over the world dropped aid packages onto the desiccated and war-torn countryside to slow the pace of death, but the Ethiopian government stood firmly against the rebels, disallowing any substantive aid to reach the hands that most needed it.

Because Gregory originally had used his 4X product to wean himself off fasting, he thought it would make a good transition food for victims of famine. In the early 1980s, Gregory made connections with high-ranking Ethiopian officials, including the most prominent pediatrician in the nation and the dean of medicine at the University of Addis Ababa, Demissie Habte.[122] Habte used his fame and political clout to run several hasty clinical trials on 4X's effects on famine-stricken children. Of the results, Habte said 4X offered "a very bright prospect," as it seemed to have the right balance between nutritional content and cost.[123] Shortly thereafter, on April 15, 1985, Berhane Deressa, the deputy commissioner of the Relief and Rehabilitation Commission of Ethiopia and later mayor of Addis Ababa, sent an urgent request to the United States for 100 cases of Formula 4X and 100 more cases of a nutritional bar of the same makeup to help malnourished children (and eventually adults) in Ethiopia recover from famine.[124] Gregory delivered. To his credit, he also recognized that one of the major barriers to ending famine was being able to distribute supplies, not merely to ship them to Ethiopia; when he responded to Deressa's request, Gregory delivered three trucks as well to assist in distributing aid. His efforts alleviating the famine did not go unrecognized; he even gave a symbolic can of 4X to Nelson Mandela when he visited the United States in 1990.[125]

At the same time 4X was undergoing its first trials in Ethiopia as a famine aid, Gregory was having rather different trials run in the United States, where he said "Black people [were] killing themselves with food."[126] He partnered with a Swedish drug company called Cernitin America as well as researchers from Xavier and Howard colleges to test his formula's efficacy as a weight-loss therapy. Gregory knew from his own experiences at Fultonia that his formula could be used to safely maintain an extended fast and lose a massive amount of weight. Nevertheless, it is remarkable that Gregory simultaneously marketed the same product (more or less) as being amenable to weight loss, famine relief, and optimal athletic performance—a true wonder drug if ever there was one. In 1984, Gregory signed a $100 million deal with Cernitin America to mass-produce and sell a powdered version of 4X as a weight loss supplement under the trade name "Dick Gregory's Slim-Safe Bahamian Diet," and he opened a weight loss clinic in Nassau.[127]

Gregory quickly found success in the weight loss business. In 1986, Gregory helped 800-pound Ron High lose hundreds of pounds of excess weight with Formula 4X. The next year, Gregory was chosen by Walter Hudson, the man who still holds the Guinness World Record for the largest human waist—and the fourth heaviest person in recorded history—to help him lose weight. Gregory credited his new product, Correction Connection, and his liquid Bahamian diet with helping Hudson lose an astonishing 700 pounds.[128] The Correction Connection formula, too, was a slight remix of Formula 4X marketed as a cure for addiction (to drugs and alcohol as well as food). Gregory credits it with helping to wean John Lennon and Yoko Ono off drugs in mid-1970s Berlin.[129] After Gregory's dramatic encounter with Walter Hudson, he founded his own company, Correction Connection Inc., and planned an entire empire around health foods and supplements marketed specifically to African Americans.[130] His new Correction Connection formula quickly became the top selling product at GNC, the largest nutrition supplement retailer in the United States, earning Gregory $3 million in its first year.[131]

Walter Hudson's well-publicized weight loss resonated with people across the country who were struggling with their size—some trapped in their homes, unable to walk—who suddenly clamored for access to Gregory's weight-loss program. In response, Gregory spent several million dollars to open another beachside resort and weight loss clinic, originally based in "a dismal facility" in Newark, New Jersey, and later relocated to Fort Walton, Florida.[132] Attendees of his weight-loss program would participate in what was, by all accounts, a grueling regimen. Not only were his clients expected to attend exercise classes on the beach before dawn every day, they were allowed nothing but fruit, fruit juice, and salad, consuming less than 500 calories a day.[133] A nutritionist from the University of California–Davis, Elizabeth Applegate, commented that the diet was "dangerously short" on minerals.[134] Gregory's staff at the resort included several nutritionists, a yoga instructor, and a psychotherapist, yet he had no physicians on location. He argued that the very presence of a physician would undermine the central concept of his resort, which was that people could lose tremendous amounts of weight through the power of diet and their own willpower alone.

For his unconventional approach to weight loss, an article in the *Los Angeles Times* referred to Gregory as "the zany commander of some madcap crew." To be sure, his tactics attracted some deeply loyal followers. One of Gregory's more notable clients, a white man named Mike Parteleno, compared meeting the former comedian to experiencing a first kiss. Parteleno gushed that Gregory was "probably one of the greatest men on the planet," and said he would "jump from the third story into a vat of pudding" had

Gregory so asked.[135] Clearly, some people were driven to attend just to be near Gregory's celebrity as some of Gregory's clients paid over $1,000 a week to participate. There were other clients, however, that Gregory sponsored himself; they could attend the program for free in exchange for giving his weight loss program positive publicity. Because Gregory encouraged the publicity, the beaches by the resort were reportedly stalked by camera crews who recruited his clients to appear on the *Phil Donahue Show* among others.

Regardless of whether his clients paid their own way or were given scholarships, Gregory had a reputation of being harsh toward them. He even likened himself to a warden: he took their keys, tried to stay away from them as much as he could, and castigated them for ordering pizza deliveries to the resort at 3:00 A.M. He even disparagingly referred to the guests at his resort as a "freak show."[136] Unsurprisingly, some of his clients began to resent him and subsequently left the program. In spite of all this, Gregory still expected his patients to succeed, marveled when they made unlikely friendships with each other, and coached some to become nutritional educators.

Importantly, Gregory's weight loss project was only a small part of his career. His explicit goal was improved health for "millions of people who can't afford it," including white people, but at the core of Gregory's activism was a desire to help realize a greater number of healthy Black bodies worldwide.[137] Gregory followed Fulton's lead in conceptualizing Black health in terms of the freedom struggle. Food was central to the plight of Black people around the world and just as central for their salvation—but not only because of nutritional concerns. Food—and thus health—was tied to immense economic, social, and political injustice as well. Gregory imagined the food products he designed (intended to stave off chronic disease and cure drug and alcohol addiction) as having both medical and social utility. But the health benefits Gregory imagined even extended into his business model; Gregory envisioned Black Americans gaining economic footholds by becoming salespeople of his products. He reasoned that if his distributors could make over $200,000 per year, he could make a thousand Black millionaires and in doing so bring more money into and improve the health of their communities at the same time, a goal that strongly resonated with Fulton's central mission.

Conclusion

Through several independent historical threads, Black people began to eat vegetarian or vegan diets in America. From the mid-1970s on, a steady rise occurred in the number of vegetarian soul food restaurants as well as a surge in the importation and Americanization of plant-forward African and Afro-Caribbean cuisines. The more contemporary movements for food justice, food sovereignty, and urban farming, while not contributing directly to vegetarianism, have helped to reshape Black foodways as a whole, making vegetarian food more accessible to more people. The animal rights movement, despite its white-normativity (and bad history of race relations), also has a long history of overlap with the fight for racial equality.[138] Some of the first public figures to agitate on behalf of animal rights were prominent abolitionist thinkers as well, including Jeremy Bentham and William Wilberforce.[139] More recently, work by such esteemed Black feminists as Angela Davis, Alice Walker, Audre Lorde, and Coretta Scott King have drawn compelling connections between animalization, dehumanization, and the way such processes of social degradation have been used to justify the mistreatment of entire classes of beings.[140]

Though she is seldom cited by name, Fulton's formative influence is most clearly visible by proxy. Many Black vegans, including the most prominent voices in the contemporary movement—Amie Breeze Harper, the critical race scholar and founder of the Sistah Vegan Project; sisters Aph and Syl Ko, the founders of Black Vegans Rock; Tracye McQuirter, the author of the best-selling vegan guidebook *By Any Greens Necessary*; and even Coretta Scott King—cite two of Alvenia Fulton's proteges, Dick Gregory and/or wellness guru Queen Afua as their primary inspiration for pursuing a plant-based lifestyle.[141] Fulton and Gregory should thus be understood as two of the most significant progenitors of the modern Black vegan diet.

The only area where Fulton and Gregory are not necessarily due credit is in the development and articulation of Black vegan cuisine. Their diet of brown rice and juice may have been good for the soil and popular among image-obsessed celebrities, but it did not necessarily appeal to the broader American palate. So when the parallel developments in vegan "soulless" restaurants and cuisines from throughout the African diaspora cross-pollinated, they gave Fulton's and Gregory's ideas a richer and more distinctive flavor. Significantly, when we weave these threads together (animal rights, food justice, food sovereignty, the rediscovery of Black diasporic foodways, combatting medical racism and health inequalities, environmentalism, and feminism), what emerges is a philosophically robust articulation of veganism that is, at its core, critical, intersectional, decolonial, antiracist, and soul*ful*. This is the vision of veganism that prominent Black intellectuals, diet gurus, cookbook authors, social media personalities, celebrities, activists, and scholars are articulating now.

Fulton herself remained vigilant in the fight to protect the health of her community until she passed away in 1999 at ninety-two, an age she would have considered a true testament to the power of the Fultonia dietary method. Her commitment to the health and prosperity of Black communities in the United States and around the globe through nonviolence and natural living spurred a vibrant antiracist and feminist Black vegan movement that flourishes today. In a 2020 interview with the *Washington Post* on the growing rates of African American vegans, Afya Ibomu, a holistic nutritionist cited medical disparities as a key motivator for the dietary shift among Black communities toward a more plant-based diet: "We have higher rates of obesity, cancer, diabetes and asthma. It's partly our DNA; we're not well-suited to a standard American diet. . . . Many of us came from West Africa where they mostly had goat's milk. And here it's cow's milk. The majority of health guidance is based on European bodies."[142] These disparities, which Fulton was among the first to recognize and combat openly, linger on.

By importing historically white notions of health and healing into her community, Fulton provided Black Chicagoans access to an otherwise inaccessible and elitist health framework. But in so doing, she performed similar cultural labor to the generations of African Americans who borrowed elements from a diverse range of European cuisines and applied them to cheap, local ingredients to create their own distinct cuisine imbued with local, Black meanings—a kind of creolization.[143] Fulton's approach to health advice was similarly adaptive, advising her readers to try to eat healthier despite the few resources they had available and to whatever degree they felt comfortable. So despite championing vegetarianism, Fulton occasionally advised her readership to consume such animal products as desiccated liver tablets, raw fertilized eggs, cod liver oil, or bone meal as stepping stones on their journey to better health.[144] Regardless of these leniencies, Fulton was still the first person to articulate a broad vision for the multiple overlapping uses of veganism to support Black communities, uphold Black values, and improve Black health, making her the clear ideological predecessor to contemporary Black veganism.

Ultimately, Fulton pioneered an affordable, accessible middle way for African Americans caught between the pressures of medical racism, unequal health outcomes, and the cultural importance of embodying civil rights politics. Leveraging her sway with celebrities, she persuaded Black communities to view food as an agent of health and healing, advocating fresh, whole foods as the path to alleviating or reversing the crippling burden of chronic disease. To improve Black health within and beyond her local community, Fulton recognized that her advice needed foremost to be accessible. Cultural ownership of healthy eating practices was more important to Fulton than the magnitude of actual dietary change because only by situating those eating practices in a firm cultural narrative could they be sustained indefinitely.

Entremets I

Ceding Healthy Food

· ·

During the first half of the twentieth century, while the US government fretted about food safety and *under*nutrition—fearing what spoilage and hunger might do to the nation's military prowess and its labor force during these peak (inter)war years—certain elements of the US public (especially young women) became widely concerned about weight loss and *over*nutrition for the first time. At the close of the nineteenth century, American chemist Wilbur Olin Atwater was promoting the calorie as a (rather exploitive) measure of energy expenditure that could help the US government and industrial barons calculate the cheapest minimum ration that adult men under their supervision needed to perform intense physical labor.[1] Not two decades later, in 1918, Dr. Lulu Hunt Peters imagined the same unit as a tool to help middle- to upper-class white women trim their waists to appear more waifish, modern, and attractive. For Peters, there was no irony in the fact that while the United States was urging the public to eat more—albeit not too much, not bread, and it had better be homegrown!—such credentialed scientific experts as herself were exhorting women across the country to eat less.[2] In fact, she thought dieting dovetailed quite well with the global obligation to ration food and end starvation. The less food adult women ate, she reasoned, the more food (and resources generally) would be available to help starving children and feed working men.[3] In her era, Peters's dictates—the likes of which would today brand her a kind of diet guru unto herself—were instead "a quintessentially Progressive Era regime touted as modern, scientific, and rational."[4]

Peters's popular book *Diet and Health* serves as a useful marker for the beginning of the seductively simple energy balance theory of "reducing" or losing weight. Imagining the body as essentially equivalent to a combustion engine, energy balance theory posits that by merely eating fewer calories than your body expends, weight will melt off naturally. This century-old logic underpins the basic diet and exercise advice mainstream nutrition science still touts today, despite the growing evidence of (and decades of personal anecdotes attesting to) its utter insufficiency. Contemporary fat activists argue that public health guidelines have taken too long to acknowledge that obesity is mediated by significantly more complex chemistry than the engine model would suggest.

The energy-centric understanding of body weight, which conveniently ignores structural issues in the industrial food system by reinforcing the neoliberal mandate for individuals to fix and control themselves, still pervades institutional biomedicine. Though harmful dieting messages have undeniably emanated from diet gurus, broader pop culture, and the media, the scientific establishment has long been complicit in amplifying the message that body weight is undesirable and amounts to personal failure. After all, the scientific method for weight loss is portrayed as so easy to understand that it should be just as easy for anyone with a modicum of self-control to enact. Energy balance is so seductively simple an explanation for obesity that it has become almost unquestionable. And in being unquestionable, energy balance theory has become merciless and unforgiving—casting those who have found themselves unable to lose weight with conventional diet and exercise as either incapable of understanding the basic logic of input and output (a laughable prospect) or hopelessly gluttonous in the face of ever-more-appealing mass-market food products (a cruel overgeneralization that shifts blame from deficiencies in the food system to its hapless victims).

What the energy balance model misses, of course, is the real possibility that obesity is only one symptom of a much more complex and braided public health crisis caused by decades of rapid and overlapping changes in the food system and the rest of the built environment. But there is a long history of motivated reasoning behind the energy balance model, too. At midcentury, for instance, credentialed nutrition scientists deeply resented the insinuation that America's world-famous food supply (let alone any other changes to our chemical environment) could possibly cause lasting harm to human health. Nutrition experts felt especially beholden to industrial food because heavy public investment in agricultural science and industrial food-processing technologies were still essential to meaningfully addressing their primary professional concern at the time: hunger and malnutrition.

At the national and global level, hunger and malnutrition had proven a recalcitrant social dilemma that shaped the agenda for American nutrition science and policy for decades.[5] Agricultural technologies that promised to dramatically boost food production were pioneered in the early decades of the twentieth century, yet they were expensive and slow to penetrate into areas with small farms or poor farmers. The United States also had been experiencing severe labor shortages on farms because two generations of young men had been called to war. What surpluses there had been in food production (or from voluntary rationing) were largely used to stock supply lines overseas or were exported strategically as food aid. Even during peacetime, growing enough food to feed the nation did not guarantee enough food would reach those most in need. Well into the twentieth century (and continuing today) huge swaths of America were plagued by hunger and malnutrition, threatening the capacity of the nation's labor force and its military. Though the hydra of chronic disease was starting to rear its many heads, ending hunger continued to be the preeminent concern in nutrition science into the early 1970s, becoming almost a singular focus at times, the consequences of which we will explore in entremets II and III.

In the name of ending hunger and achieving self-sufficiency, US farmers were not only incentivized to plant staple grain monocultures but to drown their ever-larger fields in ever-increasing doses of pesticides, herbicides, and chemical fertilizers and to harvest them with ever-more-resource-intensive machinery. Using a dizzying array of new chemical techniques, these artificially cultivated raw goods were then to be preserved and transformed en masse into an panoply of new processed foods in the 1950s. The new scientific food system worked so well to boost American agricultural production that it helped cement the United States as the wealthiest nation in the world and the only true superpower after World War II. Because of what appeared to be clear success in the US marketplace, scientific agriculture quickly became naturalized—even unremarkable—as consumers quickly adapted to its safety and many conveniences. In the 1960s and 1970s, parochial scientists like agronomist Norman Borlaug assumed they could easily export the unprecedented American successes with agricultural science around the world, bringing capitalistic prosperity to newly independent (and thus politically vulnerable) developing nations during the so-called Green Revolution. Yet as American-style agriculture spread across the globe, a cascade of interrelated chronic health conditions (not to mention interlocking environmental and economic disasters) followed close behind.

Expectedly, not everyone was enamored with the unprecedented growth and promise of industrial agriculture and food processing. In the United States, one of conventional agriculture's most formidable opponents was author and publisher Jerome Rodale, who in the 1940s became the leading figure of the so-called natural food movement, a major component of which he dubbed "organic" farming—a term that has since irked many a chemist.

Rodale preached (baselessly) that food grown in hearty soil fertilized with compost and animal manure free from synthetic chemicals was not just less dangerous to consume but actually contained more nutrients than food grown by the now-conventional methods.[6] Growing crops without synthetic chemicals would also preserve the fragile soils and soil ecosystems necessary to support human civilization. Rodale propagated his controversial vision for alternative agriculture through his own media outlet, the Rodale Press, which grew steadily into one of the most influential publishers in the genre of natural and healthy living in the twentieth century.

In the postwar period, the promise of Rodale's radical luddite agriculture began to resonate with proponents of the "health food" movement, a separate radical food tradition with roots in temperance. Prominent nineteenth-century health reformers thought such stimulating consumables as meats, spices, and alcohol inflamed the passions and led inexorably to moral decay: self-abuse (onanism), crime, and vagrancy. Exhibiting dietary self-control was, for them, a marker of dignity and civilization; for this reason, their attitudes thus cannot be easily divorced from white supremacy (see chapter 1). The most esteemed American proponents of health foods were Sylvester Graham and John Harvey Kellogg, whose bland, processed grain products—Graham bread, the Graham cracker, and the corn flake—were deployed for their intertwined physiological and moral effects: to calm the nerves, subdue the passions, and bolster frail constitutions. After the scientific articulation of the vitamins and minerals in the late 1910s and early 1920s, health foods were more commonly marketed for their energy-yielding or "protective" properties.

Insofar as food has served as medicine to some degree in every human culture, the US natural and health food movements were nothing special. The more remarkable transition, historically speaking, was orthodox medicine becoming more heavily reliant on laboratory science than clinical experience, leading credentialed physicians to gradually distance themselves from the otherwise universal tradition of diet therapy. With the exception of treating vitamin deficiency syndromes—efforts that yielded many Nobel Prizes for men in the field's early history and secured their predominance in the field's most prestigious posts in the decades following—dietary intervention was ultimately neglected as a therapeutic or preventive avenue among biomedical institutions. Once the vitamins and minerals had all been discovered and synthesized and overt nutrition deficiency syndromes mostly laid to rest, nutrition was considered a complete—and thus dead—science. Efforts to solve hunger shifted their center of gravity away from the laboratory-based biochemistry model of nutrition toward industrial food processing and agronomy.

The social and cultural devaluation of nutrition science was also due, at least in part, to the fact that nutrition was interwoven with the gendered labor of feeding and caretaking. Dietetics—once the exclusive province of nurses à la Florence Nightingale—was harnessed in the Progressive Era by home economists and domestic scientists, who aimed to rationalize the home using scientific principles.[7] Though dietitians quickly became essential to the functioning of hospitals, the predominantly male physicians who ran those hospitals consistently undervalued the dietitians' unique clinical expertise. Dietetics, despite being a critical element of patient care, was relegated to women perceived to be administrative subordinates and was given as much respect. Meanwhile, members of other female-dominated specialties such as nursing feared the dietitians' professional competition and helped edge them (and their expertise) out of the clinical setting. Though nutritional concerns were (and are) central to maintaining the body's proper functioning and mediating its recovery from injury (including surgery), the science of feeding lacked prestige. As elite orthodox medicine retreated from dietary modification, heterodox healers took control and infused their versions of healthy eating with antiestablishment politics.

Both the health food and natural food movements resented that hegemonic medicine presented itself as objective when its success was so clearly tied to the profits of industries that were assumed (and later confirmed) to be damaging human health and the environment.[8] Both movements lacked infrastructure and institutional protections, shared a mutual suspicion of conventional expertise, and simultaneously developed interests in alternative publishing, food processing, and distribution. These similarities served as the basis for a strong alliance between health nuts and the natural growers. In the 1960s and 1970s, through the efforts of people like Fulton and the gurus of the macrobiotic collective (featured in the next chapter), the unified natural health food community developed its own grassroots network of dedicated natural health food stores, co-ops, and other specialized grocers. The movement's inherently anticorporate stance attracted other radical and alternative cultures, and eventually their stores and magazines became indistinguishable mélanges of mostly liberal, mostly White-coded identities and health politics. Natural health food communities are now perceived as being so white, in fact, that academics and other analysts have been blinded to the underlying diversity of people using food as medicine.

In the next chapter, we will see how a movement that looks, on the surface, similar to Fulton's (in terms of its non-white leadership, its overarching message of nonviolence, and its deep cultural history of resistance to white Western oppression) developed a different audience and a different relationship altogether with its patients. Rather than promoting authentic cultural ownership of the diet, as Fulton did, the next chapter's diet grappled instead with its clients' appropriation of a foreign culture for their own philosophical and dietary use.

2 Zen and the Art of Macrobiotic Maintenance

Michio Kushi, World Peace, and a Cold War
Treatment for Cancer

· ·

On the evening of October 13, [1965] Sess and Min Wiener came to
visit their daughter in New York. When Sess glimpsed her lying on
a mattress in a corner, he gasped and visibly turned color. Beth Ann
was a living skeleton. Her legs were no longer yang, they were skin
and bones. Her eyes, still sanpaku, were sunken in their sockets.
She could barely sit up. She could not have weighed more than
80 pounds.

—*New York Herald Tribune*, 1966

Less than a month after Beth Ann Simon, a twenty-four-year-old from Clif-
ton, New Jersey, was admitted to the hospital, she died from malnutrition,
incurred, allegedly, from following a bizarrely strict diet called Zen Macrobiotics. Simon's death was the subject of a 1966 grand jury trial and was
featured in a 1967 editorial for the *Journal of the American Medical Association*, which stated that she had been on the diet for over nine months when
she entered the hospital with scurvy and severe folic acid and protein deficiencies.[1] The revelations brought forth by Simon's death and the subsequent
trial horrified the medical community, which issued a hardline rejection of
this dangerous new dietary philosophy. The public health warnings they
issued were continually recirculated around the country for the ensuing
five years. So what was this dangerous new regimen?

In its most basic terms, the macrobiotic diet sought to foster balance and
harmony (expressed in terms of yin and yang) inside the body, in broader
society, and in the fabric of the cosmos itself through the proper consumption of mostly plant-based, mostly Japanese foods. According to the
philosophy, foods are (based on a complex series of logical deductions) dif-
ferentially imbued with qualities along the binary spectrum of yin and
yang, contributing their respective forces through transmutation to the consumer's bodily equilibrium. Foods with greater yin properties were associated with feminine, passive, cold, expansive, and quiet qualities, while those

with more yang tendencies were thought to embody masculine, aggressive, hot, contractive, and loud qualities.[2]

Macrobiotics reached commercial success and national notoriety in the United States with the publication of guru George Ohsawa's first English-language book *Zen Macrobiotics* (1960) and its successor *The Book of Judgment* (1965).[3] Though the Greek roots of the word "macrobiotics" suggest that it means "long" or "great" life—and indeed every version of the dietary lifestyle/healing philosophy emphasizes longevity—the more specific principles of the diet-cum-lifestyle were and are widely variable between different practitioners and ideologues who affiliate themselves with the macrobiotics movement.

Like many other ancient medical philosophies (or those based on ancient ideas), macrobiotics teaches that every living body is a microcosmic reflection of the larger macrocosm in which it is situated. What this means is that both personal illness as well as social ills may be addressed with the same, predominantly dietary, actions; the act of healing individual bodies can, en masse, heal entire societies. One of Ohsawa's chief disciples, Herman Aihara, summarized this attitude in his book *Basic Macrobiotics*: "Individual cells make up the whole body but each individual cell is unique, separated by a membrane from each other and making up the community of the body. Each person's body is separated by a membrane called skin, and many bodies live in communities that make up humanity on Earth. And maybe our planet, separated by its atmospheric skin, combines with others, forming communities that then make up the whole universe. Individuals, whether cells or people, are separated by a membrane, but in reality we are all One."[4]

In its earliest American formulation, macrobiotics promised to quell the yang tendencies of the West and usher in a global era of peace and understanding through humility, following the Buddhist ideal. And it was not to be taken lightly. The *New York Times* admonished its readers that "to dismiss macrobiotics as merely another in the long list of American food fads is to misunderstand its true nature and to underestimate its appeal to many young Americans today," further explaining that macrobiotics was "a spiritual, social and psychological way of life, a life-style with a mutant form of Zen Buddhism as the sky above and a cereal-based diet as the ground below."[5]

The No. 7 Diet

The diet that earned Beth Ann Simon's hospital admission in 1965 was a variant of the macrobiotic regimen called the "No. 7" diet. The No. 7 diet was first outlined by founder George Ohsawa in his book *Zen Macrobiotics*.[6] It consisted primarily of brown rice and other grains—flavored with a sesame seed-based seasoning called *gomashio*—with little to no fluid intake save for some bancha twig tea. From the perspective of nutrition scientists at least, the No. 7 diet was the ultimate stage of macrobiotics: the goal toward which each person following a macrobiotic regimen strove. With so many young people beginning to experiment with the lower stages of the diet, some media commentators publicly feared an epidemic of (perhaps fatal) malnutrition. In response to Simon's death, Fred Stare, the founder and chair of the nutrition department at Harvard University, penned a public service announcement proclaiming that "macrobiotic diets are *the most dangerous fad diets* in the current market of food fads" [emphasis added].[7]

Stare's harsh warning was not without justification. According to the Food and Drug Administration (FDA) report, the diet rapidly led its adherents to severe anemia, bone and tissue damage, dehydration, and organ failure. When a Passaic County grand jury investigated Simon's death in 1966, they also investigated the cases of five similar individuals that local doctors had brought to their attention.[8] Among the five, three of the adherents had died. The other two had been hospitalized, and doctors reported they would have died without emergency medical intervention. Beyond this trial, there were many other such stories of premature death or extreme illness connected with the diet. In 1972, for instance, the *New York Times* reported on a young San Francisco woman who switched her infant child from breastmilk to a macrobiotic all-cereal regimen, and shortly thereafter the child's hair fell out, and it nearly died.[9]

Simon's father, Samuel "Sess" Wiener, was a prominent lawyer who mobilized an FDA investigation into the Ohsawa Foundation in New York City pursuant to the fact that Ohsawa's book falsely promoted macrobiotics as a cure for "anemia, arthritis, appendicitis, cancer, cataracts, tuberculosis, diabetes, epilepsy, heart disease, hernia, leprosy, leukemia, meningitis, polio, paranoia, and schizophrenia."[10] The FDA launched a search and seizure for "eight thousand dollars worth" of foods, promotional books, and pamphlets promoting Zen Macrobiotics at the Ohsawa Foundation, acknowledging that while "the foods are harmless in themselves . . . the diets are dangerous."[11] The raid, which shuttered the New York branch of the Ohsawa Foundation, was among the highest profile takedowns of the National Congress on Medical Quackery, the coalition assembled by the American Medical Association to crackdown on health fraud (see entremets II).

The Simon case had a chilling effect on the public reputation of macrobiotics, and less than a year later George Ohsawa passed away in Japan at the age of seventy-three from a heart attack, which his followers attributed to his lifelong penchant for heavy smoking.[12] With the parallel investigation of Simon's death and the death of Ohsawa, the movement was in danger of collapsing altogether. The work of maintaining and promoting the macrobiotics cause in the United States fell to Ohsawa's top students, Michio Kushi and Herman Aihara. Far from disappearing after Ohsawa's death, under Kushi and Aihara's leadership macrobiotics flourished. It became a global movement with branches all over the United States, Europe, and Japan, with its own restaurants, natural food stores, and processed food brands. Macrobiotics attracted thousands of dedicated teachers, who published hundreds of books in dozens of languages and taught hundreds of thousands of students from all over the world.

Despite the inordinate amount of negative attention Simon's case attracted and the image nutrition scientists projected that macrobiotics was an extreme rice fast, the macrobiotics movement extended far beyond the No. 7 diet. In part due to racism and cultural ignorance, the macrobiotic dietary principles were widely misrepresented as punishingly austere. After all, many of the program's most ardent devotees easily maintained a diverse and apparently healthy diet for decades. As a social movement, macrobiotics tapped into popular anxieties about the speed and direction of modern society, offering one of the most coherent alternative lifestyles to fast-paced American consumerism. For macrobiotics adherents, it represented an entirely new code by which to live. However, there were a number of followers who were attracted to macrobiotics for other reasons (like the promise of quick health benefits), who had varying levels of understanding and commitment to the underlying philosophy and its politics. This chapter examines the relationship and tensions between macrobiotics as a social movement and as a medical miracle.

From before its introduction to the United States, macrobiotics was motivated by geopolitical conditions on a global scale. Its success and peculiar progression from hippie diet to cancer cure can only be understood in the light of the medical context of the Cold War. Macrobiotics leaders, haunted by the atomic bombing of Japan, appealed to the white guilt that followed World War II and inflamed existing Cold War anxieties around further use of nuclear weaponry.[13] As the United States attempted to find peaceful applications for its nuclear reactors, including potent new cancer therapies, macrobiotics cast such attempts as fundamentally wrongheaded and positioned its simplistic lifestyle program as an appropriate antidote to cancer instead.

Sagen Ishizuka and the Japanese Origins of Macrobiotics

Though it entered the American zeitgeist in the early 1960s, macrobiotics constituted a much older philosophy of eating, having begun formally in Japan with the writings, teachings, and political activities of Sakurazawa Jyoïchī, the man who came to be known in the west as George(s) Ohsawa (1893–1966).[14] Ohsawa first used the term "macrobiotic," or "macrobiotique," in a 1956 French-language book entitled *Guide pratique de la médecine macrobiotique d'Extrême-Orient*, and served as the concept's leading figurehead and chief popularizer.[15] Macrobiotics was strongly rooted in Ohsawa's Japanese heritage and his early political thought. Ohsawa's parents were both members of the samurai class, and they had fostered in him a deep respect for traditional Japanese culture from a young age. But his parents divorced, and his mother died of tuberculosis shortly thereafter. After a brief, unpleasant stint living with his father and stepmother, Ohsawa's younger brother also fell ill and died of tuberculosis in 1911. Fortunately, when Ohsawa, too, developed early symptoms of the disease, he stumbled on an obscure book at a local library entitled *Kagakuteki Shoku-yo Chojuron* (A Chemical Nutritional Theory of Long Life), an 1897 text by an army doctor named Sagen Ishizuka, which outlined (in scientific terms) the healing benefits of reinstituting an authentic, traditional Japanese diet.[16]

According to religious studies scholar and macrobiotics disciple Ronald Kotzsch—whose work explores Ohsawa's life and the origins of macrobiotics thought—Ishizuka based his dietary restrictions on a patchwork of overlapping Eastern and Western traditions, at once epidemiological, historical, and philosophical.[17] From these experiences, Ishizuka is said to have developed a powerful new holistic theory of healing that synthesized what he knew of Eastern and Western medicine. Exploiting his station as an army doctor, Ishizuka meticulously plotted epidemiological data from throughout Japan, paying particular attention to the correlation between the prevalence of certain diseases and the displacement of the traditional Japanese diet by Western tastes and ingredients. Using what he knew of the methods of Western chemistry, Ishizuka reduced his observations of varying disease prevalence to a simple ratio between two dietary salts: sodium and potassium. He noted that high sodium consumption corresponded to concentrations of diseases like cholera and fevers, whereas too much potassium was linked to outbreaks of such scourges as beriberi and chills. Though each individual's ideal salt ratio was dependent on the geographic and climatic conditions of their birthplace, their unique bodily characteristics, and their temperament, Ishizuka thought that on average people should strive to maintain a ratio of 3:7 parts of sodium to potassium salts in their diet.

Though it ran counter to the hegemonic Western medical logics in which he was trained, Ishizuka also read widely in Asian history, medicine, and philosophy, including such classical Chinese and Japanese thinkers and texts as Kaibara Ekken, Mizuno Nanboku, Confucius, Mencius, and the *Yellow Emperor's Classic of Internal Medicine* (*Nei Ching Huang Ti*). Based on his reading of Asian history and mythologies, Ishizuka concluded that— contrary to the prevailing cultural wisdom in Japan that positioned polished white rice as the major staple food of the country—it was actually roasted and steamed brown rice that had served as the historical basis for the Japanese diet.[18] Ishizuka therefore condemned what had been passing as a traditional diet in Japan, favoring what he understood to be a more historically accurate and healthful regimen.

In *Kagakuteki Shoku-yo Chojuron*, Ishizuka laid out the historical, philosophical, and epidemiological evidence he had gathered and provided a simple guide to lifestyle changes that he argued would assist in maintaining health by achieving the appropriate salt balance in the body. Chief among his recommendations was the consumption of an unprocessed, traditionally prepared, grain-centric diet consisting principally of local, naturally grown and climatically appropriate ingredients.[19] Like his cultural antecedents, Ishizuka recognized that certain foods, like meat, could still be heavily imbalanced no matter how animals were raised because meat inherently contained too much sodium. He reasoned that meat could still occasionally be consumed because the negative effects of extreme foods could be tempered with specific cooking techniques.[20] To further moderate the body's internal salt balance, Ishizuka argued for the reinstatement of traditional Japanese therapeutic bathing and exercise to encourage salt excretion by sweating.

During the Meiji period (1868–1912)—the political power shift that reinvigorated Japanese imperialism and first opened Japan to Westernization— traditional medicine was banned, and the progressive government energetically promoted the principles and practices of Western science (including nutrition), welcoming in both Western food staples and dietary habits. Ishizuka's nutritional guidelines, though partially couched in scientific research and techniques, subtly subverted the prevailing ideology of Westernization by using scientific techniques to vindicate a traditional, conservative Japanese lifestyle and culture. By tying his salt ratio theory to individual and regional temperament, for instance, Ishizuka did more than locate food as the root of all human disease; he also opened the door to conceive of nutrition (and other lifestyle changes) as a curative force for *all* human disorder—especially the kinds of social, spiritual, and political disorder ushered in by the West. Through his guiding philosophy, food consumption became the primary determinant of events and qualities in the world as well as the main lever of power to alter or control those events and qualities.

The Shoku-Yo Kai

After learning about Ishizuka's dietary philosophy and trying the grain-centric diet for himself, macrobiotics legend tells us young George Ohsawa found relief from his tubercular symptoms. His miraculous recovery coupled with the premature loss of his family inspired him to pursue his dream of traveling the world; he promptly moved to the bustling port-city of Kobe where he took a job on a trading vessel in 1914, exporting weaponry and silk for the British. From this position, he caught his first glimpses of the broader Asian continent, North Africa, and coastal Europe. Yet he quickly became disillusioned with the world he had so long yearned to see. Everywhere Ohsawa went, including around his native Japan, he witnessed the creeping spread of Westernization and the predictable cultural flattening and erasure that ensued. These changes conflicted with Ohsawa's deep regard for traditional Japanese culture. He became radicalized in opposition to what he (and many other "Japanists") saw as Western debauchery, greed, and "progress." When Ohsawa resettled in Japan in 1916, he sought community among the followers of the guru whose book had healed him of the disease that killed his family.

In 1908, Ishizuka's followers—who, at the time, included powerful Japanese political officials and cultural figures—created an organization called the Shoku-Yo Kai, or "Food Cure Society," naming Ishizuka as its primary advisor. Despite having used scientific reasoning and practices to develop his dietary program, Ishizuka later shunned all Western medical ideas and treatments in favor of his own healing philosophy. Ishizuka attracted legions of patients deemed untreatable by Western methods. From all across Japan, helpless patients wrote to him under a variety of playful monikers ranging from "Dr. Daikon Radish," and "Dr. Miso Soup," to "Dr. Anti-Doctor." He became so popular that he allegedly had to limit his patients to 100 per day.[21]

Ishizuka passed away in 1909, but when Ohsawa discovered the Shoku-Yo Kai in 1916 the group still shared the dietary philosophy and ideological leanings that had so thoroughly shaped Ohsawa's early thought. He became an avid member, rising through the ranks to become the group's leader in 1923. He expanded the group's radical reaffirmation of traditional culture to specifically condemn what Ohsawa increasingly saw as the narrow, spiritless machinations of Western science and medicine. As the society's leader, Ohsawa also subtly reshaped the group's purpose and redefined its thought. For instance, Ohsawa saw strong parallels between the "antagonistic yet complementary relationship" Ishizuka described as the basis for his salt balance theory and the ancient divine principles of yin and yang as outlined in the *I Ching*. In making these comparisons explicit, Ohsawa transformed Ishizuka's narrow dietary guidelines into a full-throated cosmology.[22] Ohsawa was particularly fascinated with a few offhand remarks in Ishizuka's text suggesting a proper diet could lead to spiritual fulfillment. He perhaps took the concept too literally: in Ohsawa's teachings, diet became a potent force that could align the body with the underlying organizational principles of the universe, providing a backdoor to Buddhist enlightenment, so to speak.

Ohsawa Goes West

For several years, the Shoku-Yo Kai tried in vain to nationalize their neo-traditional diet, offering the Imperial Japanese government a feeble ultimatum to adopt their regimen or watch the empire fall slowly into ruin. In 1929, however, Ohsawa felt his efforts to persuade the Japanese government to endorse his program were increasingly futile. So, he reasoned, if he could not stop Westernization in Japan, he would challenge it at its source: he moved to Paris. Ohsawa was unique among Japanese men of his generation for his exposure to a variety of Eastern and Western cultures, and he "hoped that the achievement of mutual understanding would be the first step in the development of a new, synthetic, harmonious world culture, one that incorporated the best elements of both."[23] Though his primary intention was to educate Westerners about the wisdom of Asian philosophies, he was also intent on learning the basis of Western ideology— if only to better grasp the barriers that prevented the germination of his own ideas.

In Paris, Ohsawa tried and failed to become an influential writer. With little money and few prospects after his first few months in Europe, he was apparently desperate enough to eat bird seed and plants he harvested from city parks just to survive. Eventually, he began attending lectures at the Sorbonne, where he mingled with French intellectuals whom he tried to teach the principles of Japanese cosmology.[24] After several failed attempts, he was beginning to think that Westerners would never understand Asian philosophies on their own terms. He changed tactics, converting his ideas into a Western analytic style. In doing so, however, Ohsawa developed a deeper understanding of Eastern philosophies for himself. Rather than simply translate Asian philosophical concepts for a Western audience then, his 1931 book the *Le Principe Unique* (The Unique Principle) blended every major Eastern philosophical tradition he knew (Buddhism, Hinduism, Taoism, etc.) into a unified cosmological tapestry centered around the essential dualism in Chinese philosophy between yin and yang. This formulation laid the philosophical groundwork for modern macrobiotics.

For the next twenty years, Ohsawa lived in Japan where he wrote polemics and manifestos, which oscillated wildly between unqualified pacifism and self-interested ultranationalism. By 1943, when the systematic American bombing campaigns began on the lower reaches of the Japanese archipelago, Ohsawa had become firmly disillusioned with war, moving to a remote prefecture to focus on his philosophical writings.[25] Living in isolation left Ohsawa feeling bored and powerless though, so after one last doomed attempt to get the Imperial government to adopt *shoku-yo* ideology, he hatched a radical plan to move against the war effort himself. In 1944, Ohsawa smuggled himself across the border to Japanese-controlled Manchuria where he had connections with Japanese police who could permit him to cross the border into Russia illegally. From there, he planned to charter a boat and hire two horses to ride across Russia to Moscow, though he had never ridden a horse. Once there, he hoped to personally persuade Stalin to intercede in the Pacific theater since Russia's allegiance was, as yet, undeclared.[26] Unfortunately, hostile authorities quickly learned of his quixotic plot. Ohsawa barely managed to cross the border into Manchuria before being seized by the Japanese police and thrown in prison. Then, when he promptly escaped his cell, he was put in front of a firing squad, where, at the last moment, his friend in the Japanese guard interceded on his behalf and spared his life.

As Ohsawa languished in prison a second time, the United States deployed the world's first nuclear warheads on Hiroshima and Nagasaki, and

Japan unconditionally surrendered the war. Upon his release, Ohsawa devoted himself to promoting world peace and became a spokesperson for the World Federalist Movement, an organization that envisioned a global president with binding authority over member states as a more powerful version of the United Nations.[27] In his softening toward the West, Ohsawa forged from his old traditionalist shoku-yo ideology a new, Western-infused macrobiotics movement that could speak across international traditions to foster global peace through mindfulness and self-improvement.

In 1949, Ohsawa revisited Paris to found a center to foster his ideas called the Maison Ignoramus. For the next few years, Ohsawa wrote letters to everyone he considered a major world leader, asking to connect with them about his philosophical and dietary teachings. He received several notable replies, including an invitation from Nobel laureate and physician Albert Schweitzer to visit him in Gabon, which Ohsawa did. In 1953, he and his new wife Lima sold all their belongings and became self-professed citizens of the world, dedicating the rest of their lives to the international spread of macrobiotics.

Cold War Fusion: A Japanese Alternative Comes to America

Macrobiotics first came to the United States in a trickle from those who had studied at the Maison Ignoramus in the 1940s and 1950s and who had followed the lifestyle to the best of their independent abilities. Nearly all these early acolytes settled in New York City, including Ohsawa's chief disciples Herman and Cornelia Aihara and Michio and Aveline Kushi. Other important early American followers included Alcan Yamaguchi, the founder of the first macrobiotic restaurants, Zen Teahouse and Musubi; French-born actress Irma Paule, who cofounded the New York City branch of the Ohsawa Foundation; and Michel Abehsera, a French-Moroccan rabbi who established several other early macrobiotic restaurants and who also wrote several major macrobiotic cookbooks.[28]

The movement did not start spreading until Ohsawa made his inaugural trip to the United States, published *Zen Macrobiotics*, and founded an outpost in New York City called the George Ohsawa Foundation. Initially, he went to Buddhist enclaves on the Upper East Side to woo Japanese Americans with little success.[29] Soon after, Ohsawa seized the coattails of Zen Buddhism leader Daisetz Teitaro Suzuki's success, electrifying young, radical musicians and artists in New York City by selling his own Zen-branded philosophy. Though it bastardized some of the religious framing, Ohsawa's

Zen Macrobiotics fulfilled a similar cultural niche to its namesake. For instance, Japanese Americans pitched Buddhist philosophy as a "Middle Way" or "Third Power" situated between the major Cold War powers and ideologies. Ohsawa promoted his program as playing a neutral, global peace-brokering role, too.[30]

Although Ohsawa was, in some limited respects, selling religiosity like many other Asian spiritual leaders operating in the United States during the same time period, he was ultimately neither a religious leader nor a scholar. Despite situating his program in quasi-religious terms, Ohsawa understood that macrobiotics was not merely an updated, transnational interpretation of the teachings of the Buddha. Rather, he considered it the "biological foundation of Buddhist meditation and spirituality."[31] Macrobiotics was supposed to bring the body into alignment with Ohsawa's expansive conception of Buddhism as represented by his Unique Principle. Yet this "biological" conception of Buddhism bled easily into more overt mysticism.

Ohsawa apparently believed that the macrobiotic diet, when executed properly, could afford the user "powers of clairvoyance and foreknowledge" and the ability to see "beyond time and space," a capacity Ohsawa deployed when he predicted the imminent collapse of what he called the American "Gold World Empire."[32] In 1961, just after the Soviet Union began construction on the Berlin Wall, Ohsawa had another psychic vision that New York City was the target of an imminent nuclear attack.[33] Despite Ohsawa's assurances that "if an atomic bomb or a hydrogen bomb were dropped, only those practicing macrobiotics would survive," he urged the immediate evacuation of the macrobiotics community and implored them to seek out new, fertile territory where they could grow organic brown rice and thrive.[34] Ohsawa's message resonated especially strongly with the former Beat movement adherents who had been left behind when Allen Ginsberg and Jack Kerouac left Columbia University for San Francisco.

After some research, the stalwart macrobiotics enthusiasts followed the path of the Beats' own migration—choosing Chico, California, as their destination. Chico was ideally situated in the Sacramento valley, buttressed to the south and east by the Sierra Nevada range, which they thought would insulate them from the devastation of imminent nuclear war and fallout. The caravan of "atomic age refugees" consisted of thirteen families with thirty-six total migrants. Members of the group included "Broadway musicians, a Columbia University professor, a couple of Japanese immigrants, a Harvard-educated economist who'd helped formulate the Marshall Plan, and . . . Teal Ames, then one of the stars of the popular soap opera *The Edge of Night.*"[35] The trek, which Ohsawa himself called "a modern parallel to the Israelite Exodus from Egypt under Moses," attracted national media attention.[36]

Once in California, macrobiotics gained several different major followings. Its explicit antiviolence posture garnered it a sympathetic audience with the antiwar movement. Historian Warren Belasco has speculated that "perhaps simplifying one's diet to a few 'Oriental' staples symbolized solidarity with poor but spiritually strong Vietnamese peasants."[37] Similarly, macrobiotics' commitment to growing Japanese staples on local farms with organic farming techniques resonated with the budding environmental movement, especially in its hostility toward the industrial food system. This attitude proved important for macrobiotics' eventual domination of the natural health foods sector.

For several years, macrobiotics was distributed as a "cleansing ritual" among former Beats and subsequently attracted many who were tired of heavy drug use and sought to alleviate their addictions. The *New York Times* described these various stripes of macrobiotics adherents as "young (in their early 20s), white, middle-class, smooth-faced with short-cut hair, lean, ex-drug users, candid, somewhat lonely, slightly righteous and more than a little disenchanted with contemporary American life."[38] There were even rumors among doctors and nutritionists that the macrobiotic diet was popular because it yielded an equivalent "natural" high that could lure users away from hallucinogens.[39] Testimony from a Chicago-based macrobiotics leader, Tom Swan, bears these suspicions out: "For a couple of years, I'd eaten different diets. . . . I went thru various stages, but it didn't come together until I did 10 days of brown rice. I felt fantastic. It was the highest experience of my life. I dropped weight, but evenly. I got more relaxed. I'd have the strongest, clean sleep. I'd close my eyes and go right out into the Universe. It was like meditating all night."[40]

The fact that one ate macrobiotically was not necessarily a guarantee of a drug-free lifestyle, as the reports of Haight-Ashbury hippies "dealing macrobiotics along with marijuana and other drugs" would attest.[41] The relationship between macrobiotics and drug use was not necessarily straightforward. Although the diet became known for its use in drug detoxification, *Chicago Tribune* journalist Mary Daniels interviewed employees at a macrobiotic store in Chicago and found that "most are not ex-drug users . . . some are straight people who made themselves sick in other ways. . . . Alcohol, birth control pills, or just plain coffee and cigarets [sic], for example." One of her interviewees, Loren McCune, reportedly said,

"I never took psychedelic drugs, but I did take a lot of medicine."[42] Daniels's interview suggests that what macrobiotics considered to be drugs may not necessarily have aligned with the ubiquitous drug detox narrative in the press, and perhaps even included products of mainstream medicine.

Racial and Religious Politics in the Popular Reception of Macrobiotics

By importing macrobiotics to the United States under the auspices of an authentic Japanese culinary and religious tradition, Ohsawa quickly ran afoul of the extant culinary and religious practices other Japanese Americans had been developing for decades in the United States. In the decade before Ohsawa's arrival, Japanese Americans had already been struggling to protect their domain over Buddhist culture from white appropriation by the "Beats and elites," who found inspiration in the teachings of Daisetz Suzuki.[43] For many American convert Buddhists, such as Alan Watts, Zen philosophy resonated with their deep desire to reject the predominating Cold War ideologies and institutions, especially those most associated with materialism.[44] Yet for Japanese American Buddhists who had suffered the profound racial prejudice of the US government, such a radical rejection of American life ran counter to the intense political pressures of assimilation. As Japanese Americans worked to integrate Buddhist practices and values with their adoptive culture, white convert Buddhists increasingly understood their efforts as compromising the integrity of Buddhist teachings. Troublingly, some white American convert Buddhists saw themselves as having a more disciplined and "authentic" Buddhist practice than Japanese immigrants who had been raised Buddhist.[45]

That Ohsawa came to the United States in the 1960s to sell what by all appearances was an Asian religion places him in conversation with a host of other so-called Oriental Monk figures.[46] In her book *Virtual Orientalism*, religious studies scholar Jane Iwamura argues that the way white Americans "[wrote] themselves into the story" of Suzuki and other Cold War era Oriental Monk icons created a "modernized cultural patriarchy in which Anglo-Americans reimagine[d] themselves as the protectors, innovators, and guardians of Asian religions and culture and wrest the authority to define these traditions from others." Insofar as Ohsawa "represent[ed the] future salvation of the dominant culture," and embodied "a revitalized hope of saving the West from capitalist greed, brute force, totalitarian rule, and spiritless technology," he epitomized the Oriental Monk stereotype.[47] In several important ways, however, Ohsawa differed sharply from Suzuki and others in the monk mold. Whereas many other Oriental Monk figures became known in American mass media through images in which they draped themselves in traditional Asian dress and other cultural iconography, Ohsawa preferred to wear an American suit and tie and "forbade his students to address him with the traditional title of Sensei."[48] Perhaps because he did not fit into all of the tropes of the Oriental Monk, Ohsawa was not widely understood in the American press to be an authentic mediator of his own Japanese culture.

Scientific and medical experts in the media loudly proclaimed the diet's inherent conflict with its namesake, Zen Buddhism, hoping to undercut Ohsawa's credibility as a philosopher, spiritual leader, and, bizarrely, as a Japanese man. In a statement he prepared for Harvard University Health Services, nutrition scientist Fred Stare quoted his "Oriental scholar" colleagues at the Massachusetts Institute of Technology as saying that "Ohsawa has perverted Buddhism" and "such a rigid diet would be a deterrent for spiritual growth in Zen Buddhism. Food cultism is abhorrent to real Buddhists."[49] Stare, a major opponent of diet gurus who will reappear in subsequent chapters, continued, "One might be led to believe that Ohsawa's diet formulations are based on the great ancient philosophies. This is not true. The diets seem to be no more ancient than Ohsawa himself. . . . Macrobiotic eating is an excursion into make-believe Oriental cultism."[50] The narrative stuck: seven years after Ohsawa's death and the Beth Ann Simon incident, Stare's claims were still circulating in prominent newspapers. As an example, Dr. Walter C. Alvarez—physician, writer, and father of renowned nuclear physicist Luis Alvarez—quoted Stare in a scathing piece against macrobiotics for the *Los Angeles Times* asserting that, in addition to being dangerous, the diet was a "bogus version" of Zen Buddhism with no "authentic" connection to Japanese heritage. This was despite the fact that Ohsawa and many of his most loyal disciples were themselves indisputably Japanese.[51]

To undermine the cultural authority of Ohsawa's Japanese heritage, Stare and his allies positioned themselves as gatekeepers to an essentialized caricature of "authentic" Asian culture. Their critiques were not limited to Ohsawa's spiritual or health claims either. Stare inveighed against the foods central to macrobiotics in writing "the advocacy of brown rice is not Oriental. . . . Japanese, Indians and Chinese, do not prefer brown rice, they place a high priority on white rice."[52] By defending a narrow vision of *the* traditional Asian diet, critics like Stare collapsed the great culinary diversity of Asia to generalizations based on relatively recent cultural transformations in isolated geographic areas. Polished white rice had only become a popular alternative to whole grain rice in parts of Asia during the second half of the nineteenth century, its rising availability the result of industrialization. Cruelly, this processed staple's popularity led to devastating epidemics of beriberi, a vitamin deficiency syndrome. Like Ishizuka before him, Ohsawa justified his preference for brown rice by invoking its history as the predecessor of modernized Japanese cuisine: the artificial, industrialized food culture macrobiotics had been originally designed to replace during the Westernizing Meiji era.

There was a modicum of truth behind Stare's and other critics' skepticism though: Ohsawa admitted to having added the "Zen" to macrobiotics as a shallow marketing gimmick.[53] The Unique Principle underlying macrobiotics had but a passing resemblance to real Zen Buddhism. Ohsawa admitted that he admired Daisetz Suzuki's success explaining and advertising Zen Buddhism in Europe and the United States and thought he might be able to take advantage of the cultural current—as had Eugen Herrigel in 1948 with his popular book *Zen and the Art of Archery*, the first book that purported to explore various leisure activities to gain insight into Zen philosophy.[54]

Regardless of how and why Ohsawa used the language of Zen Buddhism in recruiting followers and framing his diet, the ways in which Stare used Zen Buddhism as a weapon to dismantle Ohsawa's credibility reveals a more incisive agenda. Stare's and others' early statements about macrobiotics demonstrate a willingness to deploy racial stereotypes and scandalmongering to defend an idealized Western culture and diet from intercultural challenges and cross-pollination. The critiques were not even internally consistent. In 1966, Stare said—despite his admonition that "the Zen Macrobiotic Diet *in all of its various forms* is a dangerous diet and if followed for any length of time can lead to ill health and death" [emphasis added]—that the "initial program" offered such presumably nonthreatening foods as "chicken, fruit, vegetables, with emphasis on brown rice."[55] To his credit, Stare recanted his earlier intolerance of macrobiotics in 1978, grudgingly admitting that it was little more than a traditional vegetarian diet on which users could expect to lose between ten and fifteen pounds. His admission came too late and did little to reverse the damage of his earlier caricatures in the court of public opinion.[56]

Instead of intervening in a way that respected the spiritual or political convictions of the diet's followers, nutrition scientists and physicians chose to depict macrobiotics as coextensive with its most extreme pronunciations and adherents, thereby dismissing the entire lifestyle and its associated philosophies as hopelessly dangerous. Medical professionals' bad faith and racialized dismissal not only failed to deter people from experimenting with macrobiotics, it further isolated macrobiotics followers and apologists from mainstream medicine and nutrition as well. With this in mind, it is worth revisiting this chapter's opening vignette.

Death by Restriction: *Sanpaku* and the No. 7 Controversy Revisited

From within the macrobiotics community, the Beth Ann Simon case looked very different than it did in the Passaic County courtroom. Rather than concede that Simon's death signaled an implicit danger in the promises of their shared dietary program, macrobiotics leaders largely attributed her death, and those of many others, to user error. Despite the implausibly numerous health miracles Ohsawa said were possible through the transformative No. 7 diet, and the misleading manner in which Ohsawa framed the purpose and duration of the diet and, therefore, the likelihood of the fulfillment of those promises, other macrobiotics leaders insisted that the No. 7 diet's intended function was far more limited. While Stare described the intent of the program to "move from diet No. 1 to diet No. 7 in set stages," for instance, countless macrobiotics lieutenants insisted this was a radical misinterpretation of Ohsawa's text. For one, Ohsawa's formulation actually had ten stages, ranked from −3 to 7 (each permitting varying amounts of yin or yang foods), which adherents could shift between as they pleased. Moreover, these leaders argued vehemently that the No. 7 diet was only intended as a fast and should be reserved for moments of heightened spiritual clarity or "special healing purposes," and it was only "to be followed for about ten days at a time," not endured as a long-term regimen.[57] They cited numerous examples from their personal experiences and those of their students of the successful (but substantially more modest) deployment of the No. 7 regimen.

Yet acknowledging the difficulty of properly interpreting Ohsawa's text does not fully account for the particular problems of Simon's untimely death. Like other macrobiotics converts, Beth Ann Simon and her husband, Charlie Simon, had been heavy drug users looking to get clean.[58] Additionally, both of the Simons sought relief from chronic pain—Beth Ann from back pain and Charlie from migraines. After Charlie tried No. 7 and reportedly relieved his migraines with a single dose of *gomashio* (the mixture of sesame seeds and salt that is the only seasoning allowed on No. 7), he implored his wife to try the ultrarestrictive regimen as well. After just days, both Simons had weaned off drugs and resolved the worst of their chronic pain. Yet as Charlie relaxed into a more liberal regimen, Beth Ann remained uncompromising.

After reading Ohsawa's 1965 book *You Are All Sanpaku*, Beth Ann Simon continued to believe herself seriously ill and remained on No. 7 for several more months with the hope that the rest of her health woes would eventually dissipate.[59] The book outlines one of the major methods Ohsawa taught to identify hidden signs of ill health. Based on physiognomy, the book explored the consequences of having a peculiar physiological defect Ohsawa dubbed *sanpaku*. The term, which translates literally as "three whites," describes the condition of having a third visible patch of sclera (the white part of the eye) underneath the iris (in addition to both sides). Ohsawa thought this defect portended a serious health crisis. In a 1972 *New York Times* article explaining this macrobiotics concept to the broader public, Ohsawa's followers were reported to have diagnosed President Richard Nixon as sanpaku, adding his name to the long list of figures (including Ngo Dinh Diem and John F. Kennedy) for whom Ohsawa had already successfully predicted early demise based on that principle.[60]

Tormented by the disturbing third white patch she saw in her own eyes, Beth Ann Simon stayed on No. 7 far longer than macrobiotics leaders recommended, and Charlie Simon watched in agony as his wife's health gradually deteriorated. In desperation, he called Irma Paule. Paule had been a French actress and student at Ohsawa's Parisian school, the Maison Ignoramus; because of her language skills, Paule became Ohsawa's assistant and translator during his first trips to the United States. After Ohsawa left the country and his chief disciples each abandoned New York to establish macrobiotics institutions elsewhere, Paule single-handedly ran the city's branch of the Ohsawa Foundation in their stead. Her position meant she was the go-to authority for all things macrobiotic in the New York City area. Though it was a position she adopted somewhat begrudgingly, she gave lectures and served as the coordinator for the local macrobiotics community while maintaining a relatively low profile. Nevertheless, under her leadership the foundation attracted notable attention from dancer Carmen de Lavallade, actress Gloria Swanson, and her husband Bill Dufty (who cowrote *You Are All Sanpaku* with Ohsawa).[61]

Just before Beth Ann Simon died, her husband Charlie informed Irma Paule that she "had drunk three-fourths of a bottle of ta-man [sic] soy sauce and eaten a big chunk of gomashio" but refused to take any other food until they reached the hospital, where, under Paule's recommendations to feed her "anything sweet," they force-fed her the only thing she would tolerate: carrot juice.[62] This was not Paule's first encounter with Beth Ann Simon, however. Paule understood that Simon had been using the diet improperly long before her hospitalization. Though Paule herself claimed the No. 7 diet had healed her paralytic arthritis, she would have been aware of two previous cases where people had allegedly died from stubborn adherence to the No. 7 diet; Monty Schier and Rose Cohen had both passed away after following it in 1961.[63] Paule did not recount these stories to Simon, but she offered appropriately stern rebukes. It did not matter. According to the *Herald Tribune*, "Beth Ann was unmoved. Irma, she said, a little self-righteously, was a coward—afraid to 'encounter the deep change' which continued adherence to Diet No. 7 entailed. Instead of widening her diet, she fasted altogether—four times for a total of about fourteen days in September."[64]

Paule was not the only macrobiotics veteran who had attempted to sway Simon down a different path. Simon's sister and brother-in-law had both been more liberal macrobiotics followers for years; along with Charlie Simon (who solicited letters from Ohsawa himself), they had tried in vain to persuade her to relinquish her commitment to the No. 7 diet. Still, she had refused, unwilling to accept any food or medical treatment until she expired. Her steadfast commitment to food refusal in the face of explicit contrary advice from the macrobiotics experts who had allegedly inspired her to eat in this manner, coupled with the obsessive dysmorphia that inspired the belief she was sick for reasons beyond starvation, support the possibility—raised first in the *Herald Tribune*—that Beth Ann Simon (and perhaps several of the other plaintiffs) may have died of anorexia nervosa rather than the ultrastrict No. 7 diet itself. In other words, she had followed the diet with excessive zeal as an extension of a pre-existing eating disorder.[65]

Nevertheless, for her failure to reroute Simon, Paule's office and its partner in California were raided by the FDA after the ruling of the Passaic County grand jury, despite the fact that the Ohsawa Foundation was not found responsible for her or any other death.[66] Instead of punishment, the jury recommended public health warnings be issued, so for the ensuing decade following Simon's death newspapers across the country stoked fear in the parents of would-be teen diet rebels that their children would die if they began showing inclinations toward brown rice. These warnings also undermined the natural food movement in which brown rice played a central role. Following Fred Stare's unequivocal denunciation of macrobiotics—then still a fledgling dietary lifestyle—the confusion surrounding Simon's death was simplified into a narrative with a clear villain and elevated into a public bogeyman. One could be forgiven for thinking that such an obvious oversimplification was aimed to suppress not only the eating habits but the politics of the recovering youth counterculture and the Asian customs with which they were flirting as well.

Changing of the Guard

Whether or not Simon actually died from the No. 7 diet, the media narrative nevertheless seriously wounded the reputation of macrobiotics around the country for years afterward. And even though macrobiotics' chief spokesperson died at the same time, the community remained vibrant, if hidden. Though many macrobiotics followers described going underground and despite its lower public profile, the late 1960s and early 1970s were a time of enormous growth for macrobiotics thanks to Ohsawa's two chief American acolytes, Michio Kushi and Herman Aihara.

Kushi and Aihara arrived separately in New York from Japan in the late-1940s. On a scholarship from the Japanese government—and perhaps facilitated by Ohsawa's connection to journalist and world peace advocate Norman Cousins—Kushi continued his education in political science from Tokyo University at Columbia University.[67] Aihara attended a technical college in Brooklyn to study helicopter manufacturing. Through the early 1950s, both men worked odd jobs to support themselves while trying to secure citizenship and establish families. In the mid- to late 1950s, Kushi and Aihara began opening their own Japanese import companies, first R. H. Brothers selling woodblock prints and nylon stockings, then two Japanese gift shops, Azuma and Ginza, where they sold food, textiles, and other basic commodities.[68] They used the success of these small ventures to convince a Japanese department store, Takashimaya, to open its first location in the United States in 1958, and Kushi later became the president of a branch.[69]

By that point, Kushi and Aihara's primary exposure to Ohsawa's thinking had been through the World Federalist Movement. Kushi found the movement after his harrowing experiences in a military regiment facilitating the recovery at Nagasaki; Aihara joined after his first wife committed suicide.[70] Neither knew much of nor cared about macrobiotics before

Ohsawa's first trip to the United States. When George Ohsawa met the pair in New York in 1959, they quickly abandoned the import business to pursue macrobiotics full time and to build institutions that would help realize the lifestyle's broader ambitions.

After Ohsawa predicted that a nuclear strike would destroy New York, Aihara served as the anchor point for macrobiotics on the West Coast, where he founded a branch of the Ohsawa Foundation and a training program named the Vega Institute. There, Aihara quietly devoted himself to the education of macrobiotics students. With his support and guidance, Aihara's student-pilgrims founded the Chico-San health food company, which—in addition to importing and helping to popularize such Japanese and vegetarian staples as miso, tamari, tofu, tempeh, and seitan—grew the first organic brown rice in the country, from which they manufactured and popularized the first rice cakes sold in the United States. The company went on to make important deals with other natural foods giants: with Eden to manufacture soy milk, with Lightlife to make the first commercial tofu in the United States, and with Lundberg Farms to grow more organic brown rice, significantly fortifying the natural health food industry.[71]

While Aihara led his band westward, Kushi remained in New York. In 1964, he moved his family to Massachusetts, and the following year he established his own macrobiotics headquarters in the suburbs of Boston, where he and his wife Aveline founded Erewhon Trading Company in 1966.[72] Like Chico-San, Erewhon also became a multi-million-dollar health food business.[73] From their Boston compound, the Kushis also founded the Kushi Institute, the East-West Foundation, the One Peaceful World Foundation, and a latent (but prolific) publishing business spearheaded by the *East-West Journal*.

More than any other macrobiotics guru, Michio Kushi was responsible for the global spread that made macrobiotics into an empire. While both Kushi and Aihara trained students, gave lectures, and generally fostered the development of their regional macrobiotics communities, Kushi developed the apprenticeship aspect into a well-oiled machine. Despite his ambitions, descriptions of Kushi portray him as demure but never surprised. Like Ohsawa, he often wore a three-piece suit and offered a smile and a handshake to everyone he met.[74] Students trained at the Kushis' home in Brookline (and later the 600-acre farm they purchased in Becket, Massachusetts) and worked in their stores and restaurants until they left to found their own macrobiotics communities. Kushi's students added substantially to Ohsawa's international infrastructure, setting up over 600 independent macrobiotics centers—satellite operations to teach the macrobiotics lifestyle—all over the United States and around the world in such diverse cities as Lisbon, Amsterdam, Paris, Rome, Florence, Antwerp, Barcelona, and London.[75] By 1973, Walter Alvarez estimated that macrobiotics had at least 10,000 devotees (not counting people experimenting on their own with eating macrobiotically) in the United States alone.[76]

The movement owed much of its success between 1966 and 1973 to its leaders' embrace of American capitalism; both Kushi and Aihara exploited the skills they had gained importing goods from Japan when they founded their respective natural health food companies. During this period of quiet growth, macrobiotics leaders were careful to avoid another national scandal as well. The years following the Simon debacle and Ohsawa's death were marked by a gradual retreat from some of Ohsawa's more extreme claims, like those undergirding the controversial No. 7 diet. For some this was a long-awaited opportunity: before the 1960 publication of *Zen Macrobiotics*, Michio Kushi reportedly tried once to warn Ohsawa about including overly severe prescriptions without an explanatory appendix for fear they could be misleading, but Ohsawa was unmoved.[77] Yet even for Kushi the most austere versions of the diet like No. 7 were difficult to retreat from because they were intricately entwined with the antiviolence posture of the movement and its curative promises. In fact, they were embedded in the core philosophy and cultural framing of macrobiotics, whether the legions of recovering Beats and hippies recognized it or not.

The Atomic Balm

The connection between such a bizarrely strict regimen as the No. 7 diet and macrobiotics' promise to quell global violence is particularly visible in a macrobiotics legend about the miraculous recovery of a victim of the Hiroshima nuclear attack. Known in Japanese as a *hibakusha*—someone marred and socially stigmatized by atomic radiation—a young woman, Sawako Hiraga, wrote positively about her experience on the No. 7 diet, which was closely facilitated by Ohsawa himself. "I had a discharge of black blood," she wrote, "even though I was not menstruating. . . . It was the tenth day of the #7 diet. After one month, I started adding some vegetables. To my surprise, my acne began to disappear. Within two months of starting macrobiotics, all the acne had disappeared and my face became beautiful."[78] Hiraga's recovery not only represented a complete fulfillment of Ohsawa's promises about the power of the No. 7 diet to rebalance the body from any ailment, including disfiguring radiation scars and poisoning, it demonstrated that macrobiotics' commitment to world peace was not merely an aspiration or gesture. Macrobiotics mobilized its success in repairing the (heavily gendered) physical damage from nuclear radiation to assert itself as the premier diet of peace: a diet whose powers were so strong they could alleviate even the most intense global conflict. Importantly, the peace that macrobiotics promised was not merely a lack of violence but a kind of restorative, embodied antiviolence that emanated from each macrobiotic individual.

That Hiraga's story bore a strong resemblance to the famed Hiroshima Maidens—a group of Japanese women scarred by the atomic bomb who were flown to the United States for reconstructive surgery, the spectacle of which attracted much national press attention—is no accident. Norman Cousins, the *Saturday Review* journalist who had orchestrated the Maidens' journey to the United States, was a major leader of the World Federalist Movement, through which he met Ohsawa on a postwar trip to Japan. Seeing the political advantages of the Hiroshima Maidens spectacle, Ohsawa decided to emulate some of the successes of Cousins's program. By reconstructing the damage done to women's bodies in the atomic blast, both the United States and Japan sought to erase the horror of nuclear war. Both the public narrative of the Hiroshima maidens as well as Sawako Hiraga's encounter with the macrobiotic diet entangle female desirability and social utility with an immaculate physical appearance.

Yet Hiraga's narrative, while so similar in its surface details to that of other hibakusha, was deployed toward different political ends. In her analysis of the Hiroshima Maidens, religious studies scholar Yuki Miyamoto emphasizes the damage that both the US and Japanese officials had inflicted upon radiation victims by essentially repurposing their suffering to justify remilitarization while upholding traditional white heteronormative Christian family ideals.[79] Even at the time, the Hiroshima Maidens spectacle was widely perceived as an attempt to defang the public perceptions of danger surrounding nuclear technologies and to help transition toward peacetime uses of nuclear materials. Macrobiotics leaders, on the other hand, pointed to Hiraga as evidence that nuclear war was incredibly harmful, but that their lifestyle was an effective vaccine against such injury.

Because Beth Ann Simon's death effectively tainted the public reputation of the No. 7 diet, it also jeopardized macrobiotics leaders' ability to draw on this key antinuclear selling point. Fortunately for macrobiotics leaders, there was an equally compelling legend that could serve as evidence of the lifestyle's alleged antinuclear capacities: the story of Dr. Tatsuichirō Akizuki, the so-called Atomic Bomb Doctor, and his experience surviving and aiding recovery efforts from the atomic blast at Nagasaki. Akizuki's heroic exploits at Urakami (later St. Francis) Hospital were outlined in his book *Nagasaki 1945*, which was first published in Japanese in 1967 and later translated into English in 1981.[80] His harrowing eyewitness account of the bomb and its aftermath has proven invaluable to historians studying the bombing at Nagasaki, an event whose horror has been all but eclipsed by its sister event in Hiroshima.[81] Of Akizuki's significance to macrobiotics, amateur food historian Lorenz K. Schaller writes,

> According to Ohsawa (and his faithful editor, the Japanese-American Herman Aihara), Dr. Akizuki was operating his hospital with a focus on macrobiotic fare as medicinal food, serving the simple plant-foods to both patients and staff. Because of this, large stocks of basic staples were stored on-site, which somehow escaped or were rescued from the conflagration. This, and Dr. Akizuki's own personal survival gave rise to the American macrobiotic myth of the 1970s and beyond, that brown rice, wakame seaweed and umeboshi plums could inoculate a person against atomic death. The myth, largely imaginative fiction, arose from a thread of truth. A strict macrobiotic diet, wisely applied and followed, apparently allows the human body to endure a sub-lethal dose of atomic radiation (not exceeding a certain range of severity) and recover intact and somewhat unscathed.[82]

Like Hiraga's miraculous cure from radiation poisoning, Akizuki's efforts and his mythically plentiful macrobiotics storehouse were highlighted repeatedly in natural health food literature, especially those publications most closely affiliated with macrobiotics, as a guide to healing radiation damage.[83] Akizuki even assisted in this promotion of his story; in 1980, he wrote an article for Michio Kushi's *East-West Journal* where he claimed that, after the bomb, "there was nothing else to do than go back to brown rice and miso soup. It was already the basis of the usual macrobiotic diet of the hospital long before the nuclear catastrophe. Thanks to this food, fortified after the bombing by even more salt and miso soup, the people living in the hospital endured and survived."[84]

By tying the macrobiotic diet to this case of miraculous human endurance, macrobiotics leaders claimed special access to immense healing power. Specifically, by establishing their program as the antidote to nuclear radiation in Japan, a country whose atomic scars were prostrated before a captive global audience, they could simultaneously capitalize on America's guilt-ridden, orientalist romance with postwar Japan while positioning macrobiotics as an essential tool to aid international nuclear war and accident recovery efforts. As the movement matured, the diet's entanglement with nuclear disaster remained strong from continuous reinforcement. After the meltdown at Chernobyl in 1986, for instance, a macrobiotics liaison was sent to meet with a Soviet agency, Union Chernobyl, to advise them on dietary solutions to radiation sickness. As word spread that macrobiotic staples could reverse radiation damage, all the stocks of miso were reportedly purchased throughout Eastern Europe, and truckloads of miso had to be imported directly to the Soviet Union from Japan.[85]

The Standard Macrobiotic Diet

To preserve the antiviolence aura surrounding macrobiotics while distancing the community from the Simon scandal, Kushi and other post-Ohsawa leaders also needed to reformulate the basic structure of the program. While some macrobiotics leaders and instructors consciously de-emphasized macrobiotics' medical claims, Kushi and his lieutenants instead reframed the narrative to reclaim and even expand the medical promises. To distance themselves from the negative media attention that Ohsawa's macrobiotics had garnered, especially the cries of obsessive restrictiveness encouraged by any mention of the No. 7 diet, Kushi rewrote Ohsawa's stepwise program into a new form he called the Standard Macrobiotic Diet (SMD), depicted concisely in Figure 1.

Kushi's pivot solved several major problems for the macrobiotics movement. It gave a baseline recommendation to absolve the diet's leaders of responsibility for any further bad faith efforts by dieters like Beth Ann Simon because the SMD was far more balanced and nutritionally apt than the No. 7 diet. The SMD had a much clearer emphasis on what people should eat rather than let them decide for themselves when they were ready for the more "advanced" levels, which at once gave leaders greater authority and less culpability. The SMD enabled Kushi and others to promote the antiradiation benefits of the macrobiotic diet without the No. 7 diet as well. Macrobiotic enthusiasts kept a careful eye on global media reports showcasing the negative effects of radiation, carefully tracing news reports on the effects of nuclear fallout, human experimentation with radioactivity, recovery from nuclear disasters, and the effects of improper nuclear waste

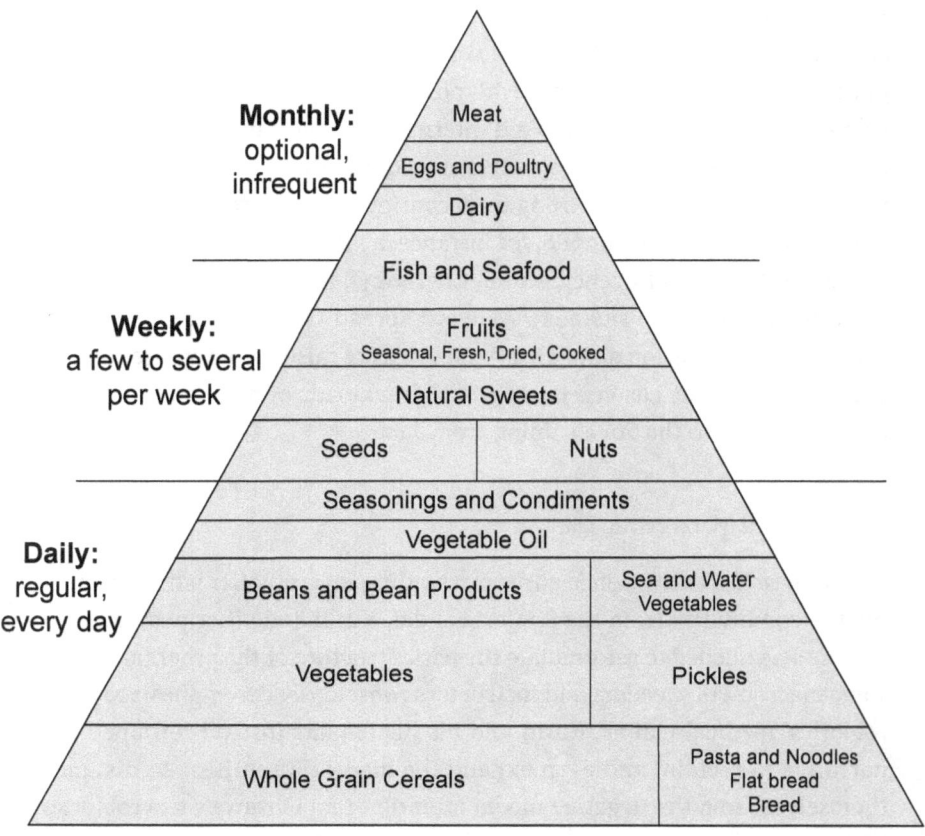

Standard macrobiotic diet as conceived by Michio Kushi.

disposal. They also combed medical literature for positive indications of their dietary promises, citing experiments that demonstrated the positive effects of such macrobiotic foods as sea vegetables on processes such as ion absorption.[86] Macrobiotic leaders soon amassed a rich bibliography showcasing the antiradiation effects (and other health benefits) of macrobiotic staples like miso soup and sea vegetables.[87]

In the mid- to late 1970s, Michio Kushi parlayed the diet's promise of nuclear rehabilitation into a full-blown medical system. Given the synonymity of the diet's early presence in the United States with premature death, such a turnaround is remarkable. Kushi's SMD proved a valuable template for the movement's increasing emphasis on medical interventions. Rather than relying on the healing power of the problematic No. 7 diet, as Ohsawa had, Kushi's SMD instead promoted the consumption of key antiradiation foods like umeboshi (pickled plums), sea vegetables, and miso soup—foods that were previously disallowed. During patient consultations, Kushi made modifications to a printed copy of his SMD to tailor the treatment regimen he recommended to each individual. In his tailored treatment protocols, Kushi relied heavily on variations of the SMD coupled with several other standard behavioral adjustments: chewing thoroughly; walking barefoot in simple cotton clothing (especially where clothing touched diseased areas); engaging in moderate daily exercise; taking long, regular baths with hot water; avoiding or minimizing the use of electronic appliances (including electric stoves); and singing happy songs daily.[88]

"The Doctor's Cure": Macrobiotics and Cancer

Insofar as macrobiotics had positioned itself as the antidote to radiation—and as radiation became the hallmark of global violence in the twentieth century—cancer, which was both caused and treated by radiation, became the ideal disease to make amenable to macrobiotic intervention in the late 1970s. From the perspective of certain macrobiotics gurus, the transition to cancer treatment was an intuitive direction to expand the movement. Herman Aihara encapsulated this reasoning in his book *Basic Macrobiotics* where he wrote, "Humanity is literally on the verge of being destroyed by the two deadliest products of modern civilization—cancer and nuclear war."[89]

It was not only for macrobiotics leaders that cancer and nuclear war held some resemblance to one another. Historians have argued that cancer became the signature disease of modern civilization during the Cold War. In her book, *Life Atomic*, historian Angela Creager demonstrates how the Atomic Energy Commission (AEC) participated in the repurposing of nuclear facilities toward peaceful applications, including the production of the radioactive cobalt isotopes that served as the basis for radiation therapy. This transition was as much propaganda as recycling. Creager shows how the AEC also, against its will, became saddled with the obligation to direct congressional funds toward using radiation as a cancer therapy.[90] Journalist Ellen Leopold argues that the US government was especially eager to redirect nuclear facilities toward medical ends (as opposed to environmental or other industrial applications) to compensate for the nuclear strikes against Japan.[91] Deploying nuclear materials and technologies toward defeating such a modern (and radiation-linked) scourge as cancer, could, in the minds of government officials, help compensate for the incalculable harm of the atom bomb.[92] In his book *Contested Medicine*, Gerald Kutcher demonstrates how the overlaps, both real and imagined, between cancer and nuclear radiation contributed to widespread public apprehension about the entire ecosystem of radioactive materials—fueling not only antiwar sentiment but also environmental concerns during the 1980s antinuclear movement, and driving cancer patients toward more "natural" alternative therapy options.[93]

The transition from Akizuki's miraculous healing of radiation victims during World War II to cancer treatment was facilitated by such studies as Fumimasa Yanagisawa's showing that certain Japanese staples (radish leaves, carrot leaves, hijiki) assisted his patients' recovery from leukemia acquired through exposure to atomic radiation.[94] Yet evidence alone was not sufficient to attract global attention or encourage cancer patients to experiment with macrobiotics. It was primarily due to Michio Kushi's bold restructuring decisions that macrobiotics became one of the most popular alternative approaches to preventing and combating cancer in the United States.[95] Spurred by the revelations of the 1977 McGovern Report, which emphasized the role of nutrition as a major risk factor in developing chronic diseases, Kushi forcefully argued that "the diet-cancer link . . . would be a vehicle through which the rest of the world, starting with doctors, would learn about macrobiotics and flock to [our] doors," and that macrobiotics leaders would need to start "establishing a dialogue with doctors and proving the validity of macrobiotics as a healing agent for serious illness."

Kushi developed a grand plan to boost public awareness and acceptance of macrobiotics by greatly expanding the visibility of its promise to prevent, treat, or cure chronic health conditions, especially cancer, founding "full-fledged treatment centers ('macrobiotic hospitals'), institutes of higher learning ('macrobiotic college'), a professional credentials and peer-review system ('macrobiotic teacher certification') and most ambitious of all, a multi-tiered system, from regional to global, of alternative government ('macrobiotic congresses')."[96] Kushi also flexed his considerable influence in the natural foods publishing sector, unleashing a tremendous number of books on the subject of macrobiotics and cancer, written by himself, his patients, his students, and his students' patients.[97]

These early efforts promoting macrobiotics' potential for cancer found only moderate interest until 1982, when, according to macrobiotics leader John David Mann, "Kushi found precisely the medical/media catalyst for which he had hoped": a Philadelphia-based surgeon named Anthony Sattilaro.[98] Sattilaro had just been diagnosed with stage 4 metastatic prostate cancer, the same cancer that had just killed his father, when he learned about macrobiotics from two hitchhikers he picked up, Sean McLean and Bill Bochbracher. After driving these young men to the home of their local East-West Foundation leader in Philadelphia, Denny Waxman, Sattilaro was welcomed and enculturated at the community dinner table, where he found his Western medical training challenged by his hosts' adoptive Asian sensibilities. Despite finding the ideas irrational, the food unpalatable, and the lifestyle unlivable, Sattilaro managed to convert to a fully macrobiotic regimen with one huge caveat. Sattilaro detested food preparation, an essential (but heavily gendered) step to becoming macrobiotic, so he had his hosts prepare many of his meals for him. After a year, he visited his oncologists who informed him of his spontaneous, permanent remission.[99] In 1982, an electrifying article detailing his cancer-curing experimentation with the macrobiotics lifestyle appeared in *Life* magazine, after which Sattilaro's book, *Recalled by Life*, became a bestselling bombshell.[100]

Though Sattilaro confessed he did not believe the regimen would work and cautioned his readers not to abandon conventional cancer treatment for something that may have been a fluke, his book, "together with his many appearances on radio and in newspapers, spurred a surge of people pouring into macrobiotic centers looking for 'the Doctor's cure.'"[101] Though Sattilaro's personal recovery was subjected to heavy skepticism and criticism from the mainstream medical community, the success of his book encouraged a flurry of similar cancer cure narratives, including from actor Dirk Benedict.[102] As the public profile of macrobiotics as a cancer cure or preventive increased, there followed a flurry of medical studies purporting to support or debunk the alleged power of this diet (and other similar programs) through the late 1980s and beyond.[103]

So what made macrobiotics so appealing to cancer patients? And of what did the "treatment" consist of? Like other medical alternatives, macrobiotics fulfilled an important niche for cancer patients by speaking directly and powerfully to widespread patient dissatisfaction with orthodox cancer therapies. In *Basic Macrobiotics*, Herman Aihara wrote, "What it seems we can expect from conventional cancer treatment . . . is a prolongation of life for about five years with a great deal of pain, agony, and fear. This is not health or happiness; it is like being sentenced to hell."[104] Sattilaro himself described the problem as follows: "At one extreme we have patients who still regard the doctor as the highest form of public servant; at the other are those who see us as a criminal elite, money hungry, and getting a certain sadistic pleasure out of putting people through torturous tests and therapies. In between the two are the majority of patients, who are increasingly skeptical of our motives, no longer fully trusting of our methods, but frustrated by the fact that they haven't got a better solution."[105]

These sorts of declarations obviously resonated with the lived experiences of those who had undergone the morale-shattering agony of chemo- or radiotherapy. But macrobiotics was hardly the only voice decrying orthodox treatment methods during this time. Its competitors in the alternative medical market for cancer during the 1960s and 1970s included such controversial concoctions as laetrile, Krebiozen, Hoxsey herbal tonic, Koch antitoxin, Glover serum, and Iscador, in addition to rival nutritional programs such as Gerson diet therapy, Linus Pauling–backed megavitamin therapy, and the Beverly Hills Diet, and the nutritional philosophies of Emanuel Revici, Johanna Brand, Edgar Cayce, and Adelle Davis.[106] There was a rising fascination and experimentation with therapies derived from Asian healing traditions such as meditation, acupuncture, and moxibustion. And, in his survey of breast cancer therapy, historian James Olson details the surprising longevity of psychotherapeutic models for cancer, including orgone energy and even cancerous personality theories.[107]

Like several of these alternatives, macrobiotics was successful not only for its well-timed and well-targeted critique of medical orthodoxy, but also for the explanatory power and coherence of its system relative to its competitors. A 1971 article in the *Chicago Tribune* explained the appeal as follows: "Modern doctors may dispute some of the macrobiotic methods, but followers of the philosophy regard modern medicine as a sham; they say physicians treat symptoms, not the root causes of diseases, which are related to the order of the universe."[108] By explaining why orthodox medicine continually failed to grasp the true nature of complex diseases like cancer (by emphasizing proximal rather than primary causes, one could say), macrobiotics opened its audience to explanations beyond the strictly scientific. Strategically, macrobiotics never undercut biomedicine entirely. In the foreword to a memoir written by a macrobiotics cancer patient, Kushi wrote, "Whenever people come to me for advice, I ask whether normal medical treatments have been sufficiently tried, and if there is any possibility that such methods can help the problem, I will suggest that the individual continue to pursue that direction. However, as with many cases that are referred to me, [the author's] was apparently hopeless according to modern medical standards."[109] Despite the movement's adamant official stance toward nuclear radiation, in practice, macrobiotic treatment for cancer patients often accompanied radiation, both diagnostic and therapeutic.[110] It should be noted, too, that when Michio and Aveline Kushi both contracted cancer later in life, both obtained conventional cancer care to supplement their macrobiotic lifestyle.[111]

As for Anthony Sattilaro, the man whose tale of miraculous recovery triggered the macrobiotic cancer craze, his eventual death became somewhat controversial. In his book, *Health Robbers*, career quack-buster Stephen Barrett writes that "[Sattilaro] died of his disease in 1989, but readers of [macrobiotic] books may not learn of this fact."[112] Macrobiotic officials countered that Sattilaro was to blame for his own demise, as Ohsawa had been. According to reporter Len Lear, who had interviewed Sattilaro in the early 1980s, in the intervening years between his second book *Living Well Naturally* (1984) and his death, the once-cured doctor had returned to his former food habits—replete with rich and overprocessed restaurant food—because he had grown bored with underseasoned macrobiotic food and had never quite mastered cooking for himself.[113]

"From Hugh Hefner to St. Francis": Macrobiotics for HIV/AIDS

In 1982, Michio Kushi was alerted to the possibility that macrobiotics could have a useful application in the burgeoning human immunodeficiency virus/acquired immunodeficiency syndrome (HIV/AIDS) crisis when patients from New York with this new, seemingly inexplicable disease began arriving at his cancer lectures in Boston.[114] During its original outbreak, HIV/AIDS was predominantly characterized by one of its most visible sequelae, Kaposi's sarcoma, an otherwise rare cancer that was being treated unsuccessfully with costly and debilitating chemotherapy and radiation.[115] The new disease fit naturally into the pre-existing schema Kushi built around cancer and macrobiotics' inherent opposition to radiation and other nuclear technologies.

Within several months of their first arrival, Kushi recruited several of his new clients to write letters to various federal and private agencies explaining the benefits of his lifestyle program for their disease in order to secure funding to run a clinical trial. Every letter writer foregrounded their experience with macrobiotics by first expressing profound dissatisfaction with extant medical care. In one letter, patient Eric Gibbs reported that before seeking help from the East-West Foundation, he "did not feel at all comfortable with the available medical approaches to recovery."[116] An anonymous writer wrote, "I decided not to submit to any of the so-called conventional cures such as radiation or chemotherapy. My reason was because none of these are cures and not only did they not have beneficial results but were frequently dangerous and fatal." In a published retrospective interview, patient Oscar Molini said after he had been diagnosed with AIDS, he was offered chemotherapy, which "promised all the comforts of a torture chamber."[117] In addition to the harrowing biological consequences of the disease, AIDS patients of the early 1980s confronted a dire social landscape that not only demonized their lifestyles but blamed them for their illnesses and fled their contact for fear of contracting the disease. Historians of the epidemic have thoroughly documented the harsh indifference AIDS patients were met with from orthodox physicians, as well as the struggle to understand the disease's etiology and find effective therapies.[118]

To survive such medical ambiguity and overt bigotry, AIDS patients formed tight social networks and relied on word of mouth about any new or experimental treatments. When the first several patients found relief, even empowerment, in macrobiotic cancer therapy, the word about this miraculous and restorative medical alternative spread quickly. In their letters, nearly every patient reported having heard of macrobiotic therapy and its potential value from a friend. As one patient explained, "I am so very convinced throught [sic] my personal involvement, that macrobiotic living is helping me to restablish [sic] my health and strengthen all aspects of life, that I can not help but urge others, with illness or not, to investigate and incorporate the principles into their daily lives."[119]

The letters Kushi collected demonstrate that one of the most valuable components of macrobiotic therapy was the emotional and psychological effects of empowerment and self-determination. Several writers emphasized the psychological benefits they experienced after starting the diet, with claims like, "My awareness has sharpened. My physical, mental and spiritual condition has definitely changed for the better. I've been able to self-reflect and have a full understanding of my condition. I feel I'm in control of my present situation." Another explained, "My strength [has] returned to a great degree since I've begun to eat macrobiotically. . . . I also find that mentally and spiritually I have become more understanding and relaxed in my dealings with work situations and family and social encounters."[120] In rejecting orthodox therapy, these AIDS patients refused to submit to their physicians' pessimistic prognoses and the grotesque deaths they felt awaited them on the other end of conventional therapy. An anonymous AIDS patient wrote in support of macrobiotics, "[Michio Kushi] said that we weren't condemned to die, that we could take control of our health and our lives. When everyone else was running the other way he came and embraced us, physically and figuratively."[121] Through macrobiotics, men with AIDS reported living longer, happier, healthier lives with greater freedom; one wrote, "If anything I have too much energy. I am very busy in my work. I swim every day. I go out dancing twice a week. I live a typical New York life."[122]

For Michio Kushi, securing the trust of AIDS patients proved substantially more difficult than with cancer, despite the philosophical similarities (and political opportunities) of cancer and AIDS therapies. Following Ohsawa's lead, Kushi dismissed microbiological evidence that infectious diseases, including HIV/AIDS, were caused by pathogens—an attitude now referred to as AIDS denialism. As with cancer, Kushi assigned the cause of HIV/AIDS to a lifestyle out of balance with nature, and his cure was, as always, targeted dietary and behavioral change. Expectedly, not all gay men who had been exposed to the macrobiotics approach and its virtues became converts of the lifestyle for fear that "macrobiotic philosophy [was] not in harmony with homosexual lifestyle [sic]."[123] Although at least one historian-participant, Karlyn Crowley, has praised macrobiotics for its acceptance of fluid ideas of gender and empowerment, others have criticized its enforcement of strict gender roles.[124] Regardless of any benevolent or relativistic attitudes macrobiotics leaders may have deployed about gender in other contexts, their openness did not originally extend to homosexuality. In an interview he conducted for the *East-West Journal*, macrobiotics leader Ron Kotzsch quoted one AIDS patient as having said, "The macrobiotic community has long been explicitly heterosexual and implicitly homophobic. It has had the idea that homosexuality is another disease to be cured. I remember back in the mid '70s when gays in the city were picketing outside Kushi's lectures."[125] By targeting the improper, "unnatural" lifestyle of gay men as the cause of their ill health, Kushi and other macrobiotics leaders alienated many of their most prized potential converts.

Even for those early adopters of macrobiotic AIDS therapy, many demonstrated a firm commitment to the orthodox medical worldview even while practicing alternative therapy. The men continued to understand the progress of their disease in strictly biomedical terms (e.g., using white blood cell counts) despite arranging their lives by decidedly extramedical tenets.

Although they found tremendous social and psychological benefits to a macrobiotic regimen for their well-being, attitude, and relationships—and advertised these benefits to their friends—they rejected Kushi's discriminatory etiological framework that essentially blamed them for their disease. Interestingly, while the medical establishment slowly scrambled to adjust its morals and epidemiology to account for the spread of HIV/AIDS, macrobiotics underwent a much more rapid adjustment. Kushi listened to the negative feedback he received from New York's gay community; in a flyer he distributed widely, he apologized:

> Such impressions [of homophobia on behalf of macrobiotics leaders] may have been conveyed through some writings and publications written in the past. However, we believe that homosexual friends, and, in fact, all people, should not be reviewed from any legal, ethical, moral, political, or social standards, unless harmful for social well-being. It is totally individual and personal exercise based upon the freedom of biological and psychological nature. . . . Those who are homosexual and those who are non-homosexual are all our brothers and sisters who share the same origin, the same planet earth, and the same future—the return to the universe. We all share the same human destiny in this world and in this century. We all must love, help, support each other for the benefit of everyone and every society. Now especially, we are confronting a critical period— one which may see destruction of the existence of the human species, either through possible annihilation by nuclear disaster or prevailing degenerative disease. We need much closer cooperation among ourselves regardless of the differences of race, beliefs, customs, cultures, including differences of sexual practice.[126]

It was a difficult sell for Kushi to intrude as an outsider, but his apology managed to appease many AIDS patients' political outrage by shifting his hardline macrobiotics philosophy to account for differences in sexuality and sexual preference. By signaling that he was, in fact, an ally of sorts, who not only understood his clients' pain but could potentially provide life-changing therapy if they would so permit him, Kushi attracted a significant early following in New York's gay communities. By 1984, Michio Kushi had reportedly seen thirty patients who self-identified as having AIDS, all from the New York City area.[127] Within two years, by one patient's estimate, the number of AIDS patients practicing macrobiotics as a treatment had doubled, while the number of healthy gay men practicing macrobiotics ballooned to over 500 in New York alone.[128]

While Michio Kushi struggled to position macrobiotics as amenable to a gay lifestyle, he softened his hostility to the biomedical explanations of HIV/AIDS as well. He began an initiative to recruit participants for medical research conducted through two New York City–based action groups called Wipe Out AIDS and the Health Education AIDS Liaison (HEAL). The first pilot study exploring the effects of macrobiotics on AIDS ran from 1984 to 1987 and was run by Kushi's son, Lawrence Kushi. The younger Kushi had trained as an orthodox medical researcher, and he recruited his medical colleagues from nearby Boston University Medical Center to help run the study.[129] In the study report, the researchers wrote, "Several individuals with diagnoses of AIDS or ARC [AIDS-related complex] have seen macrobiotic counselors for their illness, and feel that their condition is improving. Although most of the improvement has been subjective, at least two people have had measurements of their helper to suppressor (T4/T8) cell ratio that suggest improvement while on the macrobiotic diet. While these observations are only suggestive, the macrobiotic diet may increase this ratio, and perhaps influence other parameters of immune status as well."[130] Notably, the patients also reported higher levels of "curiosity" and hardiness with lower levels of anxiety and depression as a result of being on a macrobiotic diet.[131] One of the authors of the study, Elinor Levy, wrote Michio Kushi in 1985, saying, "At this point, we feel confident that the men following a macrobiotic approach are doing no worse than men receiving conventional therapy."[132] In a letter to the editor of *The Lancet*, she also claimed, "The men in our study may not be representative of KS [Kaposi's sarcoma] patients in general. Their choice to forgo medical treatment may indicate a type of fighting spirit or psychological makeup which could possibly enhance survival."[133]

What is interesting here is not whether the macrobiotic diet was the driving force behind the patients' improvement, or indeed whether the patients "actually" improved. In all of these cases, it is clear that the patients were desperate, but also that they were cogent and fluent with medical discourse enough to choose consciously and rationally to avoid (or supplement) what they perceived to be ineffectual, harmful, or even life-threatening treatment for an already debilitating and demoralizing condition. One macrobiotics leader said of her experience, "The key lesson I have learned working with AIDS patients is that a person's feelings are incredibly important in their cure. One has to feel accepted, loved, and respected without qualification. This is especially true for gay people who are almost pariahs in our society."[134] The emotional tenor of macrobiotic intervention—and the ensuing feeling of empowerment—was key. For AIDS patients, the sense of empowerment stemmed from the fact that the diet's natural healing principles (eventually) fit into patients' pre-existing expectations for what constituted acceptable medical treatment. In this way, the success of macrobiotic AIDS treatment was coproduced by patients' social needs and macrobiotics leaders' strategic flexibility and accommodation.

Fall(out) of an Empire

Though health had always been a central goal of macrobiotics, for the young white students who comprised the movement's earliest American followers the health they envisioned was holistic and deeply spiritual. More importantly, the maintenance of individual health had always been subservient to the "revolutionary social ideal": the drive to end world wars; purify the land; grow, cook, and distribute balanced food; and educate the masses to perpetuate the movement.[135] If people recovered from incurable chronic diseases along the way, it was just a fortunate side benefit.

Under Kushi's reign, however, many of these American lieutenants saw the promise of global peace and ecological harmony that originally attracted them to Ohsawa's program being increasingly sidelined for the terminally ill. When Kushi transitioned the major focus of his substantial macrobiotics organizations (including the training, consultation programs, and publications) toward alternative medical therapy, it was a major success, and the movement enjoyed wide popularity and media coverage. To the chagrin of long-time macrobiotics followers, the patients attracted by the medical promises were never being exposed to the full doctrine of global peace through harmonious living beyond a basic nod toward spirituality, nor did many of them seem to care.

Many of the white second-tier macrobiotics leaders—those who trained under Kushi and Aihara—felt the transition toward treating diseases was leading the movement astray by oversimplifying its overarching message and creating hostility in its ranks for those who resisted the new dogma of cure. As one leader put it, "Packaging the macrobiotic view of life as a 'recipe for health,' suitable for marketing to a paperback audience, squeezed macrobiotics' broadly eclectic vision into a specialized mold it was ill suited to fit."[136] Consequently, many former adherents abandoned the lifestyle altogether. Warren Belasco argues that, for these ex-macrobiotics, the lifestyle ultimately served "as a congenial rest stop on the path to Frances Moore Lappé's more secular version of ecological vegetarianism."[137]

There were legitimate reasons for macrobiotics followers to be concerned about Kushi's medical expansion. Beyond the fact that many people seeking medical advice were not being fully inculcated in macrobiotics culture, the care offered to some lacked merit, even by macrobiotics standards. For instance, Kushi regularly offered medical advice through the mail to international patients he had never met. In the early 1990s, a Turkish man with bone cancer, Dundar Kaya Buharali, wrote Kushi for advice after having lost the ability to walk and lost almost fifty pounds in three months while on the macrobiotic diet. Despite never having seen Buharali in person or observed his condition, Kushi nevertheless advised him, via his deputy letter writer Jim Sleeper, that although his constitution was strong, the reason he was unable to walk was because he consumed too much salt. In addition to curbing his sodium consumption, Kushi advised Buharali to stop taking his chemotherapy drug, flutamide, for his condition (which Buharali also variously called "zona nerves") for a trial period of two months. Kushi issued a sole caveat: if Buharali's doctor disagreed with stopping conventional treatment, Kushi advised taking the drug at a lower and less-frequent dosage instead. The patient complied, but his condition got worse despite following Kushi's instructions to the letter (including singing happy songs and walking for half an hour daily).[138] There were some conditions, Kushi admitted, that were simply not curable. But the fact that Kushi advised so many patients using only what he knew from their letters deprived those patients of the social and psychological value of in-person macrobiotic care that led Sattilaro and dozens of HIV/AIDS patients to respond positively.

The falling out of some of macrobiotics' most important members highlights several issues with the manner in which macrobiotics was originally built and sold to white Americans in the 1960s, especially across racial and cultural fault lines. As I have demonstrated throughout this chapter, examples of miraculous healing have been apiece with shoku-yo and macrobiotics philosophy since their original inception. And while those healing miracles have always been grounded in a larger sociopolitical dream (for macrobiotics leadership, at least), the contents of that dream have evolved over time in response to changing geopolitical circumstances. When the original diet was created, for instance, Ishizuka consciously rejected what he saw as damaging American imperialism and progressivism in Japan and the spiritual isolation that flourished in the wake of consumer capitalism. As Ohsawa took the reins of the Shoku-Yo Kai, however, he expressed keen interest in taking advantage of Japanese imperialism to spread his diet across Asia and the globe. It was only after Japan's defeat in World War II that the diet and its followers adopted peace (and denuclearization) as their core mission—a mission that was later expanded to encompass the ecological framework that white hippies saw as one of the diet's chief draws.

As macrobiotics spread to and through the United States, it carried Japanese political sensibilities with it. And for the Japanese-born leaders of macrobiotics, those sensibilities remained central—even as they sold the program to a wider white audience by emphasizing the *terroir*-esque elements of Sagen Ishizuka's original philosophy to appeal to the budding political concerns of their target market. But as time passed, the tensions between the nativist Japanese underpinnings of the philosophy and its pragmatic alignment with Western values grew more apparent. Despite Ishizuka's notion that people should eat the foods common to their home region, Michio Kushi and Herman Aihara first attained commercial success in the United States by importing and later growing and distributing Japanese staple foods: brown rice, soy sauce, sea vegetables, tofu, and miso. By privileging Japanese staples in their versions of the macrobiotic diet, they subsequently inculcated their students to have Japanese tastes and sensibilities. Ironically, as Erewhon and Chico-San blossomed into titans of the natural health food industry, these same Japanese staples became quintessential American health foods, independent from the macrobiotic label. Under Kushi's tutelage, these foods remained at the core of macrobiotic identity, even as he and other leaders encouraged white Americans to apply the Unique Principle to any foods they wished to eat. Kushi's attachment to Japanese foods was most obvious in his dietary prescriptions to cancer patients, where he regularly recommended such foods as umeboshi plums, seaweed, and pickled vegetables to steer patients away from the trappings of Western cuisines—including, ironically, products from his own brand of preprepared food, Kushi Cuisine.[139]

The degree to which macrobiotics retained a Japanese identity eventually became a major point of contention and confusion among white American leaders. As one leader, John Mann, wrote, "One of the myths of macrobiotics most frequently bemoaned is its identification as specifically Japanese. Yet the truth is not as easily unwrapped as it might at first seem— its skin peels off like layers of an onion."[140] This apt metaphor captures not only the ambiguous cultural authenticity of macrobiotics, but it also exposes among its white American devotees a deep ambivalence about race and Asian culture generally. Some followers clearly felt macrobiotics was not inherently bound to Japanese culture. Richard Price, an acolyte who joined the movement in 1968, argued, "The only reason macrobiotics makes such a big deal out of brown rice is because Ohsawa was Japanese. . . . If he had been German, we'd all be eating cabbage and sourdough bread."[141] While on its surface, Price's description matches the emphasis from Ishizuka on region-specific cuisine, his characterization nevertheless hints at a broader oversimplification of the diet's historical development and its lasting entanglement with Japanese politics, philosophy, and Cold War militarization.

Despite criticisms that Kushi sacrificed the environmental and global peace missions of the movement for his quasi-medical pursuits, these issues were nevertheless still demonstrably central to Kushi's efforts and were compatible with his alternative medical mission as well. Perhaps the best insight into Kushi's broader vision for the global macrobiotics movement comes from his attempts to leverage his success with HIV/AIDS in New York to create a global outreach program for macrobiotic AIDS therapy starting with the People's Republic of the Congo (PRC). In their capacity as the leaders of the Kushi Foundation for One Peaceful World, Michio and Aveline Kushi visited the PRC in July 1987 to conduct a series of macrobiotics educational programs at the World Health Organization Regional Office for Africa as part of the Government AIDS Symposium in Brazzaville. The conference brought together over 200 world health officials, medical doctors, and diplomats to discuss the AIDS crisis.[147]

Several months after the conference, in December 1987, Kushi wrote a summarizing report and outlined a list of objectives for the Congolese government. "We discussed and agreed that macrobiotic ways of dietary and nutritional approaches are beneficial to prevent and improve [AIDS and other degenerative diseases]."[148] The nutritional recommendations that Kushi outlines in the report were a variation on his SMD and included such boilerplate advice as consuming more protein, complex carbohydrates, and unsaturated fat from plant sources; fewer refined carbohydrates, saturated fat, and protein from animal sources; and more vitamins, minerals, and enzymes from natural versus artificial sources. Importantly, Kushi envisioned the Congolese government drawing heavily from macrobiotics expertise to reshape their entire government to solve the country's nutritional crisis and its AIDS crisis at once. He offered the Kushi Foundation as a source of expertise to help the PRC into a two- to three-year agricultural transition away from the cultivation of traditional African foods to regionally appropriate but macrobiotic-friendly staples like "river weeds."[149] Further, he advised the Congolese government to recruit macrobiotics leaders from Europe and North America to teach nutritional and sanitation courses and distribute educational materials.

In his report, Kushi argued that the Congolese government, after adopting his recommendations, would not only serve as a model for the development of the rest of Africa but for the rest of the world as well. For this final point, Kushi returned to his antinuclear agenda, commenting that developed countries were in particularly bad shape because not only were they overwhelmed with chronic disease, they were "suffering from environmental pollution resulting from improper disposal of chemically hazardous waste products from nuclear power plants and other industrialized facilities."[150] This report made it especially clear that Kushi was trying to harness his momentum helping AIDS patients in the United States to secure a greater role for macrobiotics on the global stage. Far from abandoning the principles of world peace and environmentalism, the Brazzaville conference demonstrates that Kushi had far grander plans in mind than his followers ever knew: to leverage macrobiotics' success in any arena (including medical applications) to gain access to state-level, and eventually international, power and policy.

Conclusion

The macrobiotics movement is far less visible today. The original companies that Kushi and Aihara founded are gone; both Erewhon and Chico-San were bought out or declared bankruptcy in the 1990s, though Erewhon has since returned. In the late 1990s, as Kushi began selling off his other assets and winding down his career, the movement itself was suffering a crisis of identity. Between the growing ruptures over racial resentment, rumors of sexual abuse, and national reports of labor disputes, macrobiotics had grown so big and so influential—and its secondary leaders so disenchanted— that no one could agree what macrobiotics was anymore.

Public awareness of the macrobiotics movement has now largely faded away; all that seems to remain of this once-mighty empire is the smattering of its signature staples at co-operative grocery stores and in natural foods aisles across the country.[151] Macrobiotics' real legacy lives on, however, in the core philosophy of the natural health food movement itself. Ohsawa's idea that good health, harmony with the environment, spiritual awakening, and world peace were inextricably linked with one another, and that to advance one was to advance all, was indelibly pressed into the hippie sensibilities that continue to fuel the alternative food movement. Though macrobiotics may have largely disappeared from the wider public consciousness, its history still helps illuminate key features about the contemporary entanglement of the food movement and alternative healing practices.

There were essentially two major branches of macrobiotics, one concerned with achieving world peace through bodily and environmental harmony, and another concerned with ridding the world of harmful chronic diseases (themselves expressions on a microscale of living in discordance with nature according to hegemonic Western logics). Each half of the macrobiotics philosophy acted to complement the other like the forces of yin and yang, each contained and depended on elements of the opposing force. In the thinking of major macrobiotics leaders, these two branches were apiece with one another, yet at times certain leaders emphasized different elements of this core philosophy to differing degrees. Practically, however, the patients invested in macrobiotics as a replacement for conventional medical treatments were a significantly different population from the adherents who sought spiritual enlightenment. Yet both halves of the macrobiotics ideology succeeded, not only out of a persistent countercultural romance with Japanese and other Asian ideologies, but because of how macrobiotics resonated with unique aspects of global culture that arose as a result of the Cold War. At first, there was robust common ground between both branches; Kushi's anticancer program specifically appealed to Cold War anxieties about nuclear war and radiation therapy when macrobiotic staples were advertised as reversing radiation poisoning.

In the late 1970s, however, these two branches of macrobiotics gradually started becoming incompatible, ultimately resulting in a schism. As Kushi invested more resources in opening clinics to train specialists to provide macrobiotic care for terminally ill patients, longtime acolytes began to question his priorities. For many of Kushi's new patients, macrobiotics was a temporary lifestyle, the limits of which coincided with the duration of their sickness. They saw macrobiotics as providing individual-level benefits, and their membership was largely guided by self-interest; in other words, these patients did not necessarily share in the expansive worldview so central to the movement's history. But their membership did much to further macrobiotics' legacy; by demonstrating a willingness to take patient complaints with Western medicine seriously, Kushi's macrobiotics became a major player in the deliverance of alternative therapies in the latter half of the twentieth century—uniting its righteous cause to heal neglected bodies with its push to globalize peace. To embrace both halves of macrobiotics as Kushi had, was to believe this narrowly construed ideal of intentional and spartan Japanese cuisine was a panacea, not only to heal the ailing bodies of the public but to quell the inherent dangers of naive Westernization, nationalism, imperialism, and of science, untethered to a cosmology that emphasized harmony above all.

Entremets II

Quacking under Pressure

· ·

When inventor Fred J. Hart's wife was dying of cancer in the early 1950s and conventional medicine had proclaimed her case terminal, he turned to an electronic device of his own making to cure her.[1] The American Medical Association (AMA), which classified products like Hart's as phony or fraudulent, allegedly intervened with his treatment plan, denying him the ability to use his machine on his wife for the cancer that would take her life. In retaliation, Hart founded an unusual organization in Monrovia, California, in 1955 that he called the National Health Federation (NHF) with the express goal of promoting the interests of "health freedom" in the United States. The group fought to protect what it claimed was the right of all Americans to reject drugs, surgery, and other invasive medical interventions and to uphold the liberty to employ heterodox therapies to whatever extent people thought best for themselves. NHF members lobbied against public health interventions like mandatory vaccination and the fluoridation of public water, and they fought for access to unproven cancer cures like laetrile and Linus Pauling's infamous megavitamin therapy.

Diet gurus and other like-minded natural health food advocates joined hands with practitioners from a spectrum of other drugless specialties like homeopathy, naturopathy, and chiropractic to swell the ranks of the NHF to more than 17,000 dues-paying members in 300 chapters around the world by the early 1980s.[2] Alvenia Fulton (see chapter 1) was a featured NHF speaker on multiple occasions, and she studied under Kurt "The Vitamin King" Donsbach, who served as the NHF's president from the late-1970s through the 1980s. Robert C. Atkins, the subject of chapter 4, served the NHF directly as a board member and advisor. Though some heterodox groups, such as chiropractors, had their own professional associations, the NHF became by far the most significant lobbying force on the collective behalf of holistic healing. Yet as grassroots healers began to organize and empower themselves, their rivals in the medical establishment—or as it was known among NHF members, the "big Medical-Government-Press Conclave"—sounded the alarm.

The AMA gathered a host of allies to conspire to torpedo this budding movement and the interests the NHF represented. On October 6, 1961, the AMA held the first National Congress on Medical Quackery (NCMQ). Between 700 and 800 people representing such varied groups as "the Post Office Department, the Federal Trade Commission, the Food and Drug Administration (FDA), the AMA, the Department of Justice, the American Cancer Society, the Arthritis and Rheumatism Foundation, the National Better Business Bureau, state medical societies and licensing boards, research institutes, women's clubs, medical and pharmacy schools, and health insurance companies," all shuffled into a large ballroom at the Sheraton-Park Hotel in Washington, DC, to vent their collective frustrations at what they perceived to be a tremendous resurgence of medical quackery.[3] During one of the opening speeches at the NCMQ, a presenter representing the AMA publicly estimated that health fraud had ballooned into a staggering billion dollar a year industry.[4] If accurate—the AMA never specified how it created this estimate—these revenues were large enough to rank health fraud in fortieth position on the 1961 Fortune 500 list.

The quackery these expert groups so feared had modernized since the nineteenth century. Gone were the days of patent medicines and snake oil salesmen; they had been replaced by the beguiling buzz of phony medical electronics and untraceable mail-order pharmaceuticals. Incredibly, in the AMA's estimate of the size of the American market in health fraud, overt medical quackery like fake devices, bogus drugs, and other treatments aping genuine medical care made up just half of the total market share. The other half—$500 million—was credited to a range of practices collectively and interchangeably labeled "nutritional quackery" or "food faddism."[5] In other words, the natural health food movement, fad diets, and their attendant dietary recommendations had worryingly become, in the eyes of these disgruntled regulators, a new kind of alternative medicine that sat just outside of their jurisdiction.

The original charge of the Pure Food and Drug Act in 1906 (which established the predecessors to the FDA) was to ensure product safety and combat food *fraud*. For example, in the late nineteenth century, it was common for commercial millers to secretly cut their flour with cheap fillers such as sawdust, borax, or chalk.[6] Unpasteurized milk was a public menace for spreading tuberculosis. As Upton Sinclair famously revealed in *The Jungle*, Americans were also regularly being fed diseased or otherwise contaminated meat, which could be injurious to consumers' health.[7] The 1906 law also required manufacturers of patent medicines—privately made health tonics, which were once completely unregulated and rife with scams—to refrain from using unproven health claims on products that crossed state lines and to alert consumers if their products contained alcohol, opium, cocaine, or the like. Deceit was so embedded in the cultures of these industries that Harvey Wiley—the first chief chemist of what would become the FDA—had his hands full just trying to prevent the most egregious of these contaminants and toxic adulterants from entering the market.[8]

Food *faddism* was another animal entirely. As an umbrella term, food faddism included all the heterodox claims, products, and services related to food or nutrition, including dietary supplements, weight reduction formulas and elixirs, foods advertised as "organic" or "natural," and even certain food staples from international cuisines such as brown rice (see chapter 2). To most of their critics, food fads were a minor nuisance—mere economic parasites—unnecessarily draining naive consumers' wallets, which only posed a serious danger to those who were already financially precarious.

But others saw darker omens in the rise of food fads. As Fred Stare's close friend and Harvard colleague Jean Mayer articulated his fear in 1963, "Nutritional quackery does not just cost money: it also systematically undermines the confidence of American people in their food supply, in their physicians, and in their universities."[9] Mayer foresaw the widespread erosion in public trust toward conventional expertise that roils our modern era and traced its roots to the food system. Once public trust was gone, anti-quackery activists feared, faddist products could be used to delay or replace vital medical care, seriously endangering people's health and undermining orthodox institutions. In his remarks at the 1961 NCMQ, Stare warned, "There are times when persons with real health problems rely on the products of nutritional quackery rather than on sound medical treatment. . . . When nutritional quackery becomes a substitute for the type of diet and care which will cure certain deficiencies, illnesses or diseases . . . [at] that point nutritional quackery becomes a health problem of considerable magnitude."[10]

For the AMA and nutrition scientists like Stare and Mayer, food faddism proved a more difficult foe to combat than other, more overt types of medical fraud because the products and services that faddists sold were not—for the most part—directly harmful. Heterodox entrepreneurs had also learned the hard way not to make unprovable health claims on packaging, which would have qualified them for censorship by the Federal Trade Commission or the Post Office. Instead, the claims of diet gurus and health food advocates for their products' healthfulness were increasingly moved to less regulated spaces. In the 1920s and 1930s, for example, instead of listing the recommended medical applications of a given product on the label, such claims were instead made on radio programs and in magazines, enticing customers to order health-promoting products with claim-free labels through the mail.

Later in the twentieth century, as the media landscape underwent radical changes with the advent of television and color photography, the new growth in independent radio, and the explosion of underground and alternative presses, diet reformers used any means at their disposal to broadcast their ideas. They hosted their own radio shows, wrote and published their own journals, and developed their own industry-specific magazines such as *Prevention*, *Runner's World*, and the *Vegetarian Times*. Lifestyle gurus' stories, products, and ideas were then picked up and featured on late-night talk shows where celebrities were grilled for their hot takes; their books, meanwhile, were obsessively dissected and ranked by periodicals of every size and reputation. All these media preserved the gurus' right to articulate their opinions—even those advocating for unproven medical treatments—under the First Amendment. The close partnerships with media outlets made the purveyors of dietary and lifestyle advice (especially the kind that challenged or undermined nutritional and medical science) into a powerful and persuasive class of public figures. Because of the slipperiness (or more favorably, wiliness) of heterodox healers and their claims, it was clear early on to anti-quackery activists that combating the fraudulent health claims that propelled heterodox health products required confronting them at their source. Yet because food faddists often broke no laws, the regulatory efforts to quash nonscientific claims about food were piecemeal and thus largely fruitless.

Credentialed nutrition experts like Fred Stare led the charge to drown out or defeat heterodox claims in the media ecosystem with what he considered to be cold scientific truth. But these experts were hardly as disinterested as they portrayed themselves. Though he was first trained in agricultural chemistry under Conrad Elvejhem at the University of Wisconsin and later secured a medical degree from the University of Chicago, Stare had industrial food processing in his blood; his father (Fred Stare Sr.) was the president and CEO of the Columbus Canning Company. In 1942, he was invited to found and fund (with lots of industry support) the Department of Nutrition at Harvard—the first such department attached to a medical school in the world. As chair of the department until 1976, he became a master corporate fundraiser and a respected national nutrition authority. He sat on the boards of countless food companies and nutrition foundations, and eventually cofounded (with his student Elizabeth Whelan) the American Council on Science and Health (ACSH), a leading think tank, lobbying group, and apologist for industrial science.

Early in his academic career in the late 1950s, Stare began investigating the relationship between diet and heart disease, becoming a prominent spokesperson for what became the standard medical recommendation of the low-fat diet. Notably, Stare was also heavily involved in international nutrition studies regarding hunger and malnutrition. Funded largely by the Rockefeller Foundation, Stare traveled to Peru, Colombia, Tunisia, Thailand, Germany, and the Netherlands to conduct studies concerning hunger and malnutrition.[11] For nutrition scientists like Stare, partnerships with industrial food manufacturers aligned nicely with scientific initiatives to combat malnutrition, like the enrichment and fortification of staple foods with essential vitamins and minerals.[12] When chronic diseases rose in tandem with the rising consumption of ultraprocessed industrial food, the corporate partnerships nutrition scientists maintained (which will be discussed in more detail in entremets III) made it that much more personally and politically difficult to change the scientific approach to health care and diet.

Because Stare made himself into such a vocal opponent of dietary heterodoxy (recall his racially insensitive tirade against Ohsawa and macrobiotics from chapter 2), he will reappear in every chapter for the rest of the book. For his role in organizing the first NCMQ, diet gurus and their NHF allies reserved special ire for Stare, branding him "the cockiest star of this Extravaganza of Slander."[13] Revealing his tyrannical impulses at that very event, Stare sought to silence diet gurus by publicly calling for a full-scale governmental crackdown on over sixty radio stations through which, he claimed colorfully, food faddists "purr their melodious incantations of nutritional nonsense."[14] Radically, he suggested that any station broadcasting health misinformation should be prosecuted for practicing medicine without a license. Such efforts would obviously have been illegal, so instead of using the tools of bureaucracy, health authorities tried instead to best these so-called nutritional quacks in the court of public opinion, where they have been hashing it out (often unsuccessfully) ever since.

The diet gurus at the center of the second half of the book took an entirely different approach to fighting back against what they saw as the flawed logic of nutrition scientists. Whereas Kushi and Fulton engaged with perceived medical gaps in the service of larger sociocultural movements or philosophies, the next two diets placed medical intervention at the forefront from the start. These diets, theorized and led by white men, cultivated different kinds of relationships with the US medical establishment and with their largely white clientele.

3 Death's Door People

The Pritikin Program and the Natural Antidote
to Aging and Debility

∙ ∙

The oatmeal and kasha tasted like wood
But we forced ourselves to say it was good
Four weeks went by, we ate all that slop
We went for the program and couldn't stop.
The instructions were followed to the letter
And we must admit that we do feel better.
Now we know what it's all about. . . .
It does do good there is no doubt.
My friends will ask me, "Where have you been?"
I'll merely tell them "Pri-ti-kin."

—Harry Oliphant, October 22, 1981

By her seventy-seventh birthday, Eula Weaver, "a tiny, wiry, tough-fibered woman" from California, had already witnessed all of her closest loved ones, including her husband and four of her five children, die.[1] After her eldest son, a Naval officer, passed away from cancer in Chicago in 1965, Weaver stayed in Illinois to take care of his daughter while she finished college. Yet Weaver was "barely able to keep a step ahead of death" herself, eventually suffering a heart attack during a routine checkup at an Illinois Naval medical center in 1969. At age eighty-one, she was diagnosed with congestive heart failure. Her doctor gave her two options: go to bed and let a permanent caregiver spoon-feed and bathe her for the rest of her life, or change her diet and push herself to exercise as much as she could bear. She confessed to her doctor that she could not walk "any length of ways" before having to sit but affirmed that she would "rather be dead than down."[2] Weaver had grown up the daughter of a south Texas cattle rancher, and she had married a semiprofessional baseball player, who, after not making it to the Big Leagues, became a rancher himself. Beef, particularly steak, had been an integral part of Weaver's identity, and her entire family's culture. Soon after beginning a daily walking regimen, Weaver found that her taste was changing, too, claiming, "Suddenly I couldn't eat the greasy, sugary, salted foods I used to."[3]

Weaver found her new lifestyle was even harder to maintain than she had imagined. After her heart attack, she was plagued with severe angina pain, high blood pressure, arthritis, and claudication (pain in the legs) for which she was prescribed a treatment involving sixteen to eighteen pills a day. Her circulation was so poor she wore gloves all day and socks all night—even in summer—to keep herself warm.[4] An article in the American Medical Association's lay magazine *Today's Health*, reported, "The heavy medication and constant chills kept her enfeebled and uncomfortable. Sometimes she could barely walk 50 feet without her calf muscles cramping so severely she had to be carried home."[5] Despite her best efforts to maintain the diet and exercise program she had been assigned by her physician, Weaver's condition was not improving. When her granddaughter graduated from college, Weaver moved back to her home in Santa Monica, California, but remained in her significantly diminished state; she was diagnosed as being "beyond hope of recovery."[6]

One fateful evening in 1973, Eula Weaver went to have dinner with her favorite grandson, Jim Weaver, a "prosperous wholesale food buyer," who was entertaining his friend, Nathan Pritikin. Pritikin—a pasty, dark-haired man whose low voice clashed with his slight appearance—was a popular health promoter and dietary reformer. His coauthored book *Live Longer Now*—through which he tried to cement a connection between diet and degenerative diseases—had just become a national bestseller, and he was talking about opening an intensive, live-in clinic in southern California to put into practice the ultrarestrictive principles outlined in his book. Weaver and Pritikin became mutually impressed with one another: "Pritikin was fascinated . . . by Eula Weaver's determination and mental toughness. She was intrigued with his theories." Reading his book reinforced her inclination, and Weaver immediately "rededicated herself to her life" and began implementing Pritikin's program to the letter.[7]

Over the next few months, Pritikin slowly weaned Weaver off of her medication while steadily increasing the duration and intensity of her exercise. What started as walking around the block soon became jogging around the track at the local high school. But casual jogging was an alarming sight even among fit people in the early 1970s, let alone for such a superannuated woman as Eula Weaver.[8] As *Today's Health* reported, "When neighbors saw Eula in jogging clothes, hobbling along, they thought the old lady had slipped a cog."[9] She was unperturbed. "Within one year," an article in *Woman's Day* gushed, "she was jogging a mile and a half every day and bicycling the equivalent of fifteen miles a day on a stationary machine."[10] As her neighbors gossiped and bragged about her unusual habits, she attracted the attention of the local Senior Olympics in Irvine, California, and was soon persuaded to compete. She was eighty-five years old at the time of her first entry, and Weaver won gold medals in both the 800- and 1,500-meter races. Following her debut performance in 1974, she won two gold medals every year for the ensuing five years for a total of twelve.[11] Perhaps most remarkably, she had accomplished all of this after stopping taking medication altogether.[12]

After Weaver "became something of a star at the senior games," her remarkable story was repeated in newspaper articles all over the world.[13] More importantly, tales of Weaver "trotting around the track in flapping pants with women 30 and 40 years younger" appeared in a wide variety of specialized publications by authors seeking to glean broader lessons from her miraculous-seeming recovery.[14] Her achievements were celebrated in running magazines, fitness publications, and other books promising the reversal of chronic disease. Her story also helped jumpstart the market for aging women's self-help, health, and fitness literature. Pivotally, Weaver's success was repeatedly cited in publications about aging. For this latter category in particular, "Eula Weaver symbolizes that the elderly can find independence of mind, spirit, and body if they eat, exercise, and, perhaps most importantly, think positively."[15] Weaver became the poster child for Pritikin's program, and he was quick to brag of her successes during interviews as evidence of his diet's promise.

Through the success stories of his patients like Weaver, Pritikin helped transform white, wealthy Americans' expectations about aging and the inevitability of infirmity from chronic disease. Though the specifics of his diet and exercise program largely mirrored recommendations from national authorities like the American Heart Association (AHA), Pritikin's approach was widely considered to be more intensive (and intense). The AHA recommended that people cut back on their consumption of dietary fat and cholesterol to stymie the development of atherosclerotic plaques, recommending a diet that was centered more on grains and lean meats. Pritikin thought these guidelines were far too lenient, advising his followers to eat a rather monotonous diet composed of 80 percent *complex* carbohydrates (not just any carb would do) with only 10 percent of calories from dietary fat and another 10 percent from protein. Commensurate with the severity of his restrictions, the claims he made about the success of his program were far grander than the AHA's. Beginning in the early 1970s, Pritikin's extremely low-fat program promised a sharp reduction in morbidity from nearly all varieties of chronic disease along with a total liberation from pills and other forms of burdensome disease management for people who had been languishing under pessimistic and oppressive prognoses from their physicians.

Pritikin's unusual ascendance to become one of the most influential, popular diet experts in the United States from the latter half of the twentieth century was a product of many factors: he had multiple bestselling books and was regularly featured in mainstream media juxtaposed to other dietary giants such as Atkins (see chapter 4) and Weight Watchers; he was called as an expert witness to testify before the US Congress multiple times during a pivotal transition period in the nation's dietary history; and he served as a personal inspiration to some of the biggest names in dieting from the 1990s to now. Though his name may have lost some of its cachet in the past several decades, publications from the 1970s and 1980s treated Pritikin so casually as to assume their audiences would be intimately familiar with him. Pritikin was squarely on the fairway of mainstream (re: white, middle-class, mass-market) dieting culture. Accordingly, Pritikin's program offers a lens through which we can put mainstream dieting culture into relief.

Pritikin's diet, though ostensibly centered around health, constructed normative models for his patients' bodies and in so doing certainly contributed to the American diet cacophony that vilified fatness and disability, glorified youth, and blamed individuals for failing to achieve bodily ideals. But to stop here would be to miss the soul of his program and its lingering effects on American health consciousness. Like the diets of the previous two chapters, the Pritikin program was self-avowedly aimed not at weight reduction per se but at the "prevention or treatment of high blood pressure, diabetes, gout, atherosclerosis, gallstones and other diseases."[16] Although many who adopted the Pritikin regimen reported moderate weight loss anyway, symptom relief and restored physical ability were the most desired outcomes of the diet. Unlike the other figures covered in the book thus far, Pritikin's success was also notable for the relatively high degree of medical buy-in he achieved given that he, like Alvenia Fulton and Michio Kushi, had no formal training in medicine. Pritikin frequently locked horns with skeptical medical authorities over his assertions that he could not only lessen but reverse America's most intractable illnesses; however, he nevertheless managed to shore up a sizable following among respected physicians.

Pritikin's ability to infiltrate hallowed medical spaces and to be taken seriously when he adopted medico-scientific ideas and language depended in no small degree on his positionality as a white man. Unlike Fulton or Kushi, whose success depended on having carefully embedded cultural hooks in their respective programs (ingredients, flavors, preparation methods, etc.) that aligned with their followers' broader values, Pritikin's success was not as transparently reliant on securing cultural buy-in for the cuisine that underpinned his dietary program. Like so much of nutritional thought in American society, Pritikin's program was largely structured around technoscientific understandings of food and nutrition that reduced cuisines to their macronutrient composition—an attitude food studies scholar Gyorgi Scrinis has labeled nutritionism.[17] With few exceptions, Pritikin's nutritional absolutism mercilessly eschewed the foods most associated with chronic disease, irrespective of their sociocultural ties. In doing so, he disregarded nearly every major American culinary tradition, eliminating many of the foods Americans found most palatable without proposing viable replacements and without situating such bland cuisine within an appealing cultural counternarrative as did the Temperance reformers who rallied around Sylvester Graham and John Harvey Kellogg a century or so earlier. Ironically then, Pritikin's performance of whiteness—exemplified by his flippant disregard of cultural identity and his subservience to the supposed culture-less facticity of science—fed into one of the most potent medical critiques of his ideology: his diet was so austere and so stripped of all cultural value that dieters struggled to maintain fidelity to his recommendations.

In spite of his assertions that people would develop a taste for his diet over time, Pritikin knew that a significant portion of his target market considered the dietary choices he was advocating too restrictive, requiring a prohibitively high degree of discipline to maintain. Yet Pritikin also knew from personal experience that his program *could* work with enough dedication. But the patients with whom he had had the greatest success were not representative of older Americans with faltering health. His success stories came disproportionately from those people most motivated to recover from terminal illness. These patients had already been subjected to intensive conventional medical programs for the management of chronic disease that required a great degree of self-discipline.

Historians of medicine have persuasively shown that, in the last decades of the twentieth century, chronic disease treatments and management strategies did not lessen the prevalence of disease so much as transform the experience of living with illness.[18] While medical intervention in these illnesses extended life without eliminating disease, the patients' improved life expectancy masked the new symptoms and complications that arose from managing an illness for an extended period of time. Even after months or years of invasive and expensive medical regimens, most patients could never expect a full recovery and often experienced a severe decline in their quality of life. Pritikin used this sentiment to justify his own intervention, arguing, "Current medical therapy for heart disease, most hypertension and adult diabetes deceives both physicians and patients. The symptoms may lessen, but the disease continues its destructive course."[19] In his mind, the austerity of his program was no more severe than the devastating medical treatments to which these patients were already being subjected. Since his program at least held out the promise of cure, he reasoned that the struggles he inflicted on patients would be more worth their efforts.

Obviously, Pritikin was not alone among diet gurus to have proclaimed an end to chronic disease. He was unique, however, in the way he made his proclamations reverberate in the halls of scientific medicine. Harnessing the techniques, language, and other trappings of medical science more successfully than his forebears, Pritikin managed to persuade an impressive number of American physicians that his program could reverse some of the worst, most intractable symptoms of the nation's top killers. Pritikin's program was also unique for its clientele: he specifically targeted illnesses that affected older Americans, which shaped the meaning of his program for his patients. Because many of the symptoms of chronic illness were often associated with aging itself (enfeeblement, frailty, pain, etc.), Pritikin's program mounted a serious challenge to the inevitability of decay or decline. In this lies Pritikin's central innovation: he redefined the possibilities and meaning of aging and age-related disability, especially for those who had expressed faith in traditional, orthodox medical authority and found it bereft of care or comfort. The degree to which Eula Weaver's story found a broader audience—especially among those new theorists of aging who, in the early 1990s, began to speculate about life extension, "successful aging," and even age reversal or antiaging—speaks to Pritikin's centrality as an architect of the life-extension movement.

Whereas living to old age was once perceived to be rare and those who attained long lives were appropriately revered, in the past century or so living well beyond seventy has become increasingly common, resulting in fundamental changes to the social meaning of aging. Much of the history of aging and old age has focused on the twentieth-century construction of elderhood (via gerontology) as a unique stage of life with its own distinct identity and challenges.[20] In broader American culture, however, aging has often been defined in contrast with youth culture, the privileging of which created images of aging that portrayed older people as irrelevant, powerless, and doomed to decline. The increased prevalence of the aged in the early twentieth century also coincided with the rise of science and secularization, leaving many older Americans struggling for meaning and against the medical system. Some scholars have argued that the construction of old age is inseparable from the medicalization of infirmity, which posits old age itself as a disease, fortifying the intense societal pressure to maintain youth at all costs with the power of hegemonic medical logics.[21] The medicalization of aging has yielded greater scientific interest in the biology of senescence and its physiological causes and has contributed to the popularization of life-extension techniques, the cultures of youth preservation, and the perennial quest to cure aging altogether. A postmodern wave of longevity-oriented science provided an opportunity to redefine aging against the backdrop of medicalization so as not to preclude the possibility of life extension and personal growth. Pritikinism was one such species of life-extension philosophy in postwar America.[22]

This chapter critically examines Pritikin's transformation from an obscure self-taught inventor to a renowned diet and lifestyle expert. He used his own body as a laboratory through which to conduct medical research and to, eventually, develop a tailored diet program for disease reversal. Pritikin struggled to gain recognition for the efficacy of his program from the medical community, which led him to concentrate his efforts on buttressing his claims to expertise and combating pernicious critiques. His eventual success, however, was only dependent in part on his claims to medical expertise—his primary success came from creating a supportive ecosystem that empowered a narrow band of people to transform their own lives beyond the limits of what orthodox medicine thought possible (or prudent). This intervention laid the groundwork for his enduring legacy.

A Self-Taught Inventor

Nathan Pritikin was born August 29, 1915, to Jewish parents who had immigrated from Eastern Europe, settling in Chicago's predominantly Jewish West Side. Pritikin disavowed his faith in early adolescence, preferring to set himself to solving complex scientific puzzles. From a young age, Pritikin displayed a keen technical mind and an entrepreneurial spirit. Though he only secured two years of formal post-secondary education at the University of Chicago, Pritikin managed to convert his high school passion for the technical minutiae of photography into a thriving event photography business, Flash Foto. In 1941, he leveraged his curiosity and photography experience to secure a lucrative military contract mass-producing cheap, high-accuracy reticles (precise etchings in eyepieces that assist aiming) for Air Force bombers, a position he held through the end of the war.[23]

For a decade afterward, Pritikin remained in Chicago developing and patenting new technologies, building businesses for their manufacture, and starting over again. Though impressive, Pritikin's life as a self-taught inventor had its share of vulnerabilities; his hard-won expertise was constantly and excessively scrutinized. In one notable instance, an engineer with whom Pritikin had gone into business sued for the intellectual property rights to their shared invention, claiming in court that Pritikin did not deserve to have the patent in his name given his lack of formal education. Because Pritikin had a robust personal history filing patents and running other successful businesses from the fruits of his intellectual labor, the judge ruled in Pritikin's favor. He eventually licensed forty-three patents in chemistry, physics, and electronics to companies such as GE, Corning Glass, Bendix Aviation, and Honeywell.[24]

Though his livelihood came from engineering, Pritikin nurtured a side passion for medicine that mirrored his love of technical puzzles generally. His first definitive exposure to rigorous medical thought was, serendipitously, through his photography business where he was occasionally hired to photograph medical conferences. Between shifts, he would sneak through hotel kitchens and back rooms to attend medical lectures for free, cultivating an amateur interest in a wide variety of subjects. He became an avid reader of popular scientific and medical literature shortly thereafter, and he eventually began collecting and devouring academic medical journals as well.

From as early as the 1930s, Pritikin had become especially interested in the problems of heart disease research. The prevailing medical explanation of heart disease emphasized the contributions of "regular" aging—and particularly the accumulation of stress—to the "natural" process of the hardening of the arteries. When Pritikin secured his reticle contract with the Air Force, he quietly used his high military clearance level to study the issue for himself by requesting and investigating army medical records. He expected to see heart disease rates explode across Europe during the war because it was, by all accounts, an extraordinarily stressful occasion. Yet the incidence of coronary heart disease declined, in apparent conflict

Beyond the movement's reliance on and identification with Japanese foods, macrobiotics followers had a range of reactions—from hostility to appropriation—to the diet's other Japanese ornamentation. For example, Mann describes a tendency among some white macrobiotics educators to "adopt the superficial trappings of the Japanese personality," including delivering lectures in "clipped English with all the accessory words compressed out of it" and using Japanese idioms.[142] At the same time, critics and followers alike punctuated their assessments of macrobiotics with assaults on their gurus' substandard fluency with English—assaults that became especially intense as discontent grew around Michio Kushi's medical pivot.[143] One of macrobiotics' earliest and most prominent white American followers, Bill Dufty, was quoted as having said, "The people around Georges Ohsawa had not a sufficient command of their own language, let alone a second one."[144] Yet despite his critiques, Dufty was sufficiently impressed with Japan to attend a 1920s-Paris-themed ball, with his then-wife Gloria Swanson, dressed as Ohsawa himself—in apparent yellowface—wearing a full ceremonial Japanese costume.[145] Some leaders, like Michel Abehsera, recognized the racial tensions between the Japanese leadership and white follower base, which he described as "reverse cultural arrogance" on behalf of the Japanese leadership, and a "cultural inferiority complex" on behalf of white devotees; taken together, the assumption was that "the modern Westerner is fundamentally a barbarian, and that all things Japanese are good." These "love-hate cultural dilemma[s]," he said, sometimes yielded "a cathartic binge of Japan-bashing."[146]

Concurrent with this latent racial prejudice were widespread (and ironic) calls to "Americanize macrobiotics," ignoring the degree to which macrobiotics was already uniquely American. The movement as it came to be under Kushi and Aihara's leadership could have only grown to such a remarkable capacity in America. To build their movement, Ohsawa, Kushi, and Aihara used American financial tools and techniques, appealed to American political pressure points during the Cold War, and evoked the widespread dissatisfaction with the American health care system. They also self-consciously appealed to the particular vision of Japan held by white Americans, capitalizing on the new special relationship that was forming between the two countries. Ohsawa's failure to successfully sow macrobiotics ideology in 1920s and 1950s Paris—under the pretense that it then served as the intellectual seat of the West—precisely demonstrates the dependency of the movement on the special fertility of American cultural soil.

with medical theory.[25] As he followed the problem after the war, he also learned that heart disease incidence fell dramatically among victims of the Holocaust, one of the most stressful events in recorded history; however, after the war, as life returned to normal, heart disease rates not only recovered, but they also swiftly rose past prewar levels.[26]

Though Pritikin was far from the only observer to note this predictive failure of medical theory, it stoked his voracious interest in the technical problems of medicine, and he, along with many other medical researchers, began hypothesizing correlations between the decline in cardiac morbidity and interrupted food rations. Among Pritikin's greatest sources of inspiration was Nazi refugee and Duke University physician Walter Kempner, who developed a diet of mostly rice and fruit to treat patients with chronic kidney disease. Despite the rice diet's narrow application and monotony, Kempner's program earned notoriety in the 1940s for significantly improving patients' health on a range of metrics, from cardiac to retinal.[27] Although Pritikin was inspired by Kempner and kept himself busy theorizing his own connections between diet and heart disease, he had not yet attempted to change his own habits. Pritikin continued to enjoy international cuisines, steak, lobster, eggs, and ice cream—even putting "six pats of butter on his baked potato"—for the next ten years.[28] Clearly, these early experiences with medicine were not the sole inspiration for his eventual diet program, but he continued to follow trends in medical research, and especially the heart disease problem, as a curious amateur while returning to his life as an independent inventor.

Eschewing the Fat

In 1955, tired of the subarctic cold and worried about the pollution in metropolitan Chicago, Pritikin set himself upon yet another new puzzle: locating the healthiest place to live in the United States. In a striking resemblance to George Ohsawa's early American followers (see chapter 2), Pritikin wrote letters to meteorologists in dozens of cities across the country asking them to send him detailed reports on their respective local climates—demonstrating again the high level of scientific literacy he had achieved thus far. After weighing the various factors that concerned him, Pritikin decided to uproot his family and his latest engineering business to move to healthful Santa Barbara.

Once settled, he wasted no time in arranging a meeting in a Los Angeles hotel with a heart disease researcher, Dr. Lester Morrison. Born in London,

Morrison earned his medical degree from Temple University in 1933, staying in Pennsylvania for several years afterward to practice gastroenterology and to teach. Later in his career, Morrison would teach in the medical schools at the University of California–Los Angeles, the University of Southern California, and Loma Linda University; he served as an investigator for the US Department of Health, the National Institutes of Health, and the American Cancer Society and became the chief of staff at Cedars of Lebanon Hospital.[29] Morrison had had the same intuitions as Pritikin about the origins and causes of heart disease. Like Pritikin, he too found inspiration to investigate dietary connections to heart disease from the anomalies in medical data during World War II. Morrison was among the first researchers to show, using experiments on rabbits, the connection between arteriosclerosis and cholesterol.[30] As of 1946, he had placed fifty patients on an experimental regimen (and another fifty in a control group) to bear those intuitions out, where "he began finding evidence that America's fat-rich diets were fostering heart and artery disease."[31] Pritikin had been following Morrison's study closely since its inception and was well aware of his conclusions ahead of their meeting. The night before their rendezvous, Pritikin claims to have ordered an ice cream sundae through his hotel's room service, a treat he dramatically swore to himself would be his last.

During their fateful meeting, Morrison and Pritikin discussed the role of cholesterol in promoting and measuring the progression of heart disease. As they chatted, Morrison casually inquired if Pritikin knew his own cholesterol values—he did not. Morrison insisted he have his blood examined and to take a Master's Step stress test in his laboratory. Pritikin agreed. When the tests were completed, Pritikin discovered to his great surprise that his functioning was considered "barely normal," and that despite his slender frame his cholesterol level was an eye-popping 280. Morrison told Pritikin that his cholesterol was in the high range of normal, but based on his own reading of the literature, Pritikin understood that figure to be dangerously high for long-term arterial health.

To curb his risk of developing heart disease, Pritikin started changing his lifestyle. First, he stopped eating "obvious" sources of fat: butter, eggs, the visible fat on meat. Within the year, his cholesterol had dropped to 200. After another year, he sought a different doctor's opinion on his arterial health where he was diagnosed with "posterial wall myocardial ischemia, with ST depressed leads"—still at high risk of having a heart attack.[32] Like Fulton, Pritikin was advised to avoid what he considered healthy behaviors, including any strenuous physical activity (exercise, climbing stairs, etc.). He

lamented that the advice was "everything consistent with a sedentary exis-
tence."[33] Instead of following his doctor's recommendation, Pritikin stopped
eating red meat in April 1958; within the month, his cholesterol had
dropped another 40 points. His stress test in December 1959 remained unfavorable, however, so the next month, undeterred, Pritikin began a moderate exercise program and cut animal protein from his diet altogether. His
next stress test—a more rigorous treadmill test—indicated he had finally
returned to normal functioning and his cholesterol had dropped to 120,
just slightly above the levels he maintained for the rest of his life. Pritikin
had cured himself of heart disease.

Concurrent with his struggle against heart disease, however, Pritikin's
health took another, more dramatic turn. In 1957, plagued by anal itching,
Pritikin sought relief from scientific medicine. Finding none in the various
topical creams and ointments and reacting poorly to the antifungal medicines he was prescribed, Pritikin's physician convinced him to undergo three
rounds of unfiltered x-ray therapy (two at 88 rem, one at 44 rem) to kill off
what his doctors presumed were unwieldy gut flora.[34] After this therapeutic exposure, Pritikin's blood showed abnormalities in his white cell count
for the first time, a precursor to the leukemia (first diagnosed in 1958) that
would eventually lead him to take his own life. Indeed, Pritikin would later
blame the X-rays he received for the mutation in his lymphocytes, a cruel
side effect of excessive medical therapy.

After his first test with Morrison in 1955, Pritikin turned his obsession
with medical literature and puzzles inward, hoping to use his prodigious
mind to solve his medical problems. He began actively interrogating every
step his doctors took in his diagnosis, making detailed notes and copies of
every medical record he ever received about all the different parts of his
body. He also began collecting impossibly detailed information about his
own health, including taking his own measurements and keeping meticulous records of his health-related data, even tracking his daily blood counts
manually on graph paper. He would then compare the notes he kept on his
blood chemistry with the records he made of his diet and exercise routine
in an attempt to suss out possible effects.[35]

To make time for his newfound passion for learning about and monitor-
ing his own health, from 1955 to 1967 Pritikin sold off all of his patents,
stock, and prior business interests. It was a blessing in disguise for his family.
Pritikin's son reflected, "My dad was a horrible businessman. Our family
was always sitting on the edge economically with the way he would run
things. He was a wild man in business—a wild man with a pen, I used to

call him."[36] This time, luckily, the collective deals were lucrative enough to allow Pritikin to take an early retirement and to begin independently funding medical research. During this time, he also began corresponding with a wide network of physicians through which he earned limited recognition as an authority on a variety of medical topics—but especially nutrition—in certain sectors of the medical establishment.

The Pritikin Program for Diet and Exercise

From his years of meticulous research and self-experimentation, Pritikin eventually settled on a complicated dietary formula to combat his own illnesses that emphasized the intake of complex carbohydrates, fruits, and vegetables while abstaining almost entirely from salt, sugar, cooking oil and margarine, animal fats, caffeine, alcohol, and nicotine. Included in his list of foods to avoid were many other cooking staples: all but nonfat dairy products (including nondairy substitutes), egg yolks, honey, molasses, all refined carbohydrates, all but lean meat and only then in limited amounts. His crusade against fat drew no distinctions between saturated animal fats, monounsaturated vegetable fats, or polyunsaturated fats (like omega-3s), as all were liable, in his mind, to "create havoc by raising triglyceride levels and creat[e] metabolic suffocation by the resultant sludge in the blood."[37] In fact, Pritikin was so convinced of the negative effects of dietary fat that he even avoided such high-fat plant products as avocados, olives, soybeans, and nuts (except low-fat chestnuts). Not only was this a diet that was virtually free from all refined ingredients, most dairy, and most meat, but the preparation methods he considered acceptable even for grains and vegetables were severely limited as well, ruling out much of Western cooking culture in one fell swoop. Although there were many forbidden foods and flavors on the Pritikin program, the one upside was that anyone following his program was permitted to eat to their heart's content with no limits on portion size.

Pritikin found that his program worked so well on himself that he decided to proselytize. In a 1991 *Vegetarian Times* interview, Pritikin's son Robert said his father soon became a "rabble-rouser," claiming, "He'd go around talking to anybody who would listen to him. My dad became an evangelist. He was seeing millions of people dying from all of these diseases, and no one would listen. He finally started talking to these really off-the-wall longevity groups of the 1960s and 1970s, the pseudo-science groups."[38] His involvement in life-extension circles eventually led to his being appointed

Director of Nutrition Research, in 1972, for a nascent organization called the Longevity Foundation. Pritikin had befriended the organization's president, the mathematician and fellow longevity enthusiast Jon Leonard.[39]

Pritikin's first major national exposure came two years later, in 1974, when he and Leonard coauthored the bestselling book *Live Longer Now*.[40] The book proposed a strict diet—similar to the Pritikin plan outlined above—entitled the 2100 Plan. The authors of the book claimed that the program was the product of collaboration between twenty scientists.[41] Though it was a lie, it presaged Pritikin's lifelong quest to garner a medical seal of approval for his ideas. Regarding the purpose of their diet plan, Leonard said that people were "not afraid of the now, but of the future. They confuse living a long time with being debilitated a long time. That's what we're avoiding."[42] Unlike most diets that emphasized the speed of results—particularly with respect to weight loss—Pritikin advertised his diet as a long-term, holistic, preventive lifestyle that could ensure a rich, active life well beyond median life expectancy. With the success of the book, Pritikin was granted appearances in magazines, newspapers, national TV spots—most notably two slots on *60 Minutes* from which came his greatest surge in popularity. His first solo-authored book, *The Pritikin Program for Diet and Exercise* in 1979, sold nearly 2 million copies and became a bestseller.[43]

After the release of *Live Longer Now*, Pritikin gave a presentation on his theories at a 1974 conference for the American Academy of Medical Preventives in Miami, which was, by all accounts, sensational.[44] His controversial ideas were received with enthusiasm, and he began receiving letters in the mail asking him about the finer details of his program, how it could be implemented, broadened, or more thoroughly assessed by medical institutions. Among the flurry of inquiries he received was one from a physician from the Long Beach Veterans Administration (VA) Hospital, John Kern, dated July 27, 1974. Kern had become excited about the potential of conducting a study with VA patients to evaluate the results of Pritikin's diet and exercise program on severe cardiovascular disease—a program Kern hoped would revolutionize cardiac care at his hospital. In his first letter, Kern said, "We are planning on putting your diet to [the] test at the Long Beach Veterans Hospital. We plan angiography before and after your diet as well as the noninvasive studies. Our patients will be men suffering from atherosclerotic peripheral vascular disease. . . . We are interested to see if we can reverse the atherosclerotic process with your diet."[45] Excited by the potential to underpin his program with real science, Pritikin enthusiastically accepted the offer and began making plans to design and execute the study in cooperation with staff from the Long Beach VA Hospital.

The study was to be a preliminary test comparing the AHA's diet (which allowed nearly 40 percent of daily calories to come from dietary fat) with the Pritikin program in thirty-eight men with advanced cardiac conditions over a period of five months. Because the hospital lacked sufficient facilities to entertain and feed such a large group of men for so long, Pritikin rented a house near the VA hospital where the men were supposed to come every day to exercise, to have basic measurements taken, and to collect and eat premade meals (including taking home doggy bags with late night snacks). Kern, who was supposed to be the lead author of the study, found himself preoccupied with his duties as the Acting Chief of General Medicine at the hospital. There was so much work to run everything for the study that Pritikin hired his son Robert, who took a leave from his research job at a diabetes foundation to supervise the activities in the house—or, as he also once said, "to babysit a bunch of older men who acted like children most of the time."[46] The elder Pritikin spent much of his time shuttling between the study house and the hospital to consult with medical staff, set up testing at neighboring hospitals and clinics (including Loma Linda University Medical Center and the Orange County branch of the California Heart Association), and solicit food donations from local businesses and corporations alike to feed his patients (including, notably, from Erewhon, Michio and Aveline Kushi's natural food company).[47]

The hard work paid off, from Pritikin's perspective at least, when the final results were tabulated, and they showed substantial improvement in the physical condition of the men on the experimental Pritikin program. On average, their exercise capacity increased tenfold, several of them had weaned themselves off of or were taking substantially reduced doses of their medications, and their collective arterial stenosis (cholesterol blockage) was estimated to have been reduced by more than half.[48] As a nonscientist, Pritikin felt understandably vindicated by these results, which were especially important to him because they provided the first evidence (beyond Eula Weaver) that his program could work for more people than himself. His team had difficulty publishing their spectacular results, however. They submitted their write-up to the AHA, but were rebuffed to Pritikin's great chagrin. He cynically assumed the AHA was merely buttressing their own dietary program against criticism and competition. After a few other rejections from medical journals and conferences, Pritikin was finally accepted to present his findings from the Long Beach VA Study at the 1975 session of the American Congress of Rehabilitation and Medicine in Atlanta.[49] It was there that "the real fireworks began."[50]

In his own telling, Pritikin's presentation was not only honored as the most important paper at the conference, but his presentation also earned him an interview with a local science reporter.[51] His son later contradicted this version of the story, suggesting that Pritikin himself had "got a few science editors down there and pumped them up" before the presentation to make a splash.[52] Regardless, the interview led to the publication of a front-page news story about Pritikin's claims to have reversed heart disease with diet, after which the "wire services picked it up and made it a national rage." Though many had experimented privately with Pritikin and Leonard's 2100 Plan, after the bombshell talk in Atlanta "Pritikin returned to Santa Barbara to discover hundreds of letters inquiring about where the nutritional treatment could be obtained. He resolved to start such a facility."[53]

The Longevity Center

The crown jewel of Pritikin's operation was to be a magnificent, luxury clinic-cum-health resort called the Longevity Center, but it took several years to come to fruition. The first iteration of the rehabilitation clinic was founded in January 1976 and required that guests stay at a rather lackluster motel, the Turnpike Lodge in Goleta, California, for the duration of the program.[54] Pritikin moved his enterprise to its first independent location in Santa Barbara—at the more sophisticated Mar Monte Hotel—shortly thereafter. However, Pritikin and the owner of the Mar Monte had a dramatic falling out when the owner put a "financial squeeze" on Pritikin.[55] In fairness, Pritikin also had a reputation for being difficult.[56] Finally, in May 1978, Pritikin relocated his clinic to its permanent address in Santa Monica with a newly renovated space designed specifically for his purposes.

Despite the difficulties of moving and scouting locations in these early years, the Pritikin program proved remarkably popular. After finding success in California, the Pritikin Foundation opened two additional locations in Downingtown, Pennsylvania, and Surfside, Florida, with unrealized plans for another in Maui. At each satellite center, Pritikin sought to replicate as nearly as he could the program to which he subjected himself. Just as Pritikin detached from his work responsibilities, collected mind-boggling amounts of health data about himself, studied physiology and medical literature, exercised, and strictly monitored his eating, so would his patients—at least, approximately. And they would do so in the relative lap of luxury.

Pritikin's flagship Longevity Center in Santa Monica was a health and wellness resort similar in function to John Harvey Kellogg's nineteenth century Battle Creek Sanitarium but updated to fit contemporary tastes. It was "an immense building furnished in the plush carpet, natural wood look and stained glass that shouts of California modern," located on a prime stretch of unspoiled golden beaches. His guests stayed on-site in the resort's 107 rooms, and their supervising physicians lived next door in the resort's other fourteen rooms. The "tall, tinted windows" of the large, quiet dining hall, according to one commentator, overlooked a stand of "palms flapping in a stiff onshore breeze," which "give the impression one is watching a sepia film of the idyllic California beach life."[57]

Would-be Pritikinites from across the country (and the world) signed up to stay with him for an entire month; they attended nutrition and physiology lectures, group exercise classes, and Pritikin-approved dinner parties while their bodies turned back the clock.[58] Expectedly, this immersive, life-altering Pritikin experience was not cheap. The entry cost to the Center when it opened in 1976 was $2,750, the equivalent of $13,500 today adjusted for inflation. Interestingly, patients only paid this hefty admission fee after having their applications accepted, and the application required an additional $1,100 panel of medical tests, bringing the total cost of attendance to $3,850, almost $19,000 today.[59] "In return," an article in *Women's Wear Daily* suggested, Pritikin's patients "expect that their future which, before the center, included a certainty of pain, surgery or a lifetime of drugs, will be considerably brighter."[60]

Because the program was not initially covered by insurance, the high cost, both financial and temporal, of attending a month-long getaway at the Longevity Center was borne entirely by the patients themselves. This meant that, more often than not, Pritikin's clientele was retired, white, and affluent.[61] That Pritikin became a bestselling diet book author with this group as his primary target demographic challenges the standard picture of twentieth-century American dieting as the exclusive domain of young and middle-aged women obsessed with a trim waistline. Rather, Pritikin's most enthusiastic followers were people who had been stricken by unmanageable chronic disease and who reported feeling abandoned by or powerless in the face of mainstream medicine. As one reporter wrote after attending a session himself, most of Pritikin's patients "were suffering from advanced artery disease. . . . They ranged in age from the mid-forties to eighty-four, and most came armed with pills—especially nitroglycerine tablets, used to allay the attacks of severe chest pain known as angina pectoris, which physical exertion produces in many heart patients."[62] But as a biographical article about Pritikin cheerfully argued, "For many, this is far cheaper than the alternatives—bypass surgery, long convalescence in a hospital, extensive treatment by conventional means, or that most costly of options, death."[63] Despite the steep entry fee, Pritikin's centers had no shortage of customers. In a 1982 PBS interview, Pritikin claimed that his centers had hosted over 10,000 guests.[64] By 1986, Pritikin's son and the heir to his foundation, Robert Pritikin, suggested that over 20,000 people had attended either the thirteen- or twenty-six-day live-in programs at one of the three Pritikin Longevity Centers.[65]

One commentator outlined the benefits he saw in the immersive Pritikin rehabilitation experience: "the launching program . . . has obvious advantages for those with little willpower. For one thing, at the institute you'd have to go out of your way to cheat. Since you are served eight meals a day, you are not likely to get hungry. There is also the added incentive of having a daily record kept of your improvement in terms of reduced weight, lowered blood pressure, increased stamina and the like."[66] But this is too pragmatic and cynical an assessment for the exhilarating spiritual experience the Longevity Center provided for many of its guests. Attendees found meaningful support and community in the other patrons who had experienced similar struggles with their health and with finding adequate care in regular medicine. The main appeal, however, was a far grander kind of transformation: a lifting of the heavy constraints of daily life. Pritikinites took solace in being away from their homes and the pressures of their day-to-day lives—and the picturesque subtropical locale did not hurt either.

By the end of the program, many of Pritikin's patients "were able to suspend most of their cardiovascular, arthritis, diabetes, and hypertension (high blood pressure)—medications by the thirtieth day. Some were able to go off medication completely."[67] The most common stories were about people who had been confined to their houses from an inability to walk unimpeded by pain who soon found themselves, rather suddenly, much more mobile and capable of living independently. Though not every patient became an international-headline-grabbing athlete like Eula Weaver, for many just regaining the capacity to walk empowered them rejoin the social sphere of their friends and families from which they had been excluded too soon by their declining health. Some patients underwent such a dramatic turnaround in their health that they likened their experience to contact with the divine, Pritikin's own atheism notwithstanding. Some exalted the center as "the Lourdes of the West"—a reference to the French town known for having water with miraculous healing abilities—and one patient simply referred to the center as the "miracle place."[68] Guests referred to Pritikin himself as a "medical messiah" and wrote poetry for him suffused with religious ecstasy.[69] In this vein, one commentator wrote that "the spirit at the Longevity Rehabilitation Center here is not unlike the atmosphere at fundamentalist revival. Like their counterparts who find God, the patients at the center are finding cures—or so they believe—and they bounce around the converted seaside hotel in brightly colored jogging suits, anxious to tell you of their mysterious discovery."[70]

The Makings of a Medical Expert

Pritikin was less interested in the revelatory enunciations of his followers than he was in documenting their medical progress to leverage his claims of expertise against the wider world of dietary skeptics. Revealingly, of his transition from engineering to medicine, Pritikin said, "What I'm doing now is no different from what I've done all my life. I'm still in research and development. But now I'm working with animate instead of inanimate objects, so I have to be more careful."[71] Though the culture of the Longevity Center was crucial for patients, it was at best a fringe benefit for Pritikin. Despite the Longevity Center's core function as a rehabilitation clinic, the constant influx of patients along with their detailed medical screenings, regular check-ins with Longevity Center medical staff, and their general captivity during their stay at the Center made it easy for Pritikin to record and compile patient data. One reporter noted that the Longevity Research Institute kept "thousands of records documenting functional improvement of circulatory problems that often lead to high blood pressure and heart disease; reversal of diabetes, hypoglycemia, arthritis, and other degenerative disorders; case histories of angina patients who are set free of pain or physical symptoms; and those who have discarded drugs, vitamins, even insulin."[72] When the Center was first founded, Pritikin even published a monthly newsletter detailing the improvement statistics from each thirty-day session or "class." The abundance of data enabled Pritikin to utilize his Longevity Center not only to provide care but to conduct his own medical research aimed at demonstrating the efficacy of his program to a more discerning medical audience.

Because Pritikin thought he had stumbled on the secret to reversing chronic disease, he was justifiably eager to promote his ideas at the highest level. But getting his ideas to the widest possible audience while maintaining credibility meant he would have to avoid the pitfalls of other faddish dietary promoters; he would have to successfully convince the gatekeepers of the nation's health that his ideas had real merit. The most obvious such gatekeepers were his patients' own caregivers: the physicians and hospitals with whom they sought treatment. Accordingly, Pritikin carefully built and maintained relationships with his patients' referring physicians (some of whom worked for such prestigious institutions as the Mayo and Cleveland Clinics), sending supporting documents when requested and even delivering personalized patient progress reports from the data he collected at the Center.[73] Pritikin also buttressed his claim to medical expertise by recruiting physicians to work at the Longevity Center—to teach classes, review patient records, design treatment protocols, and, perhaps most importantly, serve on the advisory board of his research institute.

In addition to befriending individual physicians, Pritikin began to expand his outreach to entire institutions. To forge a stronger relationship with hospitals, Pritikin placed his son, Robert, in charge of a program that aimed to connect hospitals interested in modifying their dietetic programs for patients with chronic diseases with resources about how to institute an approach similar to the Longevity Center. Initially, Pritikin would provide physicians at interested hospitals with copies of favorable medical studies and lecture slides so they could present the Longevity Center approach to their peers. This strategy managed to pique several hospital administrators' interest; in 1980, he had requests from six hospitals in Utah alone, including the Utah Valley Hospital and the Cottonwood Hospital in Provo.[74] In 1981, the financially strained Centre City Hospital in San Diego converted an entire twenty-five-bed unit to provide in-house Pritikin therapy, charging patients $4,000 each for a ten-day stay.[75] Centre City had followed the lead of a hospital in New Orleans that had made the switch in 1980 to offer the "Pritikin Hospital Plan," under the direction of the New Orleans-based health maintenance organization Qualicare, Inc.[76] Today, the program is known as Pritikin Intensive Cardiac Rehabilitation, and, according to the program's website, it has recruited nearly fifty participating clinics including St. Luke's Hospital, Arkansas Heart Hospital, and Baptist Memorial Health Care.[77]

In hopes of engaging the medical community more broadly, Pritikin recruited physicians to design, conduct, and publish experimental trials testing his program (or related concepts) to gain visibility in peer-reviewed medical journals.[78] The trials were mostly self-funded (they mostly cost between $60,000 and $150,000) or were conducted in cooperation with allied institutions with deeper pockets such as Loma Linda or Brigham Young. In designing their experiments, Pritikin's allies cast a wide net; they searched for effects of the Pritikin diet on a range of conditions beyond hypertension, including diabetes, gout, breast cancer, and colon cancer. Some of the trials (many not ultimately published) were designed to respond to his critics' complaints that his program was too low in fat, iron, and protein, and too high(!) in fiber. In addition to publishing papers, Pritikin continued to present his results at conferences and to give invited lectures to physicians at prestigious medical institutions ranging from Sloan Kettering and Cornell Medical to the Rockefeller Institute and Mount Sinai.[79]

Dietary Goals for the United States

Pritikin's forays into orthodox medical terrain provoked excitement, curiosity, critique, and alarm. But regardless of their opinions about Pritikin or his program, physicians were unable to sideline him altogether. The excitement he generated with his presentation in 1975 caught the attention of Congress at a critical juncture. Pritikin was one of thirty expert witnesses (and the only diet guru) called to submit testimony to the pivotal Senate Subcommittee Hearing "Diets Related to Killer Diseases," which partly established the influential 1977 report *Dietary Goals for the United States*.[80] The report, nicknamed the "McGovern Report" after committee chairman Sen. George McGovern (D-South Dakota), was a major turning point in the federal government's nutrition recommendations. Though McGovern's team had originally been tasked in 1968 with investigating hunger and malnutrition in the United States (their work motivated significant revisions to the Food Stamp Program, for example), after several years they transitioned to investigating all the nutritional problems of the country, focusing especially on overnutrition.[81] Based on years of sprawling subcommittee testimony from esteemed nutritional experts such as Harvard's Mark Hegsted and National Heart, Lung, and Blood Institute (NHLBI) Director Robert Levy, *Dietary Goals for the United States* became the first government publication to draw an explicit connection between diet and chronic disease. It is also credited with being the first national report of vilifying dietary fat (especially from animal products) and establishing the controversial low-fat paradigm that reigned in American nutrition through the 1980s, 1990s, and beyond.[82]

The hearing for which Pritikin's testimony was solicited was intended to establish causation between poor diet and chronic disease. Interestingly, Pritikin's expertise had been requested by McGovern himself.[83] Citing their common aims of reducing preventable death, McGovern said of Pritikin, "We became friends, mutual admirers and fellow crusaders."[84] Though it was not within his purview, Pritikin attempted to use his moment in the congressional spotlight (and again in 1980) to not only prove that diet caused disease but to advertise the success of his specific approach in reversing chronic disease with therapeutic diet and exercise, and to sway national recommendations to reflect his program at the Longevity Center as well.[85] This was hubris.

Impressed with Pritikin's disease reversal claims, in December 1975 Congressman Robert Leggett (D-California) urged the director of the NHLBI, Dr. Levy, to independently investigate Pritikin and his center to see if the hype held up. Levy had a long, decorated career. He started at the National Institutes of Health (NIH) in 1963 where he directed clinical research, led the Division of Heart and Vascular Diseases from 1973–75, and served as director from 1975–81. He oversaw the Coronary Primary Prevention Trial, the first study to prove that lowering blood cholesterol reduces heart disease risk, before leaving for academia to become vice president and dean of Tufts Medical School and later vice president at Columbia University College of Physicians and Surgeons. After Leggett's prodding, Levy sent a small team to investigate the Longevity Center in Santa Monica to assess the accuracy of its claims and its viability as a model for national nutritional recommendations. Despite the fact that Pritikin's studies had been designed and executed by respected medical scientists who worked in his clinics or served on the Longevity Center's advisory boards, some of their work was difficult to disseminate through wider medical channels because the informal, patient-centered setup of the Longevity Center chafed against more exacting study protocols. These and other irregularities undermined the study results in the peer-review process, and subsequent review committees were hesitant to believe the impressive results that Pritikin and his allies trumpeted. A prime example, and one that Levy and Pritikin disputed at length in written testimony before Congress, was the 1974 Long Beach VA Study.

Soon after Pritikin's presentation of the Long Beach VA study results at the Atlanta conference in 1975 (the presentation from which he garnered enough public enthusiasm to found his Longevity Center), Pritikin's progress was halted by an internal investigation launched by the Veterans'

Administration that threatened to significantly undermine his credibility as a medical authority. Specifically, the national office of the VA claimed that it had never given authorization for Pritikin's study and opened an official investigation into the operations of the Long Beach branch.[86] Both Pritikin and his research partner, Dr. John Kern, were deposed and gave testimony about their involvement with and the overall trajectory of the study they had designed and executed together. Although there were substantial disparities between their accounts, there were serious red flags even where their testimonies agreed.

The study itself was rife with design flaws. The most fundamental oversight was the uneven treatment of the experimental and control groups, a fact which rendered the trial's results largely meaningless. The eighteen patients in the experimental group were regularly monitored by Dr. Steven Kaye and Pritikin's son, Robert—who was not a physician but conveniently volunteered to live at the house his dad had rented so he could monitor all the patients and prepare their meals. Troublingly, one patient counted in the experimental group only read Pritikin's book and executed the program on his own from home. Even worse, the fifteen patients in the control group (though the published report listed nineteen) were told to follow the VA Hospital's recommended diet on their own, from home, but were not given the same kind of prepared meals or even detailed meal prepreparation instructions.[87] The control group was only told how and when to exercise, but, crucially, they were not rigorously monitored during the study period like the experimental group. Only at the end of the study were all the patients given angiograms at Loma Linda University and plethysmography at the Orange County California Heart Association to track the overall progress of their disease.

As the investigation of the Long Beach VA proceeded, national VA representatives discovered yet more glaring concerns about the execution of the study. Bafflingly, Kern originally claimed to have been unaware that the study had been conducted at all. He later amended his statement to say that he had abandoned the project after having difficulty identifying suitable patients at the hospital within his and Pritikin's target demographic. Other records showed, however, that Kern had visited the study house Pritikin rented on at least four separate occasions, contradicting his plea of ignorance. Kern clearly wanted to dissociate himself from the project out of fear for his reputation. Pritikin told investigators that Kern, swamped with his other hospital duties, gave Pritikin direct access to patients' records, instructing him to select and recruit them into his study by himself—a serious lapse of professional judgment and stark violation of medical ethics for which Kern was subjected to a separate disciplinary hearing.[88] Kern later admitted having felt intense pressure to get the study underway because their funding—from an obscure organization called the Kirsten Foundation—was only available for a narrow window of time.[89] Importantly, even with this mysterious outside funding, Pritikin was responsible for covering a significant portion of the study costs himself and for soliciting donations from local businesses for the food his patients consumed daily.

During his own deposition before the national VA investigatory committee, Pritikin claimed to have learned—at the hearings themselves—that Kern had never formally submitted the study to the Long Beach VA Hospital for approval, nor had he obtained permission to allow Pritikin, let alone Pritikin's son, to work with the hospital at all. Oblivious to Kern's negligence in securing adequate approval from the hospital, Pritikin simply assumed (from casual interactions with Kern's colleagues that took place while Pritikin was in the hospital) that people were generally informed and accepting of their study. What most troubled the VA's investigators was that Pritikin—as a private citizen—had not only viewed sensitive hospital records, but regularly worked in Kern's office and was present for much of the experimental testing done at the hospital. Ultimately, the VA investigation concluded that the study had not actually been surreptitious because many of the Long Beach Hospital physicians had known about it and had even sent patients to participate.

The results of the study itself were, according to Kern, ambiguous at best. During the first few months of the trial, he admitted that the results looked impressive: "The men lost weight, blood pressures returned to normal, exercise tolerance increased from a few feet to a few miles, and the men felt well."[90] But problems emerged later. Both the experimental and control group had a death from myocardial infarction by the end of the study period. The man from the experimental group who died had even seen marked improvement in his exercise ability. Nonetheless, he developed severe angina several months into his new regimen. According to Kern, Pritikin insisted the man's death could be explained away by his having smoked a corncob pipe and eaten a hamburger the day of his death. Pritikin countered that he had actually attributed the man's death to the fact that the patient had developed a six-month habit of smoking and eating hamburgers, not just on his death day.[91] Of the other patients, Kern said a third of the remaining patients did slightly better, a third had no noticeable improvement, and a third suffered a marked decrease. He conjectured that the benefits he and Pritikin witnessed early on could be explained away by the low sodium content of the experimental diet (the positive results of which were allegedly undone after a single salty meal) and adherence to the incremental exercise routine. In other words, Kern thought Pritikin's key intervention—the extremely low fat content of the diet—was irrelevant to the study results.

Despite Kern's reservations about the study results and despite never having seen a single draft of the report while it was being written, Kern was still listed as the study's principal investigator.[92] The Long Beach VA Hospital was also named as the source of the study's patients in the publication—which resulted in substantial "unfavorable publicity" for the hospital.[93] Under the fierce gaze of his interrogators, Kern lamented having ever been involved in Pritikin's Long Beach VA study and mailed a notarized request to Pritikin to have his name removed from the study and any material Pritikin printed advertising its conclusions.[94] His concerns were not unreasonable—the investigation risked severely damaging Kern's credibility as a researcher and jeopardizing the public reputation of his employer.[95] But he was also shirking responsibility for his own lapses by throwing Pritikin under the bus. Kern lamented, "With Mr. Pritikin, the diet is almost a religion and it is above scientific scrutiny and the negatives are overlooked and you only look at the positives which may be the way you do things in business but in medicine you have to look at the things that were unexpected and you have to be able to explain them and therein might lie the key to some important discovery."[96]

Kern was right: Pritikin was not a disinterested scientific researcher and had a clear vested interest in his study results. Pritikin clearly hoped not only to vindicate his dietary ideology but also to see that his substantial personal investment in the study bore fruit after Kern's significant fumbles. Having felt abandoned by Kern in the study process only to find that he disagreed with Pritikin's interpretation of the study results, Pritikin decided to circumvent him and publish the study anyway, feeling that the results merited the attention of a wider medical audience. Predictably, the report touted the diet's efficacy, even offering it as an alternative to coronary bypass surgery. Though Pritikin's actions would violate contemporary medical sensibilities, and even skirted the ethical norms of the time, Pritikin (unlike Kern) was not a physician and was therefore not bound to enforcing these standards. Pritikin defended himself at his own deposition by pleading ignorance:

I wasn't aware at first how studies had to be done in the VA and I wasn't aware of our status. I just assumed that we were, that we were given whatever authority we had to have, else I wouldn't ever have wandered into the kitchen to ask them to prepare our diets or made all the other arrangements. The idea that we weren't part of a VA study just slowly came to me after many months . . . when the Blood Laboratory started to destroy our blood [samples]. . . . The first knowledge I really had clearly that we were an unknown project, was when Aronow called me . . . either a month or two months [prior to his deposition hearing].[97]

Despite these many flaws, in letters submitted to the Senate Subcommittee on Diets Related to Killer Diseases, Pritikin nevertheless heralded his Long Beach VA study as evidence that his program worked. Dissatisfied with Pritikin's explanation of the flaws in the study, Robert Levy took Pritikin to task though he recognized that these imperfections did not necessarily rule out the promise of his program altogether. Levy wrote that he would "love to see [Pritikin's] studies proven true," but he cautioned against accepting promising trial results prematurely, saying, "We must keep in mind when somebody's cholesterol goes down it doesn't mean he no longer has a diseased heart. And the fact that someone can do more, or walk more, doesn't mean his atherosclerosis has regressed."[98] For Levy, symptomatic improvement was hardly more than an illusion, masking the real likelihood that the underlying disease may be as severe as ever, but having flawed results merely indicated the need for a more rigorous and earnest trial. Yet when Levy pushed Pritikin to submit his program for review by a federal research agency, Pritikin became defensive, citing bad experiences having his team's abstracts repeatedly rejected from major medical conferences and journals. He felt that federal evaluation mechanisms were systematically biased against his work and that this bureaucratic barrier represented a disingenuous commitment to pharmaceutical profiteering on behalf of Robert Levy.

Levy's interrogation of the ethical foundation (or lack thereof) for Pritikin's VA study is illustrative of the longtime love-hate relationship that Pritikin had with the medical profession. While the health benefits of Pritikin's program were never outright dismissed by the medical community, the appeal of his program was marred by his utter lack of humility. A physician from southern California was quoted in a local paper saying, "I have no doubt [Pritikin's] progress can make people feel better. Any doctor would have to approve of a sensible diet, the elimination of cigarettes, and that sort of thing," but, he continued, "Pritikin acts as if he's reversed coronary artery disease when no conclusive scientific evidence is in yet."[99] Pritikin clearly believed in his own work and made an admirable effort to master the techniques of medicine to persuade physicians to follow him, but to them it was clear he simply lacked the temperament for the slow march of science.

Tasteless Critiques, or the Delectability Crisis

Curiously, one of the most pernicious critiques by medical professionals of Pritikin's diet program was not rooted in its scientific merits at all but centered instead on questions of taste. Despite the medical community's insistence that nutritional recommendations be made with the highest standards of evidence, Pritikin's program (and most other diets for that matter) was judged harshly against a decidedly nonscientific benchmark: the imagined likelihood of people being able to stomach the diet beyond the plush walls of the Longevity Center. The notorious nutrition scientist Fred Stare—that staunchest of diet gurus' opponents—opined that "Mr. Pritikin has exaggerated the American Heart Association's recommendations and our National Dietary Goals to a point where the average person in real life (not domiciled in a Pritikin clinic) would find this diet too impractical and rigid."[100] Stare's colleague and frequent coauthor, Elizabeth Whelan, founder of the conservative research and advocacy organization the American Council on Science and Health—a pro-industry group founded to combat what it called the "junk science" being deployed by the environmental and consumer advocacy movements—bemoaned Pritikin's diet as "restrictive, austere, and dreary."[101] Driven by this same skepticism, in an exchange of letters submitted to the Senate Select Committee on Nutrition and Human Needs, Robert Levy challenged Pritikin to produce even a single patient who had used his program for a year after leaving the Longevity Center because he did not believe anyone could sustain such a cumbersome diet for that long.[102]

The sentiment that Pritikin's diet was unpalatable was echoed colorfully by his rival gurus and in the popular press as well. One observer wrote that Pritikin's was "a diet so severe that calling it bland would be complimentary."[103] Al Martinez, a columnist for the *Los Angeles Times* and former Pritikinite, having recently attended a Pritikin-themed white-tie dinner at Chasen's, a swanky West Hollywood restaurant, lampooned the diet at length. He whined, "There is scant allowance for fun . . . no T-bone orgies or bacchanalian delights of rare prime rib" at a Pritikin dinner composed "primarily of rice crackers and of soy beans cooked in rainwater." He skewered the meal served at the dinner itself, sarcastically speculating that "the chicken [was] actually bred skinless and boneless through a secret Pritikin formula that alter[ed] its DNA and render[ed] it tasteless." The writer then quoted his wife as having said, "They will no more offer you a martini at Pritikin than they will serve you a cup of hog fat." Of the raw melon slices served for dessert, Martinez joked that "it was probably necessary to handcuff the Pritikin dietitian to prevent him from boiling it."[104]

In some respects, these "tasteless" critiques of Pritikin—who was once quoted as having said curmudgeonly that "Mom's apple pie" was "an ingenious way of destroying the food quality of apples"—were well-earned.[105] Yet the broader concerns about his diet's restrictiveness were not—from medical professionals at least—purely out of concern for the subjects' taste buds or their quality of life per se, but rather centered on the imaginary likelihood of recidivism. A cardiologist was quoted in the *Chicago Tribune* as having said, "Whether [Pritikin's] kind of diet and lifestyle can be conducted readily or in significant amount by people outside (of the center) is a serious question. Recidivism runs rampant."[106] Many doctors who took no issue with the essential nutritional structure of the diet still argued that, without the possibility of mass compliance, the diet was useless. Ironically, the preferred diet of the medical profession, the AHA diet, was itself burdensome to follow. Though dieters were allowed to eat a wider array of foods, the AHA program nevertheless required dieters to keep detailed logs of their daily food intake and learn how to accurately track and compute dietary value through the language of nutritional percentages (e.g., percent of daily calories from saturated fat)—a difficult and tedious chore.

To his critics, Pritikin usually responded that it was Western taste, conditioned by unhealthy, heavily processed industrial foods, impeding the widespread adoption of his diet. Pritikin elaborated in one interview, saying "The idea that it is difficult for people to eat like this just isn't true. This is the way a majority of people on this Earth are eating right now, but tailored to be pleasing to Western tastes."[107] Besides, he argued, his dietary program already included several major concessions to flavor. For instance, despite stating that "dairy products are not natural to man" and that the animal protein in milk is "the principal cause of osteoporosis," Pritikin included nonfat milk and other modified dairy staples in the program because "we don't want to alienate the whole world."[108] Likewise, he advocated eating grass- or range-fed cattle in the early 1980s, but he really only included beef in his program at all so that people would not feel that the diet was too distant from what they had been used to eating, even though he assumed that people would lose their taste for animal products over time. He insisted, and his followers provide some limited anecdotal support, that it took patients two weeks just to get used to his diet, they would tolerate it for another month, and after that their compliance allegedly became easy because they had "trained their palate."[109]

In spite of his faith in the adaptiveness of the human palate, Pritikin highlighted yet other benefits of his program to compensate for its relative flavorlessness. In one interview, when challenged about recidivism, Pritikin replied, "Compliance—that's a sick question. When people try the diet, they like it. It costs about a third less. Besides, if a person knows his diet is destroying him, he'll change his ways. Most people don't know what it is to feel optimal—suddenly they have a glorious feeling—less fatigue, more energy, better concentration."[110] In other places, he doubled down on claims that flavor was less meaningful to those in dire straits with their health. Of diabetics for instance, he proclaimed, "If they could get rid of insulin . . . they'd eat cardboard and water."[111] While such claims demonstrate Pritikin's attention to and sympathy for excessive or burdensome medical care, they simultaneously reflect a cold, even crass misunderstanding of the experience of being chronically ill and the importance many patients place on retaining connections to familiar foods, especially those central to cultural practices and social networks, as a matter of preserving their quality of life.

Branching Out

Because taste (or lack thereof) was the chief complaint from Pritikin's medical detractors, and because his patients had, despite his insistence to the contrary, also complained about their limited options in the complex everyday food environment, adherence became the major thorn in Pritikin's side. The skepticism he encountered toward the flavor and adherence components of his dietary program—which, from Pritikin's perspective, smacked of allegiance with the aggressively manipulative, nutrient-pulverizing food industry—pushed Pritikin to circumvent medical channels altogether. In a major concession to his followers' gourmet sensibilities, in 1984 he and his wife, Ilene, published *The Official Pritikin Guide to Restaurant Eating* to give Pritikinites some leverage when dining out.[112] Like other books in this genre, the Pritikins' restaurant guide decoded common menu pitfalls, gave suggestions for "safe" items to order, and armed their devotees with stock questions and responses to use in their everyday encounters with industrialized food peddlers and service workers.

But as Pritikin himself knew well—even if he would not directly admit it—restaurant dining was not altogether compatible with his lifestyle. On one embarrassing occasion, Pritikin accompanied a Dallas reporter to a local Mexican restaurant, bragging that he could find something suitable to eat at any restaurant in the world—implying that his diet was flexible enough to accommodate any taste anywhere. Yet after repeatedly tussling with the server over the ingredients the restaurant had on offer (including forbidden cheeses, fatty meats, and salt) and their preparation methods (nearly everything was fried in oil, prompting an exasperated Pritikin to decry the restaurant as a "Spanish McDonalds"), he treated himself and his guest to twelve unseasoned, steamed tortillas topped with nothing but raw diced tomatoes and shredded lettuce.[113] To the reporter's amusement, he even ordered seconds. Pritikin's press coverage includes tales of his having encountered similar hurdles with other regional cuisines as well.[114]

Frustrated by the incompatibility between his vision of a nutritional utopia and the health-destroying business model of food service in America, Pritikin decided to inject his ideology into any food context that could make it easier for people to adopt his program. For instance, Pritikin was appointed to the first Governor's Council on Wellness and Physical Fitness in 1980 under California Governor Jerry Brown and started a dairy-free children's lunch program.[115] In 1979 he persuaded Edwin Edwards, the governor of Louisiana, to put the entire city of Natchitoches on his diet. When the experiment ran in 1981, he failed to recruit the entire city, but over a third of the residents tried the program.[116] In an attempt to make vacation more accessible for his followers, he hosted wellness cruises and crafted their menus himself. Pritikin was also once appointed "Honorary Nutrition Consultant" on a ship where he conducted an experiment on nine crew members to "emphasize the benefits of Pritikin Nutrition in techniques of survival."[117] He had even sponsored designs for a proposed Pritikin Pantry fast casual restaurant, getting as far as having a menu, T-shirts, and branded promotional material, but the project never took off.[118]

When plans for his own restaurant crumbled, Pritikin worked with lawyers from his foundation to develop a licensing program so chain restaurants could have Pritikin-approved selections on their own menus. This was meant to work in favor of both the restaurant and the dieter. Restaurants could advertise their Pritikin-appropriate fare to signal their willingness to accommodate dietary restrictions and attract customers, while dieters would have a smoother experience finding acceptable restaurants and/or menu items. Pritikin personally wrote to a number of major food outlets proposing his licensing program. First, he gave them the outline of his diet and asked them to send a reply with a comprehensive list of their products that fit his specifications. Once they had been generally approved, Pritikin's legal team then provided the restaurants with carefully crafted verbiage they could use to indicate their products' compatibility with the Pritikin program without having Pritikin specifically endorse any of them in case they had been misidentified or improperly prepared (to avoid liability).

One of Pritikin's more ambitious proposals was to contract with airlines to offer in-flight meals based on his own recipes for all their domestic flights. He managed to secure a deal with United Airlines to start providing Pritikin meals in May 1980.[119] His diet was attractive as a basis for an in-flight meal plan because of its severe restrictions on multiple dietary fronts, so customers wanting low-fat or low-cholesterol options and others wanting low-sodium could all be satisfied by a single dietary meal. When flying United himself, Pritikin ordered from their Pritikin menu but often without success.[120] He was deeply worried by these failures because he had already advertised his United deal to over 10,000 of his supporters.[121] If Pritikin himself had difficulty securing these meals, undoubtedly many of his acolytes would be similarly stranded in the air without acceptable fare. After several misfires, the vice president of operations at United, Richard Arnold, personally oversaw that Pritikin was provided with an adequate meal—a noodle dish dubbed "Turkey a la King"—on one flight, but on later trips the problems continued. Letters between Pritikin and senior officials at the airline revealed that the difficulty stemmed from the fact that certain regional kitchens that United Airlines hired to stock their planes initially abstained from preparing Pritikin-type meals.[122] In response, the airline took Pritikin's diet plan a step farther, including his dietary meals in their special "Preventive Medical Diet Program for Crews."[123] Because many crew members were on diets and because they ate airline meals more regularly than any given passenger, this ensured that any kitchen stocking United would have to adjust their procedures. Pritikin tried the same maneuver with American Airlines, Delta, PanAm, and others to no avail.

Pritikin expanded his ambitions to the grocery store aisles by tinkering with his own line of breads, baked foods, and frozen or preprepared foods developed through several different companies to be sold at grocery stores around the country. He was heavily involved in the research and development of novel, Pritikin-branded foodstuffs. Pritikin would develop his own recipes and send them to bakers, restaurateurs, food scientists, and others who could make them in relatively large batches. However, legal difficulties frequently arose because his prospective partner companies wanted full profit from his products while still capitalizing on the Pritikin name. In 1981, for instance, Pritikin sued a grocery store over the use of his name in their products and promotional materials despite having given them consent to sell his products in their discount health food section. For this and other reasons, Pritikin Foods and much of the other preprepared Pritikin food business was sold in 1995 to Quaker Oats, after which its sales flagged, amounting to a disappointing $10 million per year.[124]

The Dieters' Perspective

The actions Pritikin took to expand the reach of his program betray his fundamental misconception about how, why, and with whom his program found success. His incessant demands for the absolute, nationwide recognition of his program as a scientifically proven solution to chronic disease—evidenced by his interactions with Levy during the McGovern Report hearings—blinded Pritikin to his program's steep cultural limitations. When he finally acknowledged and attempted to remedy this gap, he focused his efforts on making his food available in more places—though not at the expense of his brand name—rather than making his recommendations more flexible or accessible, especially for the different kinds of dieters he hoped to attract. Ultimately, his singular focus on the scientific merits of his program prevented him from recognizing the specific conditions under which his program thrived; as a result, he dramatically underestimated the role that his patients played in the success he witnessed at the Longevity Center.

Likewise, the attitudes espoused by nutrition scientists—especially those who were critical of the Pritikin program's therapeutic potential—revealed an essential contradiction in how medical experts understood dieters' behavior. Clouded by assumptions that most commercial diets were too difficult, too restrictive, or too joyless to maintain for the average American, nutrition scientists failed to recognize that the governmental nutritional recommendations, while visibly milder than some of their commercial opponents, were no less difficult to manage—especially when coupled with a lifelong disease management routine. Pritikin was criticized heavily for his program not being realistic, but many of his patients at the Longevity

Center were already observing extensive health care regimens that required complex and cumbersome lifestyle modifications.

The irony of the accusations that Pritikin's diet was neither appealing nor manageable for a broad base of ailing Americans is perhaps best demonstrated by a unique collection of testimonials from Pritikin's patients themselves, whose perspectives offer valuable context and texture through which to understand Pritikin's own perspectives on his program and success. Like other popular health promoters, Pritikin's program accrued hundreds of patient testimonials during its peak, but the most interesting of these is a collection of semiprivate letters written to Pritikin directly. For her husband's sixty-fifth birthday and on the occasion of the 100th session at the Longevity Center in 1981, Ilene Pritikin solicited congratulations and well-wishes from every living Pritikin alumnus in which they were instructed to recount their health narratives—from woes to triumphs—in the form of personal letters to the guru himself. Unlike typical testimonials for fad diets (which can be requested selectively, heavily edited, or outright invented), these letters of testimony were not written expressly for public consumption; Ilene Pritikin's stated intention was to bind them together in a book for her husband so he could appreciate the magnitude of his own accomplishments.

In their letters, Pritikinites report having been weary of taking drugs, disappointed in the limitations—especially the physical immobility—of their ailing and aging bodies, and pessimistic about their futures.[125] Many of them wrote that they had found following their doctors' orders for the long-term management of their chronic health conditions difficult, and their quality of life had rapidly waned. They had been shuttled between countless doctor's offices, suffered hospitalizations and surgeries, obsessively monitored their "numbers" (shorthand for all the different physiological measurements, from blood sugar to cholesterol, that these patients needed to track for themselves), and navigated complex regimens of medication and medical devices daily with no end in sight. But their physicians, just like those who were critical of Pritikin's regime, failed to recognize that their own recommendations had been too complicated or interfered meaningfully with their patients' quality of life.

In their letters, Pritikinites reported wild success and unbridled enthusiasm for the new lives they credited Pritikin—whom many familiarly called "Nathan"—for helping them to achieve, and they thanked him with near-religious fervor. To believe their stories is to believe that Pritikin did not merely change their health but their entire way of interacting with the world. These writers reported feeling liberated from their bodies and from medications, and feeling more adventurous than ever, taking trips across the globe and showing off to their friends and families.

Yet from their accounts, it becomes clear that Pritikin's program succeeded not because people believed he had cracked the science of nutrition but because he placed listening to his patients at the heart of his program. The solutions he created, while challenging to implement, took to heart the global concerns that people had with their bodies; rather than giving his patients coping mechanisms and measured pessimism or small technical fixes to alleviate their daily pain, he helped them to change their entire lifestyles and attitudes, all the while providing them opportunities to motivate and educate themselves, socialize with like-minded people, and find new meaning in their lives. With this understanding, it becomes clear that the Longevity Center functioned less like a health spa and more like a mini-college. His student-patients felt respected (and felt they had earned respect) from the time their applications to the program were accepted through to the graduation ceremony at the end of each session where student-patients donned homemade mortar boards with parsley tassels.[126] Pritikin made finding health fun and invigorating for his attendees, a sharp contrast with the depressing, pessimistic, and shame-inducing medical science to which they had been subjected before.

His followers' stories reveal how Pritikin set himself apart from orthodox medicine. The community he built extended beyond the particular Longevity Center session his patients attended. Many recounted stories of Pritikin's willingness and ability to support patients whenever they called him for years afterward; he consistently answered his phone calls directly, and he made a point of remembering everyone's names from every session, along with their detailed medical histories.[127] Unlike Michio Kushi, Pritikin also responded to all the mail from his prospective and former students himself. Though Pritikin may have understood himself to be keeping track of valuable medical data that spoke to the efficacy of his program, it was the personalized touch and socialization—in short, the feeling that Pritikin knew them and cared for them—that was most persuasive to Longevity Center guests.[128] And this was a sentiment that transcended generations of Pritikin alumni through a chain of personal recommendations, new friendships, and shared experiences. Remarkably, even those patients for whom Pritikin's treatment did not fulfill their expectations reported overall satisfaction with Pritikin's program and cited themselves and their bodies as outliers.[129]

The main discrepancy between Pritikin's idea of the power of his own diet and the dismissal of his claims by physicians comes from the fact that Pritikin believed that his dietary protocols were not overly restrictive because he saw his patients maintain them and thrive. But he failed to realize that his patients were a self-selecting group of people who had already experienced (and become jaded) with medical discipline and who actively sought a more optimistic sort of care (in contrast with the general population). By seeking the implementation of his ideas into national dietary recommendations, or even into medical protocols for all people suffering from or at risk of developing chronic conditions, Pritikin underestimated the centrality of his personality and the generous community he had built for the success of his program.

Conclusion

In 1985, Pritikin checked into a hospital in Albany, New York. He had had a sudden, severe relapse with his leukemia, and his treatment options were dwindling. The doctors treating him were unaware of his identity while he was a patient because Pritikin had checked in pseudonymously as Howard Malmuth, a fictional persona he had created and whose medical records he had been fabricating for the previous twenty years.[130] This fact alone suggests the staggering pressures he felt about his public image; and "Malmuth" decided to forgo treatment. According to media accounts after the fact, Pritikin had asked a nurse to borrow an X-Acto knife so he could "cut open charts and graphs for a scrapbook he used in keeping track of his experimental method of treating leukemia," but she gave him a disposable scalpel instead. Soon after she left the room, he used the scalpel to carve deep gashes into his wrists.[131] It is a sad irony that Pritikin—known for resisting, thwarting, and earning begrudging acceptance from skeptical physicians—died in a medical institution avoiding hopeless treatment for a condition he believed had been caused by medical recklessness. Upon receiving the news of Pritikin's death, the Longevity Centers were inundated with sympathetic phone calls as well as new requests to enroll in the weeks following Pritikin's death—over 2,000 calls in two weeks by one estimate.[132]

Because of the suspicious circumstances surrounding his death and the fact that his identity had not yet been recovered, the coroner decided to perform an autopsy without his family's consent. Pritikin's family discovered later that Pritikin had, in a moment of posthumous showmanship, included a note in his will requesting an autopsy anyway; further, he wanted the results to be published in the *New England Journal of Medicine* as proof that his diet worked. In July 1985, the three authors who had conducted the examination and published the paper boasted of Pritikin's extraordinary cardiac youth. They wrote that the sixty-nine-year-old Pritikin's arteries showed no evidence of raised plaques, and his total serum cholesterol was last measured at 94 (down from 280). They were amazed that such a person could have suffered previously from heart disease, as Pritikin had in his thirties, and they called his complete lack of atherosclerosis "remarkable."[133] Pritikin was vindicated: not only had he survived as a result of his diet, but he had actually undone decades of cardiac damage. And it was his autopsy, ironically, that demonstrated the health value of his program.

In spite of the incredible claims from his autopsy, however, many diet hopefuls were left unimpressed, since Pritikin—immaculate circulatory system or not—was dead nevertheless. His dietary crusade for total health and longevity was insufficient to ward off his cancer, and what good is a diet that saves your heart if you die of cancer anyway? On top of the skeptics who found Pritikin's childlike heart to be inadequate evidence for the cardiac benefits of his diet, his worst critics attributed his plaque-free arteries to the cholesterol-fueled nature of his blood cancer rather than his painfully low fat consumption. In this most ironic of theories, not only was Pritikin said to have died of cancer, but his cancer was cast as the miraculous agent that cleaned his heart and proved (falsely) the alleged health benefits of his diet. Contending with these criticisms, Pritikin's successors and his supporters argued that Pritikin's diet helped postpone his inevitable death from leukemia for thirty years. Without the dietary innovations Pritikin pioneered, they reasoned, he would have succumbed to cancer much sooner.

Regardless of the specific meaning of Pritikin's autopsy results, the outpouring of support from prominent figures after Pritikin's death signaled his remarkable influence. Years after Pritikin's testimony for the McGovern Report hearings, George McGovern and his wife Eleanor reportedly enrolled at Pritikin's center in 1983 to get the senator into shape for the 1984 presidential election.[134] When Pritikin died shortly thereafter, McGovern delivered his eulogy, comparing him with other such esteemed inventors and visionaries as Louis Pasteur, Marie Curie, and Thomas Edison. Of Pritikin, he said, "You show me a man who usually lives by the power of his convictions and I'll show you a man with a reputation of a fanatic."[135]

McGovern's original faith in Pritikin—and his decision to ask Pritikin to testify—was motivated by concerns that have proven especially prescient. In a closing statement during one of the 1977 hearings, McGovern praised Pritikin's unconventional approach as necessary for the health of the nation:

> It is time that nutrition research receive[s] an emphasis commensurate with its potential. We have been too timid in promoting nutrition research, both in the scale of resources invested and in the breadth of research priorities.
>
> It is important to continue the current emphases. . . . But we also need to break out of the old research ruts we have been deepening over the last 10–15 years.
>
> We must be more imaginative and more balanced in our approach. . . . I realize that the Pritikin hypertension data is preliminary and is subject to a number of legitimate scientific criticisms. I only use it to make a point. This committee understands there is a way to properly do scientific research in order to obtain valid results, but we don't want to see that used as a guise to denigrate research initiatives, which for whatever reason are not being pursued by the mainstream of scientific thought—be it hypertension, diabetes, heart disease or cancer. We must not limit the great potential of nutrition research. If we had spent as much time and resources on human nutrition research as on livestock nutrition, we would be much closer to solving today's major health problems. . . .
>
> We are training our physicians and biomedical research scientists in a way which insufficiently emphasizes nutrition.

McGovern's plea for scientific humility in the face of a national health crisis with few clear answers resonates strongly with testimonies from Pritikin's other patients. When medical science fails to forge a clear path—for the health of individual patients or an entire nation—insistence on methodological purity or theoretical rigor may unnecessarily constrain practical and humane policy innovation.

McGovern's sentiment was also echoed by prominent physicians. In 1984, a physician from Northwestern University, Jeremiah Stamler (who also testified during the 1977 hearings), had described the Pritikin program to the *Chicago Tribune* as "the most advanced wing of nutritional recommendations for promoting health in the United States."[136] In another of Pritikin's eulogies, Dr. William Castelli, the influential Harvard physician and director of the Framingham Heart Study, emphasized the importance of medical pragmatism, saying, "To his critics, let me say that when you get your patients' cholesterol down to 175, then you can begin to complain about Nathan Pritikin."[137] For his part, Pritikin merely wanted the nation's chronically ill to feel optimistic in the face of long odds and to be aware of all the fruits of medical thought, regardless of whether they were profitable or whether the public would find those recommendations reasonable or manageable. The Pritikin program was meant to give patients the option to decide what course of action to take for themselves without needing to filter their options through either the blurry lens of political interference or the overly conservative requirements that scientific gatekeeping applied to national nutritional recommendations. Patients could decide for themselves the lengths to which they would be willing to go to preserve their own health.

Epilogue: A Plant-Based Legacy

He died prematurely in an ambiguous state of bodily health, but Pritikin's nutritional philosophy has maintained relevance and developed a lasting legacy by inspiring a new generation of diet gurus. Interestingly, many of these newcomers were firmly positioned within the medical community and were equipped with credentials and credibility that Pritikin had only pretended to have. After Pritikin's death, his close friend and fellow diet guru, Dr. John McDougall, wrote to Pritikin's wife, "For me the loss of your husband was more than anyone, I'm sure, realizes. He was the most important person in my medical career. Mr. Pritikin was my teacher, as well as my leader and defender. He was always on the forefront of change; battling for the health care values that care for people in a humane manner. Now I feel exposed to his opponents. I hope I can do a fraction of the good he accomplished."[138] Like McDougall, other physicians inspired by Pritikin's work emphasized not the low-fat, high-carbohydrate diet or the studies showing its efficacy per se, but the ways that Pritikin advocated for his patients and for comparatively humane behavioral changes to be taken seriously as medical therapy.

Perhaps most notable among these testimonials is that of Dr. Michael Greger, a popular and influential diet guru and author of the *New York Times* bestselling books *How Not to Die* and *How Not to Diet*.[139] Greger credits Pritikin with inspiring his entire medical career. In a striking parallel to Eula Weaver, Greger's grandmother, Frances, to whom Greger refers grimly as "one of the death's door people," displayed many of the classic symptoms common to Pritikin's clientele by age sixty-five. She was confined to a wheelchair from the pain of angina and claudication associated with end-stage heart disease. Greger recalls that "she already had too many bypass surgeries, was so scarred up inside, there was nothing more the surgeons could do." After three weeks at the Pritikin Longevity Center, however, Greger says his grandmother had abandoned her wheelchair and could walk ten miles a day. "Thanks to a healthy diet," suggested Greger, "[she] was able to enjoy another 31 years on this earth, until age 96." Greger concludes the introductory video to his popular website, NutritionFacts.org, saying, "I hope I can do for your family what Pritikin did for my family."[140]

Pritikin's program, his personal evangelism, and his spectacular results inflamed the passions and excited the imaginations of a new generation of physicians who turned their careers toward the promotion of healthy living. These physicians-turned-gurus ultimately championed a shift in the national dietary landscape, fighting for the recognition of dietary choices as a viable path of treatment for patients suffering from chronic disease. Pritikin's specific influence on these guru-physicians, however, is challenging to trace because many of the dietary choices promoted by his acolytes do not clearly map onto the Pritikin program. Nearly all the physicians who credit Pritikin as an inspiration, including Greger and McDougall, became staunch advocates of a vegetarian—even vegan—diet. To understand why these shifts occurred, it is important to first understand the general trajectory of the low-fat diet in the years following Pritikin's death.

Although Pritikin's interventions were specifically targeted at preventing and recovering from chronic disease, his legacy is often reduced to or conflated with that of the low-fat diet more generally. Though it had been the major recommendation of the AHA for decades, and had had the support of the federal government since the 1977 McGovern Report, low-fat diets saw a resurgence in the late 1980s and early 1990s. Historian Ann La Berge attributes some of this renewed energy to Dr. Dean Ornish, a diet guru with an MD (specializing in internal medicine) who, like Pritikin, developed a low-fat, high-carbohydrate diet aimed at the prevention and treatment of patients with chronic heart disease, and who, also like Pritikin, conducted medical studies to advocate for the efficacy of his diet program.

Unfortunately, nationwide recognition of the efficacy of a low-fat program proved hazardous, especially when its recommendations were over-simplified in the press and by the food industry. La Berge notes that the food industry used Ornish's studies as justification for a continued onslaught that capitalized on the fad diet craze by introducing ever more heavily processed low-fat or nonfat versions of their products in the early 1990s. But instead of introducing more complex carbohydrates in accordance with the actual Pritikin or Ornish diet plans, many food manufacturers simply replaced calories from fat with simple carbohydrates like sugar—a trend that misled countless Americans and significantly damaged their health.[141]

Though the nutritional composition of Ornish's diet was nearly identical to Pritikin's and operated under the same dietary logic (10 percent fat, 10 percent protein, 80 percent complex carbohydrates), Pritikin is absent from La Berge's account of the low-fat diet. This is likely because Pritikin's medical studies had been plagued with institutional irregularities, whereas Ornish gave a close approximation of Pritikin's diet several favorable (and more credible) tests in the late 1980s and early 1990s.[142] Most notable among these was the 1990 Lifestyle Heart Trial, which suggested, through quantitative coronary angiography, that an extremely low-fat diet could potentially reverse atherosclerosis.[143] Despite Ornish's insistence that his ideas were his own, his study vindicated Pritikin as well. The fate of both programs has since continued enmeshed, as evidenced by the 2010 decision to allow Medicare to cover simultaneously both Pritikin's and Ornish's intensive diet therapies for hospitals.[144]

To understand Pritikin's or Ornish's dietary program as important only for helping spur the low-fat craze is to significantly flatten dietary history. Ornish was also notable for emphasizing such lifestyle changes as stress management and emotional support systems in his approach to medicine. While Pritikin's program made similar—albeit more informal—interventions in patient lives through community building at the Longevity Center and through Pritikin's interactions with his patients, Ornish's program was more explicit about the medical potential of lifestyle changes writ broadly—he even pioneered the idea of making "Lifestyle Medicine" a distinct medical specialty. It should be noted, too, that Michael Greger was a founding member of the American College of Lifestyle Medicine in Loma Linda, California, an organization that is vying to be but has not yet been recognized by the American Board of Medical Specialties.[145] Despite the fact that Pritikin never used the term "lifestyle medicine," Greger has hailed Pritikin as "one of our early lifestyle medicine pioneers."[146]

Although Ornish far surpassed Pritikin in his efforts to secure support for his program from the medical community, Ornish's diet was still plagued by concerns about adherence. However, while the cuisine that Pritikin promoted lacked flavor, flexibility, and internal coherence, Ornish—by highlighting the health benefits not only of a low-fat diet but a *vegetarian* one—helped inspire others to tap into the long, rich food culture American vegetarians had been developing for over a century. By signaling that vegetarian diets—regardless of the specific nutritional composition he advocated—could reverse chronic heart disease and potentially other conditions, Ornish created new enthusiasm for skipping meat, although he was unable to fully capitalize on this cultural wave he helped create. Nevertheless, this transition was critical for the success of a Pritikin-style program in the United States, helping to set the stage for a kind of cultural cohesion that Pritikin's program was never able to realize on its own despite the fact that Pritikin's program was not, itself, vegetarian.

Pritikin-esque vegetarianism was different from its American predecessors in its singular pursuit of health and longevity—or at least the manner in which this pursuit was to be conducted and reified. Though previous waves of vegetarians had eschewed animal products to derive health benefits, they were inextricably tied to and motivated by other social ends first—such as human rights, environmentalism, animal rights, and world peace. Prior to the 1990s, vegetarians had occupied an uncomfortable interstitial space as cultural outsiders in the United States. Their ranks were filled variously with moral crusaders, political exiles, immigrants, and heterodox healers whose justifications for being vegetarian stemmed mainly from exotic religious or social philosophies. Importantly, though the physicians who practice lifestyle medicine all promote a mostly vegetarian or vegan lifestyle, they have long grappled with the pre-existing social connotations around the terms "vegetarian" and "vegan." Especially after the founding of People for the Ethical Treatment of Animals (PETA) in 1980 and the negative publicity the group garnered from its radical publicity stunts, veganism accrued an extremist, politicized image. There was also concern among nutrition-class vegetarians that certain other self-avowed vegans and vegetarians who were energized by the animal rights cause were eating foods irrespective of their health value, so long as they contained no animal products. This meant certain vegans were eating heavily processed foods—like Oreos—that were "accidentally" vegan (designed without vegans in mind, but containing no animal products), garnering their reputations as "junk food vegans."

To set themselves apart, and to emphasize the healthful message of their program over other forms of political vegetarianism, practitioners of lifestyle medicine—following the lead of Drs. Caldwell Esselstyn and T. Colin Campbell—tactfully renamed their spin on meatlessness the Whole Foods, Plant-Based (WFPB) diet. This new wave of vegans—though they undoubtedly shared some of the political attitudes of other meat-eschewing groups—were primarily invested in restoring and reinforcing their bodies as Pritikin's patients had been. Just as Pritikin had co-opted medical studies to his own ends, the health-centered vegetarians' justification for their lifestyle was to come from within the bastion of medicine itself. Medical research, long the foe of food faddists, was to become their salvation at last.

Entremets III

The Gastro-Medical Industrial Complex

• •

In 2016, Harvard's Fred Stare and Mark Hegsted were accused in *JAMA* of having accepted the modern equivalent of $50,000 from sugar industry representatives in the 1960s to purposefully steer dietary recommendations for heart disease toward saturated fat to obfuscate the harmful effects of consuming sucrose.[1] The article in question relied on archival findings that showed the Sugar Research Foundation (SRF) had recruited Stare and Hegsted to publish a literature review on dietary fats as culprits in the coronary heart disease debate. The SRF, an organization that was self-admittedly created with the goal of increasing the nation's levels of sugar consumption, was given early access to Hegsted's drafts and communicated with Hegsted throughout the research and writing process. After this industry tie was unceremoniously revealed in *JAMA*, serious concerns about the role of Big Sugar and other industrial interests in nutritional research and government policymaking flooded the international media landscape.

The now-familiar pattern of industry cash corrupting academic research showed Big Food going the way of other "merchants of doubt" like Big Tobacco and Big Oil. In some ways, the story was not surprising when it broke because public health advocates like Marion Nestle had been voicing similar accusations. For decades, it was an open secret that academic nutrition scientists maintained deep industry ties to fund their programs, their students, their laboratories, and their research. When the "Sugar Papers" scandal burst open in 2016, Stare's unethical relationship with industry stakeholders was so heavily publicized because the archival "smoking guns" the *JAMA* article described seemed to irrefutably confirm—as had the Cigarette Papers—the global public's long-held suspicions that their experts and governments had been lying to them. Only this time it was about the (un)healthfulness of low-fat diets. The corruption behind the US Department of Agriculture's industry-friendly nutrition recommendations had been obvious to the system's critics all along, but now there seemed to be hard evidence that the science itself was fundamentally skewed.

The hard evidence against Stare and Hegsted did not stand up well to scrutiny, however. Historians David Merrit Johns and Gerald Oppenheimer defended Stare and Hegsted's reputations in *Science* in 2018 by not only claiming that "twists and turns in science and policy are not necessarily products of malevolence" but that the standards for ethical research and the culture of funding disclosure were different in the 1960s. Johns and Oppenheimer demonstrate that corporate money could not have influenced the quality or direction of the research the nutrition scientists performed; instead, they insist Stare and Hegsted's pre-existing research into saturated fat and heart disease happened to align with industry interests, hence those industries chose to support them financially.[2] The authors note too that, although Hegsted had a history of accepting corporate monies, his research did not always benefit the body that funded it. In an earlier dispute regarding the role of saturated fat in heart disease, for instance, Hegsted's published study outwardly betrayed his financiers from the meat industry. Moreover, Johns and Oppenheimer show that the same kind of industry funding Stare was accused of receiving had been funneled—in greater amounts—to Stare's scientific opponents, such as British sugar *detractor* John Yudkin. Obviously, because its effects can cut both ways, the mere presence of corporate funding should not negate the value of research.

Yet even if we accept that Stare did not accept money *quid pro quo* to maliciously harm Americans and unfairly shield corporate sugar from a reputation of being injurious to public health, a quick look at Stare's history of dietary claims obviates the need for any archival smoking gun of explicit corruption.[3] Stare's commitment to industry interests was apparent in his vehement defense of DDT (dichloro-diphenyl-trichloroethane), in his exaggerated calls for increased public trust in processed food (which he cheerfully called "scientific snacks"), and in the tagline of his book *Panic in the Pantry*, which literally read "Eat your additives; they're good for you."[4] From his powerful perch in one of the best and most industry-funded nutrition departments in the world, Stare shamelessly trumpeted his corporate allies' private interests. "With his iron-gray hair parted just off center, his eyes twinkling behind pale shell glasses," one mocking article wrote, Stare "invites trust, like the family physician on a Norman Rockwell magazine cover."[5] But Stare used that trust to, among other things, defend the safety of known carcinogens like the food dye Red No. 2 and extol soda as a good source of phosphorus.[6] Throughout his career, he brazenly defended sugar and white bread as part of a healthy diet (even one geared toward weight loss), like so many ads for sugary cereals stealthily claiming to be "part of this balanced breakfast."[7]

Stare was not the only corporate crusader in his clique. Liz Whelan, Stare's closest student, with whom he proudly cofounded the virulently pro-corporate American Council on Science and Health (ACSH), "urged the industry to promote its products not so much for being safe as for being enjoyable, adding that junk food might better be called fun food."[8] Another outspoken anti-quackery nutrition scientist, Vanderbilt University's William Jefferson Darby, advocated for the United States to fortify sugary soda with vitamins because it was so commonly consumed.[9] Darby was on the American Medical Association (AMA) Council on Food and Nutrition, helped create the Food Protection Committee of the National Research Council, served as president of the industry-funded Nutrition Foundation, and, like Stare, persuaded corporate donors to create a new nutrition science program at Vanderbilt. On behalf of his moneyed donors, Darby bemoaned regulations that sought to limit or prohibit preservatives, additives, or dyes because safety tests threatened to slow the pace of corporate innovation. In 1963, Stare's close ally and Harvard colleague Jean Mayer succinctly summarized the attitude of his ilk: "Have confidence in America's food industry. It deserves it."[10]

In the latter half of the twentieth century, nutrition scientists regularly served on the boards of prominent agribusiness corporations and food manufacturers, where they helped protect these institutional entities from federal regulation, public scrutiny, and reform while shouting down their mutual enemies.[11] Anyone who opposed "the Stare school of pro-additive polemicists," was "lump[ed] together for purposes of ridicule," regardless of their reasoning or identity, and was summarily dismissed, "from the frauds and crackpots to the most serious scientists and consumerists."[12] Stare was as forthright about the dangers of Rachel Carson and environmentalism as he was about macrobiotics, as upset by the needlessness of Ralph Nader's consumer protection efforts as he was about the flavorlessness of the Pritikin program, and he will, in the next chapter, spare no sympathy for the Atkins diet either. His attitude demonstrates the artificiality of trying to separate nutrition scientists' anti-quackery activism from their efforts behind the scenes to bolster the food industry's public credibility. Nutrition scientists were worried (with good reason) that if public confidence was shaken in the food system—even by legitimate concerns—a disintegration in public trust toward other kinds of expertise would follow.

For the major leaders of the allied natural health coalition, it was clear that mainstream medicine and nutrition science had been fundamentally corrupted by corporate influence. Former Federal Trade Commission (FTC) Commissioner Lowell Mason, one of the featured speakers at the first National Congress on Medical Monopoly (NCMM), a counter-conference that National Health Federation (NHF) leaders organized to thwart the National Congress on Medical Quackery (covered in entremets II), publicly accused the leaders of the various agencies represented at the NCMQ of "devil quacking"—essentially manufacturing scapegoats to push forward unnecessarily stringent regulations to eliminate competition.[13] NHF board member Dr. Miles Robinson echoed Mason's sentiments, arguing that before alternative practitioners were prosecuted, the medical establishment should own up to its own sins: "Before we put any more vitamin [manufacturers] in jail, let us consider what the proper punishment should be for the perpetrators of thalidomide, Marsilid, MER/29, and many others."[14] The drugs Robinson referenced had all been pulled from the market after high-profile cases of severe side effects, birth defects, and death. Robinson's complaint points to a wider grievance of the alternative food and health network: the medical establishment's apparent double standards regarding punishment for allegedly unsafe treatments. The AMA condemned alternative practitioners and natural food advocates as unambiguously dangerous to public health on the basis of a few well-publicized failures like Beth Simon's death (see chapter 2). Yet, with respect to the larger scale failures of scientific medicine, the AMA made no such blanket pronouncements. Individual drugs were pulled, apologies were issued, but the fundamental edifice of scientific medicine that helped produce such tragedies remained unquestionable.

The peculiar proindustry, double-standard politics of the nutritional establishment are further reflected in nutrition scientists' (contradictory) reactions to two of the NHF's greatest legislative successes: the passage of the 1958 Delaney Clause and the 1994 Dietary Supplement Health and Education Act (DSHEA). For nutrition scientists, both pieces of legislation created opportunities for quackery to thrive, but the arguments scientists leveled against each law were intriguingly inverted.

In 1958, Representative James Delaney (D-New York), whose wife was battling cancer, introduced the Food Additives Amendment to the Federal Food, Drug, and Cosmetic Act of 1938 to help reduce cancer incidence from long-term exposure to toxic chemicals that were being added to the food system before being tested for safety.[15] The "Delaney Clause," as it came to be known, reflected an understanding, common at the time, that any detectable amount of a known carcinogen posed a serious risk of cancer. Though the aim of the amendment was laudable, nutrition scientists like Stare and Darby detested the Delaney Clause from its infancy because their corporate funders complained to them that the precautionary principle it invoked limited the rate of product development. Though the law only explicitly forbade synthetic chemicals added intentionally, nutrition scientists disingenuously argued that because everything (including vitamins) could be potentially carcinogenic with a large enough dose, the Delaney Clause would ban most known substances from the market. Stare and his allies insinuated, for instance, that the law would ban root vegetables for their selenium content and make rice illegal for its exposure to arsenic from the soil.[16] Stare's cohort thought Delaney encouraged Americans to doubt the miracles of the industrial food system, doubt they feared would lead Americans inexorably away from scientific modernity.

The Delaney Clause was never a perfect piece of legislation, and it has aged especially poorly—the law's threshold for carcinogenicity has not been updated since its passage despite the fact that oncological and toxicological testing capabilities have since become more sensitive by multiple magnitudes. That there should be a more sensible scientific standard for consumer safety, however, does not signal a need for the wholesale abandonment of the precautionary principle as Stare once advocated.

Notably, though Delaney was the key mobilizer of this legislation, after its passage, he partially attributed his success to the vice president of the NHF, W. L. Gleason, who testified on Delaney's behalf before the House Interstate and Foreign Commerce Committee. From the NHF's perspective, the Delaney Clause was a huge victory because it created a new barrier to protect consumers from the previously unlimited capacity of food corporations to add harmful synthetic chemicals to the food supply before such products had been tested for safety. Of their joint efforts to combat medical hegemony, Delaney said, "Many rivers flow to the sea, and many roads can lead to health. All of them should be thoroughly explored. Many an uncompromising approach has led to important scientific discovery and serious and well-considered experimentation, even if it seems unorthodox, should not be discouraged."[17] The NHF repaid the compliment by awarding Delaney its highest honor later that year.

In 1994, the conflict around Delaney played out in reverse when the interests of orthodox medicine suffered another defeat. This time, NHF leaders had organized a massive letter-writing campaign to secure the passage of the Dietary Supplement Health and Education Act (DSHEA).[18] Despite being fewer than 20,000 members strong, the NHF managed to solicit over a million letters of support from all over the nation. When it passed, the DSHEA effectively prohibited the US Food and Drug Administration (FDA) from regulating vitamins and supplements as drugs, treating them instead like other natural products such as food. Critics of DSHEA have accused dietary supplements of being untested and unsafe, arguing that since they are prescribed and consumed as medicines, they should be regulated as such.[19] For that reason, nutrition scientists understood DSHEA as unleashing quackery. The NHF's reasoning behind deregulation is easy to understand though; a grocery store does not have to prove any of the thousands of claims about the health benefits of natural products such as spinach or bananas to sell them, so how (despite the fact that they are typically consumed in the form of capsules or powders) are medicinal herbs fundamentally different? Why *should* fish oil be treated so differently than olive oil?

Though the Delaney Clause and DSHEA are in many ways contradictory pieces of legislation, they both put the NHF and nutrition scientists at odds. Yet nutrition scientists' opposition to Delaney was uncannily similar to the NHF's rationale in favor of DSHEA. In their opposition to Delaney, Stare, Darby, and other powerful scientists essentially argued that food corporations should be allowed to infuse synthetic chemicals like preservatives and artificial flavorings (which are arguably as similar to pharmaceuticals as dietary supplements) into their products without thoroughly testing their health effects so long as such products were being consumed like food (for which there was no similar proof of safety requirement). Similarly, the NHF likened dietary supplements to other processed foods with decades of health promises (such as whole wheat bread, molasses, or tonic water), undermining the notion that they needed to be subjected to efficacy trials like drugs rather than just safety or contamination tests like food. On its face though, pouring novel synthetic chemicals into the general food supply without *safety* testing (as scientists advocated) seems a lot riskier than selling processed agricultural products with centuries of recorded use in pill form without *efficacy* testing (as "quacks" advocated).

The widespread perception of nutrition scientists' flagrant, pro-corporate hypocrisy (feigning outrage with hippie brown rice but pledging fealty to corporate white bread) is a large part of what animated the gurus in this book, their allies, and their patients. Against this backdrop, the ideological contradictions of the NHF become, in some ways, more forgivable because their organization was much less sophisticated and far more decentralized than the establishment, and they were working against the headwinds of the determined antagonism of powerful scientists, governments, and corporations. Of course, the natural health movement's anger has to be understood within the broader context of the general social and political upheaval of the 1960s and 1970s and the general disenchantment with expert authority as well.

Still, it is easy to criticize the medical heterodoxy for their more extreme stances—the NHF opposed birth control, mandatory vaccination, the fluoridation of public water, and more—but much of the substance behind their concerns with medical hegemony and the corporate food world was nevertheless legitimate.[20] And many of their concerns about food and medicine (regarding refined grains, artificial dyes, synthetic pesticides, overprescription, unnecessary surgery, and other matters) have since been vindicated. Just because the NHF and the broader US network of heterodox healers, natural health food stores, and diet gurus could not form (against the determined effort of federal agencies, orthodox medicine, and the food industry) a cohesive, coherent, and legal grassroots alternative to capitalist food *and* medicine does not mean their collective political concerns with the system should be so easily dismissed.

If ever there was a poster child for mass market American fad diets, it would be the subject of the next and final case study–the Atkins diet. You would be hard pressed to find a diet that expressed less interest in natural health foods or that fed more into the psychology of weight loss culture. Because Atkins was the flagship diet of the twentieth century and the antithesis of the plant-forward, liberal-minded movements of the three previous chapters, his example will serve as a powerful contrast to the historical connections I have so far built between the natural health food movement and the alternative medical movement. If the conventional history of dieting is to be believed, Atkins would be the last person we would expect to be involved in dieting as medicine. And yet, in just this way, Atkins is the exception that proves the rule.

4 Let Them Eat Meat

Dr. Atkins's Complementary Medical Revolution and the American Blood Sugar Epidemic

• •

Vivian Coy was sixty-six years old when her terminal breast cancer was diagnosed in 1982. For seven exhausting years, she ran the gauntlet of toxic chemotherapy and was at last deemed cancer-free. Four years later, tests revealed the cancer to have made a resurgence.[1] She was not eager to resume conventional cancer treatment so, while remaining under the care of her oncologist, Coy scoured the medical marketplace for other, more experimental modes of care. On September 14, 1993, Coy—now widowed—traveled two hours from her Long Island home to a narrow six-story townhouse-turned-clinic on East 55th Street in Manhattan. Instead of submitting herself to another hopeless round of chemotherapy, Coy ventured to the city for a different, more controversial kind of intravenous injection: ozone gas, alleged by the clinic's proprietor to neutralize cancer cells. After the treatment, Coy was to come back within two months for a "simple blood test" to determine whether her cancer had recurred, at which point she would have another round of ozone injections.[2]

As Coy got off the elevator on the third floor and was ushered to a seat in "a sea of reclining chairs," she was given a "hand-held pump to inject herself" with ozone gas.[3] Alongside her sat patients with human immunodeficiency virus (HIV), some also self-administering ozone, and other patients had intravenous bags filled with vitamin concoctions. There were patients with multiple sclerosis receiving exotic mineral infusions and yet more cancer patients taking herbal remedies such as Essiac.[4] Accounts of the incident vary, but all agree that shortly after beginning her ozone injections, Coy reported feeling ill. Representatives from the clinic said Coy merely felt "a little weak-kneed."[5] Other media accounts, however, reported that Coy complained to the clinic's staff that she was experiencing blurred vision and dizziness but was told to continue the injections anyway. When she tried to walk, Coy "found her legs were weak, her balance poor. She felt clumsy, and had lost some feeling in her left arm."[6] After as many as three hours at the clinic, Coy was finally taken by ambulance to Jacobi Hospital where her attending physician, Paul Gennis, reported that she had developed an embolism in her brain.

Gennis was quoted in *New York Newsday* as having said, "I can't imagine what benefit ozone would have. It sounds like quackery to me," and he promptly reported the incident to the New York State Department of Health.[7] In an interview, State Health Commissioner Mark Chassin labeled the clinic responsible for Coy's ozone infusion "an imminent danger" to New Yorkers' health, and filed a complaint against Coy's physician, who had his medical license "summarily suspended."[8] The perpetrator was none other than Dr. Robert C. Atkins, known nationwide for the rapid weight-loss program bearing his name.

"The Granddaddy of All Low-Carb Diets"

From the beginning, Atkins was, in the immortal words of the *New York Times* writer Verlyn Klinkenborg, "the conundrum of the American diet in the flesh."[9] Scarcely any diet in American history can claim to have encountered greater public enthusiasm, skepticism, or outright criticism as Atkins's weight loss program. His controversial diet has seen unimaginable volumes of ink spilled by detractors and defenders alike. When Atkins's program was first published under the title *Dr. Atkins' Diet Revolution: The High Calorie Way to Stay Thin Forever* in 1972, it contradicted virtually all extant medical theory and experimental evidence on the etiology of metabolic disease, which blamed rising rates of obesity, heart disease, and diabetes on Americans' penchant for fatty foods.[10]

Prevailing explanations of chronic metabolic morbidity drew evidence from grain-based cultures (or living experiments like the Dutch Hunger Winter of 1944–45, where animal products became scarce) to suggest that the less fatty meat and more whole grains people ate, the lower the overall rates of obesity and chronic disease they would experience. Atkins's thinking flew directly in the face of this received wisdom, salvaging the healthfulness of meats and other fatty foods and instead villainizing sugar and other refined starches. He roguishly insisted that people could lose weight and improve their health just by avoiding carbohydrates (popularly shortened to "carbs"). By wholly eliminating the consumption of the body's chief source of fuel (glucose, or products that directly metabolize into glucose including all carbohydrates), Atkins posited that a low- or no-carbohydrate diet would force the body to mobilize its energy reserves stored in fat deposits through glycolysis, leading to a rapid loss in the body's stored fat.

More radically—one might even say heretically—Atkins challenged the fundamental scientific consensus about the centrality of energy balance to maintaining body weight. Since Dr. Lulu Hunt Peters first popularized the calorie as a domestic measure of food energy in 1918, scientists and medical professionals have instructed the public that to lose weight one must simply adjust the body's energy balance (see entremets I). Energy balance theory taught that weight loss would result from reducing daily caloric intake below the number of calories expended—by eating less, increasing physical activity, or both.[11] One of Atkins's chief appeals, however, was the promise that people on his program could theoretically eat an unlimited number of calories from fat or protein and still lose weight. Depleting the body's stores of glycogen instead of glucose meant none of the extra calories from fats or proteins would contribute to the production of new fat cells or to the storage of glucose therein. The precise mechanisms Atkins proposed for accomplishing this bit of bodily trickery will be elucidated in greater detail later.

Atkins was hardly the first to suggest limiting carbohydrates to reduce body weight. In the nineteenth century both the famed French lawyer and politician Jean Anthelme Brillat-Savarin and British undertaker William Banting had written at length about the benefits of restricting the consumption of starches and sugars.[12] In the twentieth century one of the earliest to suggest the idea was the well-known Arctic explorer Vilhjalmur Stefannson; he admired the Inuit diet and, after experimenting with the nearly all-meat regimen in 1930 himself, published several books outlining the diet and praising its healthfulness.[13] Toward the middle of the century, the low-carb idea began to pick up steam again after Dr. Alfred Pennington earned notoriety with his low-carbohydrate diet, known popularly as the DuPont diet, introduced in 1953. Across the ocean, British physician Richard Mackarness published an updated version of the Banting diet called *Eat Fat and Grow Slim* in 1958.[14] That same year, fellow British nutritionist John Yudkin (famous for his 1972 book decrying sugar: *Pure, White and Deadly*) published *This Slimming Business*.[15] In the 1960s—still over a decade before Atkins's *Diet Revolution* went to press—the carb-averse Air Force diet become popular.[16] American physician Herman Taller then published his own bestselling spin on the plan with his *Calories Don't Count* in 1961.[17] Unfortunately for Taller, he was later accused by federal authorities of using his diet book to advertise the sale of his own safflower capsules (he advocated taking 84 of them a day!) and was eventually convicted of "mail fraud, violation of drug regulations, and conspiracy."[18]

In his own time, too, Atkins was merely one voice in a veritable crowd of low-carb advocates. After Taller's fall from grace, the low-carb model was repackaged and resold again just three years later as the *Drinking Man's Diet* (1964), and again in 1967 as Dr. Irwin Stillman's popular *Doctor's Quick Weight Loss Diet*, a book credited (erroneously, it would seem) by the *Chicago Tribune* with "once again making the world safe for fad diets."[19] Even after Atkins published his record-breaking version of the low-carb idea in 1972, he could hardly have been said to have cornered the market. Just three years later, gastroenterologist Walter Voegtlin published *The Stone Age Diet*, a truly bizarre low-carb program that "recommended the mass slaughter of tigers, dolphins, and other carnivores."[20] Then in 1978, Dr. Herman Tarnower published his version, *The Complete Scarsdale Medical Diet*, to much fanfare before he was famously—and brutally—murdered in 1980 by a jilted ex-lover.[21]

After a brief dip in the 1980s when low-fat dieting reigned, low-carb diets emerged victorious once again after *Dr. Atkins' New Diet Revolution* was released in 1992 and reprinted in 1999. Atkins's renaissance triggered a wave of what *Time* magazine described as "the most guy-embraced diets ever, regimens with Henry VIII as a role model and beef jerky as a food group." Atkins's ostensive heirs have since included *Protein Power* (1996), *NeanderThin* (1999), *The Dukan Diet* (2000), Loren Cordain's *The Paleo Diet* (2001), *Sugar Busters!* (2003), Dr. Arthur Agatston's *South Beach Diet* (2003), and the *Bulletproof Diet* (2014).[22] This trend of grain-avoidance has continued apace with more recent (and more diffuse) trends like eating gluten-free (which became popular in the early 2010s) and the 2017 resurgence of the Keto diet.

Despite the great number of lookalikes, Atkins managed to overcome the cacophony to become arguably the most important diet guru in modern American history. In 2005 *NPR* reported, "At its peak in 2003, nearly 10 percent of Americans said they were either on the Atkins diet or had tried it. . . . The phenomenon was strong enough to bankrupt several bread and pasta makers and attract the interest of Wall Street investment bankers."[23] His name became virtually synonymous with low-carb dieting in the United States and continues to serve as the standard against which other low-carb programs are judged (or even understood).

Atkins's program signaled a break from its competitors by constructing an image of a modern dieter that was more compatible with traditional masculinity.[24] Food studies scholar Amy Bentley has argued that, with the Atkins diet, men who wanted to lose weight were no longer confined to ordering salads at business dinners or similar social functions with other men who might judge them for their supposed effeminacy. Treating meat as diet food meant men could bond with each other over their new lifestyles, share dieting tips, and discuss their bodies in new ways without having to sacrifice their privileged position within the social hierarchy.[25] This shift gave particular relief to white male businessmen living high-stress lifestyles after fears of heart disease permeated this demographic in the 1950s.

Ironically, despite Atkins's explicit masculine overtures, the diet's followers were predominantly women. Yet because Atkins ushered more men than ever into the dieting realm, his program also opened meat consumption to women in a way that had not been accepted before. Bentley argues that permitting women to eat traditionally masculine-coded foods increased their social status and power without sacrificing other characteristics of traditional femininity.[26] Women who were following more conventional (low-fat) weight reduction programs often reported resentment at their husbands' newfound penchant for diet foods high in animal fats.

Because Atkins is the most iconic diet guru in modern American history, his program has often been used as a placeholder (if not a scapegoat) to eviscerate the character of American dieting culture more broadly. Such critiques are not necessarily off the mark. Like other diets, the neoliberal slant of Atkins's dietary philosophy reinforced harmful notions of an ideal body type, and it also placed an unreasonable burden on individuals to reform their own nonconforming bodies. Although Atkins, in part, blamed social structures like the industrialized food system for Americans' weight problems and the rising costs of health care, his dietary solution (like most others) favored personal discipline over collective action. However, in the context of Atkins's life and career, his signature low-carb diet is better understood as a small (if lucrative) piece of his larger ideological agenda, which centered more around his unusual theories of the body and his arsenal of complementary medical remedies than on quick weight loss per se. If we agree to understand Atkins as the archetypal fad or crash diet his critics saw, then his underlying healing philosophy and obsession with complementary medicine should serve as grounds to rewrite our conception of American diet fads altogether.

Dr. Robert C. Atkins

Robert Coleman Atkins was born in Columbus, Ohio, on October 17, 1930. When he was in junior high, his family moved to Dayton where his father ran "a few little restaurants and places where people could stay overnight."[27] He was, by all accounts, a bright student, finishing second in the state of Ohio on an annual statewide general scholarship test, but he lamented that his peers "only really enjoyed people who were athletes rather than brains."[28] By the age of fourteen, Atkins had his first job selling shoes, yet he longed to become a comedian. He finally got a taste of the entertainer's life after he graduated from the University of Michigan when he spent a summer working briefly as a "comic waiter" in the Adirondacks.[29]

As the comic dream faded, Atkins discovered new passions in medical school at Cornell Medical College, not the least of which was his admiration for the state of New York, where he would live for the rest of his life. After securing his MD, he did an internship at the Strong Memorial Hospital in Rochester, followed by residencies at the Bellevue, Goldwater, and Delafield Hospitals, before finally completing his medical training as a cardiology resident at St. Luke's Hospital in New York City. Though she did not know him during this portion of his life, Atkins's wife Veronica reported that he "was a blue-blood at first; he believed in medical orthodoxy wholeheartedly."[30] In 1959, he opened his own private practice in cardiology and internal medicine on the Upper East Side. Yet Atkins quickly became disenchanted with his chosen specialty: not only did he struggle to attract patients, but the few patients he had made him feel like a mere technician. Once, Atkins saved a patient's life during a house call only to receive no thanks, merely an instruction to call the patient's primary physician in the morning. He fell into depression.[31]

By 1963, Atkins's six-foot frame had swelled from his scrawny high school weight of 135 pounds to a much sturdier 225.[32] His adult weight apparently never bothered him until, on his first day as a medical consultant for AT&T, he claimed to have been affronted by the three chins he saw on his own employee identification badge.[33] After that, he became determined to lose weight and began to research the issue in medical journals, where he found two major sources of inspiration for the plan he would follow. The first was a series of papers published in 1953 by Dr. Alfred Pennington, who had placed twenty employees at DuPont on a carbohydrate-restricted diet and recorded their moderate weight loss (twenty-two pounds) over a three-month period.[34] The other was a series of papers published in the late 1950s by British metabolic researchers Alan Kekwick and Gaston Pawan, which suggested that the presence of ketone bodies in the urine of people on carbohydrate-restricted diets indicated that their body fat was being consumed for energy.[35] Atkins ate his last donut and committed himself to a low-carb regimen, losing twenty-eight pounds in his first six weeks.[36] In interviews, Atkins claimed his choice in diet was primarily motivated by taste: "It was the only diet that looked like I'd enjoy being on it. I ate a lot of meat, and a lot of shrimp, and a lot of duck, and a lot of fish."[37] Another key component of the program that excited Atkins was the total absence of the gnawing hunger pangs he associated with calorie counting.

Excited by his own diminishing figure, in 1964 Atkins ran his first experiment with sixty-five executives at AT&T: "Of 65 patients he treated, he got 64 down to their ideal weights. The 65th made it halfway."[38] Word spread about his success, to the point that comedian Buddy Hackett mentioned it during an appearance on *The Tonight Show* with Johnny Carson in 1965.[39] Still, Atkins's signature dietary formula did not become a widespread phenomenon until after its debut in women's fashion magazines—first in *Harper's Bazaar* in 1966, then in a 1970 issue of *Vogue* as the "Vogue Super Diet."[40] After the first article ran, people began to flock to Atkins's clinic and "suddenly his practice became full-time weight-control business."[41] After the second article, "the doctor's 23-room East Side office complex was handling an average of 350 patients a week," of which 65 percent were making their first visit.[42] As they waited to be seen, patients encouraged one another with before and after photos, which they flaunted "like identification cards in some secret society." His prices were surprisingly affordable: an initial visit (including laboratory tests) cost just $185 (~$1,500 today), and each subsequent visit was only $20 (~$150 today). Low prices notwithstanding, Atkins splashed signs of his success all over his office walls; one article described the decor of his waiting rooms as "a scaled-down Museum of Modern Art."[43]

Among the influx of new patients to Atkins's office in the early 1970s was Ruth West, an author of two diet books herself, who introduced Atkins to her publisher, David McKay. West herself was not uncontroversial; Fred Stare once said that she "ranks high on our totem pole of quackery."[44] Together, Atkins and West cowrote the original *Dr. Atkins' Diet Revolution*. Atkins said he never expected the book to sell, so he gave West a 50 percent stake in the book's profits, taking 40 percent for himself (the other 10 percent went to the book's recipe creator).[45] To distance themselves from some of their competitors' books, who had loaded their pages with complex language, rules, and diagrams, David McKay instructed Atkins and West to "aim beyond medical experts," so they forwent academic trappings and extensive citations. Instead, they discussed difficult medical concepts in "chatty layman's language."[46] The book was released to the public in September 1972.

The Birth of a Revolution

Atkins's message spread like wildfire, not for the novelty of his ideas per se but because of his publisher's promotional skill and Atkins's voracious appetite for work. He told *New York Weekly*, "It has to be damn worthwhile for me to leave my office, and I expect every minute to be filled when I do." When David McKay sent him on a ten-day promotional tour in November 1972, he reportedly "visited Los Angeles, San Francisco, Denver, and New York, and gave interviews to 34 newspapers, one magazine, twelve radio stations, appeared on nine local television shows as well as on *The Merv Griffin Show*." Despite his earlier flirtation with the entertainment business though, Atkins had not yet developed his flair for showmanship. When he was rejected for early interview requests by Johnny Carson and Jack Paar, the editor-in-chief at David McKay blamed it on Atkins's lack of charisma, saying, "I think he is too serious for them," and "He's not a character, like Dr. Stillman."[47] They could not yet see the pugilist he would become.

Nevertheless, Atkins's promotional efforts paid off handsomely. According to David McKay's own reports, *Dr. Atkins' Diet Revolution* quickly became "the fastest selling book in the history of publishing," though the reported sales figures for the paperback—which sold for $6.95 at drugstores and supermarkets across the country—vary. Combining different estimates suggest that the book sold roughly 200,000 copies by Christmas, 660,000 by March, and a staggering 900,000 by April 1973.[48] Atkins's book was picked up "by sheriffs in North Carolina, by the elderly residents of retirement communities in Florida, by subway passengers in New York, and by the thin and the fat of America."[49] The diet doctor was in, and a surprisingly diverse set of Americans ate it up.

With his newfound success, Atkins began living large. Although he had lived in a rather small apartment with a rotating cast of English sheepdogs from the completion of his residency in the 1950s through the late 1980s, he loved to entertain and hobnob with New York socialites (he often ran in the same circles as the Trumps and other minor celebrities).[50] He was a notorious bachelor, who evidently "fancied himself to be in [Hugh] Hefner's league." In the early 1970s, Atkins began renting a large vacation home in the Hamptons for the summers, and he would invite young, glamorous people to stay with him, where, according to salacious interviews with his biographer, they would throw "wild parties fueled with cocaine and sex."[51] His guests in the summer of 1974 included "the man who wrote the music for *Grease*, an actress who had appeared in the Broadway production of *Jesus Christ Superstar*, the former mistress of the Shah of Iran, and numerous aspiring actresses, models, and flight attendants, all of whom were young, pretty, and single."[52] He was rumored to "hire a particular woman as a nurse or assistant based on her looks," then date them—though he also sometimes sent his female employees out during the workday to bid on art for him at Christie's.[53] There was also tawdry speculation that Atkins had a number of patients who "visited the office and became his patient solely to have sex with him." His biographer even implies, scandalously, that the only reason Atkins's diet came to be featured in *Vogue* in 1970 was because he had a fling with a young editor.[54]

The medical establishment was not just going to sit idly by and let Atkins enjoy the fruits of his labor though. Physicians were profoundly disturbed by Atkins's flagrant denial of the scientific consensus about the bodily mechanisms pertaining to body weight. On March 8, 1973, the American Medical Association (AMA) fired the first shot across Atkins's bow with a scathing review sounding a national alarm on the program's alleged backwardness. According to the report, not only was Atkins's diet unoriginal, it was "unscientific and potentially dangerous to health" as well.[55] Atkins had barely mustered a response before the New York Medical Society issued its own warning.[56]

Within a year of the diet's release, critics from throughout the medical establishment had "chewed the diet to pieces."[57] Dr. Jules Hirsch, an obesity researcher from Rockefeller University, exclaimed that Atkins's diet was "the most unutterable nonsense I ever saw in my life" and that it "borders on malpractice for a doctor to recommend almost unlimited amounts of bacon, eggs, heavy cream in coffee, butter sauce on lobster, spareribs, roast duck and pastrami!"[58] Harvard University's Jean Mayer piled on as well: "putting yourself on this faddish high-saturated fat, high-cholesterol diet is playing Russian roulette with your heart and your blood vessels."[59] And the president of the American College of Nutrition, Dr. Seymour Halpern, said, "Of all the bizarre diets that have been proposed in the last 50 years, this is the most dangerous to the public if followed for any length of time."[60] Experts from all corners of medical orthodoxy speculated wildly that Atkins's program would bedevil Americans with a range of health problems. Among the many conditions they predicted would ensue from an Atkins regimen were kidney failure, weakness, gout, apathy, dehydration, mineral deficiencies, brain damage, calcium depletion, nausea, increased risk of coronary disease, atherosclerosis, damage to unborn fetuses, and high cholesterol.[61] The list is comically reminiscent of (and had about as much supportive evidence as) the myriad conditions that so-called quack remedies claimed to be able to solve.

Unfortunately for Atkins, the critiques from nutrition scientists in the newspaper were just the beginning of his troubles. In March 1973, the same month the AMA's critique was published, Atkins was served with two major lawsuits. The first was a $1 million class action lawsuit filed on behalf of the 10,000 residents of Cleveland, Ohio, who were estimated to have purchased Atkins's book to "recover any medical expenses the Ohioans may incur from the diet's side effects."[62] Then he was sued for malpractice with $7.5 million in damages by a former patient, sixty-two-year-old Joseph Kottler, an actor and Democratic assemblyman from Brooklyn, who blamed Atkins's diet therapy (which had been administered directly through his private practice) for his heart attack.[63]

To top it all off, two weeks after Kottler announced his lawsuit, Atkins was called to defend his diet publicly before US Senator George McGovern's Select Committee on Nutrition and Human Needs. This was the same committee that would eventually call Pritikin to testify as an expert on the treatment of chronic disease (see chapter 3). The main task of the hearing was to determine whether the US Food and Drug Administration (FDA) or some other federal mechanism should have a formal role in regulating the claims of fad diets, especially with respect to their treatment of obesity.[64] Atkins's diet was one of just two programs hauled before the committee during this branch of its investigation, the other being macrobiotics, which had no representation.[65] Both Atkins and macrobiotics were considered emblematic examples of the imminent threat diets posed to the nation's public health (see chapter 2).[66]

Atkins sat before the committee with his lawyer, blithely nibbling a piece of cheese, as senators and expert witnesses took turns berating him. Much of the criticism had been regurgitated from the AMA's initial report. McGovern accused Atkins point blank that his diet "could lead to heart and kidney trouble."[67] Senator Charles Percy (R-Illinois) recounted a conversation he had had with Fred Stare in which Stare said, "The Atkins diet is nonsense. . . . Any book that recommends unlimited amounts of meat, butter and eggs, as this one does, is, in my opinion, dangerous. The doctor who makes this suggestion is guilty of malpractice."[68] Most damningly, Sen. McGovern himself confronted Atkins with the testimony of British metabolic scientist Gaston Pawan, whom Atkins had cited in his book as a primary inspiration for his diet. Pawan publicly disagreed with Atkins's characterization of his own work and assented to the AMA's warning that Atkins's program could be hazardous to public health. They wanted to shame and humiliate him.

Throughout the hearing, Atkins breezily dismissed the critiques of his medical peers as mere differences of professional opinion and suggested that any regulatory action against him would violate his First Amendment rights.[69] Beneath the surface, he seethed that the medical profession was turning a blind eye to what he considered to be the quick and obvious solution to a monumental health crisis. Atkins had anticipated some raised eyebrows, of course, but he felt that his colleagues' initial reactions to his program were disproportionate to the dangers—real or imagined—that his diet actually posed to public health. After all, his critics were keen to point out that Atkins's was certainly not the first bestselling diet book in US history, nor even the first low-carb program to claim the mantle.

But Atkins's lack of novelty raises more questions than it answers. If his program was old news, as many of his critics claimed, and if low-carb fads inevitably disappeared after people grew bored with eating meat and butter, why were physicians so uniquely angered by Atkins? Was the medical establishment so beholden to bread as the staff of life that they could not imagine forgoing grains for any length of time? Or were they offended because, unlike most other gurus in the marketplace, Atkins was a physician—even a member of the AMA—and they perceived him as betraying their cause? Why then were earlier low-carb advocates (Drs. Irwin Stillman or Herman Taller) not dragged before a congressional subcommittee and excoriated? More bewildering still, how could congressional investigators have even compared the risks of Atkins's program with those of macrobiotics on which patients were said to literally starve to death? It became clear to Atkins that he and the medical establishment understood the state of America's health in starkly different terms, but to probe the medical reaction to Atkins further we have to develop a more detailed understanding of the science Atkins mobilized in support of his program.

Fat-Melting Magic

The Atkins Nutritional Approach hinged on what many physicians perceived to be shaky theoretical ground. His theory inverted the prevailing wisdom of the medical establishment that by cutting calories, and specifically calories from fat, people could safely and gradually lose weight and reduce their risk of heart disease at the same time. Dietary fat had been particularly demonized because of its hypothesized role in raising blood cholesterol and triglycerides and for promoting obesity, three known risk factors for heart disease and an assortment of other serious chronic health conditions.

In the place of the establishment's familiar demons, Atkins counterintuitively blamed sugar and other simple carbohydrates for Americans' ailing health. His reasoning was simple and seductive: carbohydrates triggered the body to release most of its insulin whereas fat triggered almost none (protein only some). Insulin was responsible for delivering the glucose produced by the breakdown of carbohydrates to the body's cells. However, the more insulin the body produced, the greater the likelihood that the body would develop insulin resistance. If the body's cells became insulin resistant, they took in less glucose, which resulted in higher levels of blood sugar and triggered the body to store more glucose in the form of corporeal fat. As insulin resistance deepened and blood sugar levels continued to rise, the body would produce ever more insulin, compounding the problem of its own resistance and accelerating weight gain until "even the insulin receptors that convert glucose to fat start getting worn out."[70] The most straightforward result of this intensifying cycle was diabetes, but Atkins also suggested that high levels of insulin were strongly correlated with the creation of atherosclerotic plaques, high levels of triglycerides, low levels of "good" high-density lipoprotein (HDL) cholesterol, and an increased risk of estrogen-linked cancers. Tying hyperinsulinism to the signature risk factors for heart disease and cancer was Atkins's key defense when challenged about the unlimited amounts of saturated fats and cholesterol he encouraged his patients to consume.

To counteract the destructive capacity of insulin, Atkins recommended removing all carbohydrates from the diet. Not only would this theoretically stop the body from producing more corporeal fat by circumventing the production of insulin, the subsequent drop in blood glucose levels would trigger the body to start consuming its own energy stores, a process Atkins called "ketosis/lipolysis" (or ketosis for short). In Atkins's program, the dieter's main goal is to starve the body of glucose indefinitely by restricting all carbohydrate consumption to maintain a state of ketosis until the dieter's target weight is achieved. As evidence that the body was engaging the proper mechanisms, Atkins advised his followers to purchase Ketostix, at-home urine-testing kits to detect the presence of ketones (the alternative fuel to glucose created by lipolysis), to ensure they were on track. Ketosis had other telltale signs though, like breath that smelled of acetone, to alert dieters (and anyone in their vicinity) that it was working.[71] Because the body was essentially eating itself, rapid weight loss was purported to ensue, even if dieters ate as much fat and protein as they could handle, regardless of calories. By breaking the fundamental laws of energy metabolism, Atkins guaranteed that his patients would feel full—avoiding the unbearable hunger he had endured on other diets—and that they could eat all the sinful foods other diets forbid (although they would have to eat these once-taboo foods to the near exclusion of anything else).

There were several frequently cited critiques of the scientific picture Atkins painted in his dieting manuals. The most minor was a persistent confusion that Atkins created by calling his process ketosis, which many befuddled critics mistook for the similarly named but much more serious condition ketoacidosis.[72] According to Atkins, ketoacidosis was a condition reserved for diabetics who recklessly ate too many carbs, alcoholics, and those experiencing extreme starvation. Ketosis, on the other hand, was just as described: a normal (evolutionarily speaking) physiologic state of converting energy stored as body fat into usable fuel in the absence of glucose. Atkins famously described the process as "one of life's charmed gifts. It's as delightful as sex and sunshine, and it has fewer drawbacks than either of them!"[73] Because diabetic ketoacidosis was the product of consuming excessive carbs and ketosis was the product of consuming few if any, Atkins suggested the processes were in fact physiological opposites despite their similar appellations.

The second major critique centered on the identity of a mysterious compound Atkins pinpointed as being singularly responsible for triggering ketosis: a compound—the action of which Atkins claimed differentiated his program from previous low-carb diets—called the fat-mobilizing hormone (FMH). Nitpicking critics, including Gaston Pawan at the Senate subcommittee hearing, doubted Atkins's labeling of the mystery substance as a hormone, when the more conservative (and thus preferred) technical term for this entity was fat-mobilizing substance (FMS).[74] Others rolled their eyes at Atkins's whole shtick, not least because he used decidedly unscientific nicknames for FMH; he playfully referred to his unidentified, possibly imaginary substance as a "magic bullet" and "that powerful genie."[75]

The only magic Atkins's critics saw in his program was his magical ability to stretch flimsy evidence to account for a majority of America's health problems. Dr. Philip White, secretary of the AMA's Council on Food and Nutrition, dismissed Atkins's fanciful explanations: "The whole diet is so replete with errors woven together that it makes the regimen sound mysterious and magical."[76] Bonnie Liebman from the Center for Science in the Public Interest said of Atkins, "This whole ketosis thing is just a gimmick to make people think there's something to blame for weight gain and some magic solution to take it off. That's the beginning and end of it."[77] Atkins's diet was decried in the *Los Angeles Times* as preying on "millions of diet-fetish Americans seeking magic formulas for quick and easy weight loss."[78] And Ronald Deutsch, author of the self-published 1977 exposé on quackery *New Nuts among the Berries*, warned physicians to beware of Atkins's allure lest they "fall prey to the lure of easy solutions to difficult problems" because such easy solutions constituted "'nutrition magic' that promise[s] answers to obesity, cancer, heart disease and every other ill the flesh is heir to."[79] As these examples suggest, critics thought that Atkins's explanations of nutrition science were jazzed up oversimplifications of something that was, for them, an otherwise complex and sobering subject.

The chief complaint leveled against Atkins, however, was his privileging of the insulin pathway over all other physiological explanations of body weight and metabolic sickness. The aforementioned Philip White said Atkins "simply lumps together all the medical abnormalities that have been related to the body's handling of carbohydrates and says this is a problem that all people have. He's making everyone fit his book."[80] Elevating what his contemporaries perceived to be a peculiar physiological quirk (for which there was scant medical evidence anyway) over all other extant science about the underlying mechanisms responsible for producing such major chronic diseases as heart disease and cancer amounted to heresy. Almost vindictively, physicians extended their skepticism of his insulin theory to the idea that the Atkins's program could result in any tangible long-term weight loss at all. They preferred to explain the initial success dieters reported on his program as a loss in "water weight," a temporary and meaningless loss of weight that would rebound when dieters inevitably strayed from the program. Like Pritikin, Atkins's program was scolded for enforcing extreme dietary monotony, too, which undermined the idea that anyone could sustain his program for any meaningful duration of time.[81] Provocatively, when the diet ran as the Vogue Super Diet in 1970, it included a revealing protective disclaimer: "Not being able to stay on a diet is itself sometimes a symptom of low blood sugar."[82]

Beyond merely getting the facts wrong or spreading false hope, critics worried that Atkins's reductionist view that much of America's chronic disease incidence could be explained as rampant hypoglycemia in disguise would undercut faith in orthodox medicine and sway patients to shirk necessary medical care. The establishment was right to worry; upsetting faith in industrial medicine was exactly Atkins's plan.

The Great Diet War

Early in his medical career, Atkins grew weary of technocratic solutions to intractable diseases (bypass surgery, chemotherapy, risk-reducing drugs like statins, etc.). This was one of the major reasons he abandoned his cardiology practice (though he continued, misleadingly, to exalt himself as a cardiologist in self-promotions). His signature low-carb diet can, in part, be understood as a reaction to the tendency of orthodox medicine toward unnecessary, expensive, and harmful interventions. One of the first technocratic weight loss products to earn Atkins's ire was appetite suppressants, a wholly unnecessary (in Atkins's mind) drug made popular to combat the hunger associated with ill-conceived diet plans. His *Diet Revolution* was designed in no small part to alleviate just that problem but without resorting to pharmaceuticals.

Interestingly, Atkins understood the weight loss for which his program was best known as just one positive benefit among many of disrupting the body's tendency toward hyperinsulinism. By correcting this population-level blood sugar imbalance, Atkins thought of himself as obviating the need for most of the nation's pharmaceuticals and surgeries. His unconventional medical philosophy was frequently mentioned in the press, but usually as an aside; it never became a major part of the medical or media narratives surrounding his program. As his career went on, Atkins grew increasingly frustrated with his being reduced to a mere weight-loss guru. He had even planned a dedicated follow-up book to his 1972 diet revolution on his broader philosophy of hypoglycemia and health, but before he had a chance to publish, the AMA issued its damning report.[83]

The AMA's report and the avalanche of fallout that followed *Dr. Atkins' Diet Revolution* unnerved him. Instead of publishing his full take on hypoglycemia like he planned, he instead waited several years before publishing a watered-down version called *Dr. Atkins' Superenergy Diet*.[84] While the core of the diet stayed the same, Atkins's new book incorporated some modifications (mainly vitamin pills and supplements) to reverse the tiredness, fatigue, and depressive symptoms associated with carrying extra weight. By branching into psychological terrain, Atkins had clearly wanted the book to serve as a departure from the popular understanding that he was a mere weight-loss guru. Unfortunately, when *Superenergy* came out in 1977, its publication coincided with the release of the McGovern Report, which changed the landscape of federal nutrition recommendations, tilting the scales heavily toward the medical establishment's preferred low-fat dietary model, so Atkins's book was largely passed over.[85]

For the next few years, Atkins spent much time and energy fighting proponents of the low-fat diet. One of Atkins's biggest rivals was carb-fanatic Nathan Pritikin. Beyond their diametrically opposed philosophies and recommendations, the relationships that each guru had with orthodox medicine make for an instructive comparison. Atkins did not have to pretend at medical expertise, though his claims were arguably more inflammatory. Historian Steven Shapin has shown that Atkins was careful to distinguish himself from a diet doctor, instead casting himself as a cardiologist with decades of clinical experience.[86] By crediting his cardiology training for his initial ignorance in nutrition, Atkins was able to create critical distance from the nutrition establishment that Stare represented. In doing so, Atkins could appear to have one foot in the door of the cathedral of science, but not so heavily indoctrinated in nutrition or metabolic science as to be blinded by academic dogma. His personal touch, scientific credentials, and independence of thought, explain Shapin, predicted Atkins's rise in fame and influence above the credentialed experts who reviled him. Where Pritikin could criticize the medical profession as a plucky outsider gunning for a seat at the table, Atkins operated as a seasoned veteran of the establishment, and a war-weary renegade at that. His eventual dismissal from the medical community, however, is a clear contrast to Pritikin's numerous successful attempts to gain recognition from orthodox medicine for the efficacy of his dietary program.

Atkins's and Pritikin's stark ideological differences begat a vitriolic public relationship. They feuded in print, in person, and on air.[87] Both gurus traded barbs that each other's programs were unaffordable: Atkins charged Pritikin with bilking patients at his pricey Longevity Center; Pritikin chastised Atkins for assuming everyone could afford to eat steak and lobster at every meal. Atkins quipped that Pritikin's food was flavorless; Pritikin retorted that Atkins's diet was repulsive. In 1981, during a highly publicized debate between them on the Los Angeles–based TV show *Tomorrow*, Pritikin claimed outright that people following the Atkins diet had a significantly higher risk of developing heart attacks and strokes, dying of heart disease, and contracting breast cancer, colon cancer, and prostate cancer; he called the diet a threat to public health.[88] On air, Pritikin even offered to personally help anyone who believed they had incurred damage on

Atkins's diet, adding that several of Atkins's followers had already been "cured" at his Longevity Center in Santa Barbara.[89] Pritikin's wry smugness and Atkins's pugnacious arrogance were great for ratings, and commentators compared their sparring to "the televised encounter between Jerry Falwell and Larry Flynt."[90] When the interview was over, Atkins was so offended that he sued Pritikin for libel—seeking $5 million in damages for defamation—at the New York Supreme Court. He later expanded his lawsuit to include scathing remarks about high-fat diets found in Pritikin's publications as well. Pritikin pleaded not guilty to all accounts of libel and ultimately won the suit.[91]

Atkins never forgot his injury at Pritikin's hand. After Pritikin's death in 1985, Atkins continued to rage against the vegan physician-gurus who took up Pritikin's mantle (see chapter 3), vowing to become "the best enemy [they] ever had."[92] Atkins pulled no punches; in an interview with the *New York Times*, he gloated, "It is obviously clear that I am right, and the rest of the world is wrong."[93] Over the next eighteen years, he would berate Dr. Dean Ornish and spar with Pritikin's friend Dr. John McDougall.[94] At the US Department of Agriculture (USDA) "Great Nutrition Debate" in 2000, he grappled with both Ornish and McDougall at once, along with a host of other doctors and government representatives.[95] He tangled repeatedly with Dr. Neal Barnard, People for the Ethical Treatment of Animals (PETA), and the Physicians Committee for Responsible Medicine (PCRM).[96] And he threatened to sue Dr. Michael Greger.[97]

While accurate, the public image of Atkins as a brawler for low-carb lifestyles is hardly a complete representation of Atkins's activities through the 1980s because the work he most cared about rarely made headlines. Though his first attempt to articulate his broader philosophy of hypoglycemia and holistic health had been deterred (and overshadowed) by the 1977 McGovern Report, Atkins nevertheless spent much of the 1980s trying to regain traction for this idea. In 1981, he published *Dr. Atkins' Nutrition Breakthrough: How to Treat Your Medical Condition Without Drugs,* and in 1988, he published *Dr. Atkins' Health Revolution: How Complementary Medicine Can Extend Your Life,* but neither received the attention Atkins craved.[98] Meanwhile, the low-fat paradigm reigned, unleashing a tidal wave of laboratory-made low-fat or fat-free foods that promised to reduce flab.

Fortunately for Atkins, in the early 1990s the federal government severely damaged its own credibility when it linked hands with the medical establishment to proclaim that the nation's obesity had reached "epidemic" proportions. Shortly thereafter, in 1992 the USDA released the Food Pyramid, which prominently featured grains (ergo carbohydrates) as the base. That obesity continued to balloon exponentially—especially as more people than ever claimed to have followed low-fat diets and failed to lose weight—undermined public faith in official nutrition recommendations. By the late 1990s, it had become clear to many dieters that low-fat diets of the sort backed by the government and the medical establishment had utterly failed to shrink America's waistline. *Time* magazine reflected in 1999, "Carb paranoia struck when people discovered that all the fat-free food they loaded up on during the last diet craze was making them fat. Diet plans like the Pritikin Program . . . caused a run on processed low-fat food like Snack-Well's and frozen yogurt. But those treats, it turned out, were chock-full of sugar and a whole mess of calories."[99] Although Pritikin's program detested sugar—demanding the consumption of complex carbohydrates instead—the fly-by-night dieting crowd had no appetite for such nuance.

To Atkins, the impending failure of low-fat had been maddeningly obvious all along, especially because the foods modified to contain fewer calories from fat were often bolstered with sugar, Atkins's bane. He was finally fed up with what he described as "an industrial conspiracy" between the members of a "great triumvirate of Evil": the federal government, the pharmaceutical industry, and the medical establishment (but he probably should have included the food industry as well).[100] Describing the conspiracy between these villains, Atkins said, "The food industry (with the government's blessing) knowingly brings us the partitioned, less-than-optimum diet that hastens the development of our modern illnesses. Then the drug industry profits from the sickness our diet engenders. The voice of better nutrition is silenced. Nutrition is not profitable enough. Who loses? All of us. Because all of us must eat."[101] In 1992 (and again in 1999), Atkins took matters into his own hands and republished his ultrasuccessful weight loss program—now under the title *Dr. Atkins' New Diet Revolution*—to recapture the public's attention and save them from the failure of corrupt public health experts.[102]

As Atkins's diet rose from its own ashes over the course of the 1990s, he chose to fight fire with fire. To combat the high-sugar landscape brought about by a decade or more of unquestioned low-fat ideology, Atkins courted the food industry for himself, ushering in a new flood of equally dubious sugar-free and low-carb products. To keep up with the trends, popular chain restaurants from TGI Fridays to Subway produced reformulated, low-carb versions of their signature dishes; grocery stores rebranded such "Appalachian food staples" as beef jerky and pork rinds as "elite nutraceuticals";

and beverage giant Anheuser-Busch even released the first low-carb beer, Michelob Ultra, in 2002.[103] Atkins also invested heavily in his own food company, Atkins Nutritionals, which launched in 1996 and allowed dieters to purchase his signature energy bars (and eventually shakes, frozen meals, and protein powders) from its website.

The 1990s reincarnation of the Atkins diet boasted a veritable who's who of celebrity endorsers, starting a trend that continues today. Among the notables rumored to have "gone on Atkins" were actors Jennifer Aniston, Julia Roberts, Brad Pitt, Matthew Perry, Courteney Cox, Stephen Fry, Demi Moore, Renee Zellweger, and Minnie Driver; reality TV celebrities Davina McCall and Kim Kardashian; and singers Geri Halliwell, Victoria Beckham, Jennifer Lopez, Robbie Williams, and Stevie Nicks; and even US vice president Al Gore.[104] The Atkins Foundation began recruiting celebrities to serve as official spokespeople with actor Courtney Thorne-Smith in 2009, followed by reality TV star Sharon Osbourne in 2012 who convinced her husband and son, musician Ozzy and Jack Osbourne, to cut carbs alongside her. Actors Alyssa Milano in 2015 and Rob Lowe in 2018 — the latter already famous for his supremely health-conscious character on the scripted comedy show *Parks and Recreation*—signed on as Atkins's third and fourth official spokespersons.[105] Importantly, not every celebrity reported in the media had, in fact, done Atkins; after being widely reported to be an Atkins follower, actor Catherine Zeta-Jones even filed a lawsuit to have her name removed from the gossip columns' rosters of Atkinites.[106]

Parallel to the diet's rise in popularity among A-listers was concern that the Atkins diet was promoting a "skeletal-chic figure"—popularized by such ultrathin actors as Calista Flockhart, Lara Flynn Boyle, and Renee Zellweger—that threatened the physical and mental health of a generation of young women. Young women in particular were drawn to the diet's promise to quickly melt away what they damagingly perceived to be excess body fat.[107] During the second Atkins boom, teens flocked to online forums to trade weight loss tips to achieve the emaciated looks of their celebrity idols. In a startling 2003 article from *ELLEgirl* magazine, reporter Ronnie Carr explained the dark appeal that Atkins held for young women: "It's easier to hide a condition like anorexia behind the excuse 'Well, I can't eat carbs because I'm on Atkins,'" because adhering to a named program was "more socially acceptable than saying 'I can't eat carbs because I'm afraid they'll make me fat.'"[108] Though the Atkins diet's reputation was demonstrably built on rapid weight loss, the meaty fare defied the feminine stereotypes of traditional dieters, providing some young women with cover for their disordered eating in front of friends and family.

Though he once again rose to fame through the promise of quick and easy weight loss, Atkins nevertheless tried in vain (as he had throughout the 1980s) to redirect the conversation about his diet toward the necessity of adopting holistic healing practices. He wrote several more books detailing his unconventional approach to health and medicine: *Dr. Atkins Vita-Nutrient Solution* (1998), *Dr. Atkins' Age-Defying Diet Revolution* (2000), and the posthumously published *Atkins Diabetes Revolution* (2004).[109] None of these titles proved as successful as his *Diet Revolution* series. The greater American public, it seemed, was only interested in Atkins for his hottest weight loss tips, not his medical doomsaying.

Atkins's message of dieting qua holistic health was, ironically, drowned out once and for all by his greatest champion, journalist Gary Taubes, whose provocative 2002 *New York Times Magazine* article "What If It's All Been a Big Fat Lie?" made a compelling scientific case for Atkins's counterintuitive approach to weight loss. Taubes's article unleashed the most enthusiastic wave of pro-Atkins support yet; Atkins's *New Diet Revolution* rocketed up the *New York Times* bestseller charts for a third time, selling over a million more copies. Where Atkins had once been universally maligned in the medical community—Taubes even quotes a physician saying, "I was . . . trained to mock anything like the Atkins diet"—Taubes' article appeared to have totally vindicated him.[110] Atkins's longtime foe, the American Heart Association, inexplicably invited him to speak. Barbara Walters listed him, alongside Dr. Phil, as one of her ten most fascinating people of 2002. Of his miraculous turnaround, *New York Magazine* wrote, "Suddenly, this aging, beleaguered doctor with the second chin (which he sometimes hid behind a cupped hand) seemed fascinating."[111]

Meanwhile, Taubes's article became enmired in its own scandal, almost eclipsing Atkins himself. There was a swift backlash from nutrition scientists who regretted having been interviewed, accusing Taubes of misrepresenting their attitudes. Taubes was drawn into a public feud in the pages of *Reason* magazine with Michael Fumento, author of the 1997 book *Fat of the Land*, who called him a "Big Fat Fake."[112] He was taken to task for telling "Big Fat Lies" by the Center for Science in the Public Interest.[113] Taubes was even critiqued in *Newsweek*, by his friend and colleague Ellen Ruppel Shell, in an article titled "It's Not the Carbs, Stupid."[114] After his "Big, Fat Public Shaming," Taubes's public reputation was slowly redeemed over the ensuing decade and a half, not only by the continuing success of grain-averse diets (such as gluten-free, Paleo, and Keto), but also by new research, including the overblown 2016 revelations that the Sugar Research Foundation had paid to obfuscate sugar's role in heart disease (see entremets III).[115] For Taubes's stalwart opposition to mainstream nutrition advice followed by a stunning vindication, famed food journalist Michael Pollan likened him to the Aleksandr Solzhenitsyn of nutrition.[116]

"The Granddaddy of Complementary Medicine"

Atkins practiced what he termed "nutrition medicine," though his practice was certainly not limited to dietary recommendations, as the opening story of Vivan Coy attests.[117] Though his books had been flirting with holistic health concepts since the late 1970s, in 1984 Atkins finally transitioned his entire private practice away from internal medicine and helped transform New York City into the new mecca for complementary medicine. An article on the East Coast's complementary medical boom quoted Atkins saying, "New York doctors are at the head of this, because more and more people here are looking for alternative doctors. On the West Coast, the problem is a high density [of practitioners]."[118] In addition to the growing demand for complementary services, Atkins highlighted New York's more relaxed approach to medical regulation as a reason for the city's ascendance in the alternative medical marketplace.

Atkins's approach to food and medicine was unique among diet gurus and doctors alike, a fact that he recognized himself and touted. Comparing himself to California-based practitioners, Atkins posited himself to be a different species of doctor: "West Coast doctors are more vegetarian, and most of us here are more carnivorous."[119] This relatively minor cosmetic difference between food preferences encoded a range of deeper disparities. "After all," a writer for *New York Magazine* mused, "what self-respecting healer would proselytize for meat?"[120] Whereas many of his competitors had aligned themselves with stereotypically liberal political causes (demilitarization, environmentalism, anti-racism, etc.), Atkins came from a self-consciously conservative direction. As if his emphasis on expensive, luxury meats were not enough evidence of his political slant, Lisa Rogak, a popular press biographer, claimed direct evidence that Atkins was a registered Republican of a libertarian bent who sought reduced government regulation in the medical marketplace.[121] Moreover, Atkins was vehemently opposed to the government banning substances, medicinal or not, that he thought could be helpful in treating patients, and he avidly supported free market principles.

Perhaps the most important remedies in Atkins's tool kit were dietary supplements, of which he was a huge fan, taking twice his own recommended dosage of thirty vitamins and minerals a day.[122] His enthusiasm for supplements can be traced in part to his fervent admiration of Carlton Fredericks, another American health guru notable for putting patients on high-dose vitamin and mineral supplement regimes.[123] Atkins created dozens of custom supplement formulas for his patients, which he sold at his clinic where he maintained a fully outfitted in-house supplement pharmacy, though patients could also order his concoctions through the mail.[124] In his book *Dr. Atkins Vita-Nutrient Solution*, Atkins details his beliefs about the specific therapeutic applications of all the major vitamins, minerals, and amino acids (including a few extras like inositol, coenzyme Q10, creatine, omega-3 fatty acids, and biotin). On top of that, Atkins advocated supplementing with traditional herbs (e.g., ginseng, ginkgo biloba, garlic, ginger, turmeric, and tea tree oil), less familiar herbs (e.g., Venus flytrap, hawthorn, mistletoe, and yohimbe), and such wellness staples as chlorella, spirulina, royal jelly, bee pollen, bee propolis, wheatgrass juice, and charcoal. Adding to this impressive list, Atkins also trumpeted the benefits of glandular extracts, shark cartilage, and "a camphor compound called 714x."[125] When questioned about the necessity of adding supplements to a balanced diet, he responded brusquely, "Pollutants in the environment require vitamins to counteract them."[126]

In 1994, Atkins moved his lucrative practice from the Upper East Side to a six-story townhouse, renamed the Atkins Center for Complementary Medicine, located at 152 East 55th Street in Midtown. At its peak, his center was reported to have employed over ninety people. *New York Magazine* speculated that it "may have been the largest alternative medicine facility in the world."[127] The architectural difficulties that came with designing and constructing Atkins's fully customized office space were highlighted in a feature article in *Interiors* magazine: "The main challenge faced by [Atkins's architect & designer] Leeds and Feinn was how to program 21 exam/treatment rooms, an on-site lab, a chelation and IV therapy suite, a lobby, reception and waiting areas, and a retail vitamin store within a narrow 25-foot-by-100-foot lot with an overly large core containing two elevators and two staircases and only 10,000 useable square feet."[128] Atkins decorated the massive space himself with pieces from his private art collection. He actually owned so many paintings they eclipsed the walls throughout his home and office. In his new office alone, he had more than 150 unique pieces of art on display.[129]

In 1988, Atkins married his first wife, an octolingual, Russian-born woman named Veronica Kusmin Luckey, at the ripe age of fifty-seven.[130] They moved out of his tiny bachelor pad into a larger apartment together on the twentieth floor of a high-rise overlooking the East River, another home he flooded with moderately priced modern art. With his party days behind him, he fell out of sync with the new culture of wealth (though, according to sneering media profiles, he "had never been part of the fancier Hamptons set"). His vacation home was derided as "a sweeping double-towered brick house on the wrong side of Southampton" in "an area near North Sea Harbor where single-dwelling homes and trailers nestle."[131] One woman, a fellow "Hamptons socialite" who saw the house's interior in the 1990s, described its decor as "so late-seventies," though Atkins had installed an impressive "swimming pool holding ozone-enriched water, one of the therapy protocols he swears by."[132] Atkin's shameless penchant for luxe living could have lent him an air of overt fraud but for the fact that he so clearly incorporated the holistic principles he peddled into his private life.

That Atkins's self-image as a physician invested primarily in complementary medicine never became part of the cultural zeitgeist should not signal its triviality. Despite his name's synonymy with American dieting, Atkins nevertheless managed to draw a sizable clientele for his unorthodox clinical therapies. Though he had no hospital admission privileges and was never board-certified, over the course of his complementary medical career Atkins was estimated to have seen between 50,000 and 60,000 patients (including rock icon Stevie Nicks, who called Atkins a "god among men").[133] Whereas his mass-market weight loss programs had attracted millions of diet hopefuls from all walks of life and his reputation garnered more than passing curiosity from the elite, Atkins's brick-and-mortar practice appealed predominantly to the chronically ill. Aside from obesity, the patients he saw most were suffering drawbacks in their conventional care for such indistinct conditions as allergies, autoimmune disorders, and gastrointestinal difficulties, or from otherwise unassailable illnesses like diabetes, heart disease, cancer, multiple sclerosis, and HIV/acquired immunodeficiency syndrome.[134]

Atkins's medical philosophy was eclectic and nonjudgmental. He said, "If there's a voodoo doctor who is getting good results, I want to know how he's doing it. . . . That's the difference between me and other people. Good results warrant a serious look-see. I don't care if it is voodoo."[135] In concert with conventional diagnostic methods, Atkins deployed an array of unconventional testing procedures like glucose tolerance tests to diagnose his signature ailment, hypoglycemia, as well as food allergies, and hair analysis to assess patients' mineral levels.[136] His clinic also offered acupuncture, prolotherapy (treating injured joints with fluid injections), and chelation (stripping the body of heavy metals).[137] To ensure his products were safe and effective, Atkins practiced many of his alternative therapies on himself. He was regularly seen at meetings sucking on a metal lollipop, which he claimed was supposed to "build his immune system," and he had seen an iridologist to have the health information hidden in his irises deciphered.[138] Atkins took a great degree of pride in his trust in alternative cures: "I keep my mind open, and that little trick makes me almost unique among physicians. I made it a rule never to reject anything out of hand just because it didn't sound logical. I get into a lot of trouble because of my open mind," he said during one interview.[139]

Despite his enthusiasm for using trial and error on his own body, Atkins's appreciation for experimentalism did not extend to larger scale medical trials. Whereas Fulton, Kushi, and Pritikin had all displayed an eagerness to conduct empirical studies and earn the medical profession's seal of approval, Atkins was apathetic at best. As a clinician, Atkins did collect some data on his patients, but a hostile interviewer dismissively described it as "a sheaf of papers with some handwritten figures," which "looked like a grade school science project." At the time, Atkins balked that conducting large-scale research was too expensive: "a million dollars if you want to do a study," and he "just can't get anybody to subsidize a study." When the interviewer pressed him on why such obvious pro-fat corporate investors as Land O' Lakes butter had rejected his requests for funding, he dubiously insisted, "I can't even get them to answer my phone calls."[140]

Money was not the barrier to research that Atkins made it out to be given the amount he was making. In interviews, Atkins contended that his medical practice was not a revenue-generating operation: "We don't have a profit margin. What we charge our patients enables us to break even."[141] A 1994 *Allure* article bears out his claim suggesting that in 1991 Atkins's private medical practice made just $320,000. However, breaking even does not decorate a six-story Manhattan office building floor to ceiling with modern art; his medical practice may not have been revenue generating, but his other ventures certainly were. That same year Robert Atkins Professional Corp. made $3.8 million, and the Atkins Centers topped $5.3 million. Even still, despite his apparent financial success, Atkins did not use his own money to fund research until the 2000s with the establishment of the Atkins Foundation—a fact his earlier critics were keen to mention.[142] After all, Pritikin used the substantially smaller annual income of his California Longevity Center (around $750,000) to fund his studies.

The real reason Atkins resisted conducting medical trials to test his diet plan was because such studies conflicted with his holistic ideology. Complementary medicine required a lot more dedicated time for patient interaction, which allowed him to experiment in a different way. One of the associate medical directors at Atkins's complementary clinic, Fred Pescatore, described the clinic's original philosophy to *New York Magazine*: "We weren't so tied to evidence-based medicine. . . . We were into experiential medicine. We tried different things and saw what works with our patients."[143] Atkins felt that structuring medicine around the outcome of big research studies negatively impacted the quality of clinical care.[144] And he complained that "it's impossible to do the kind of clinical research that constitutes acceptable proof"; he continued, "I'm enough of a scientist to know what it would take to prove something to me, and I know I can't gather that kind of data. So I don't try. That's not my role."[145] Experiments to verify the premise of his mass-market diet were unimportant to him because they did not help him care for the patients who mattered most to him. Atkins's carefully tailored clinical experimentation was his passion, and it was a clear draw for the patients at his clinic.

Skirting the State

Apace with Atkins's love affair with supplements and his crusade to stem the tide of hypoglycemia ravaging the United States, he was an ardent supporter of sugar substitutes.[146] When his coauthor Ruth West first floated the idea of publishing a diet book together in 1970, Atkins was reportedly fuming over the recent federal ban of cyclamates, one of the earliest artificial sweeteners discovered. In 1969, cyclamates were found to cause cancer in rats when consumed in extreme amounts; the study (ironically, given Atkins's role as a board member of the National Health Federation) tripped the Food Additive Amendment (Delaney Clause) of the Food, Drug, and Cosmetic Act of 1938 (see entremets III).[147] Atkins credits his frustration with the cyclamate ban with motivating him to sign on to write his now-famous book. As part of his weight loss clinic, Atkins had developed strong ties with Marvin Eisenstadt, the executive vice president of the Brooklyn-based Cumberland

Packing Company, which manufactured cyclamates in addition to more commercially viable sugar substitutes like Sweet'N Low (saccharin). Atkins claimed it was his right as a physician to be able to prescribe a small amount of cyclamates "so a person could make a diet cheesecake."

Though he insisted that Cumberland never made much money from cyclamates, what little money they made was a direct result of Atkins's clinic and recommendations. Atkins admitted as much when he said, "Marvin [Eisenstadt] would only agree to sell [cyclamates] if I put my name on the labels. . . . I guess I'm an accomplice."[148] These words, spoken in 1973, were a harbinger of events to come; in 1974, Atkins was sued by a diabetic patient, Joseph Rizzo, alleging that Atkins did "pack, possess, offer for sale or sell a banned drug and a removed food additive: Cyclamates."[149] At trial, Cumberland officials testified that Atkins had maintained a special relationship with their company whereby they would continue to sell cyclamates to Atkins's own patients provided the patients arrived at the Brooklyn plant to purchase the substance in person. Yet the small quantities of cyclamates Atkins claimed to advocate were impossible to secure as Cumberland only sold the product in five-pound bags—far more than a lone diet cheesecake requires. Through the backdoor, Cumberland sold just over one ton of the product to Atkins's patients in three years (another 500 pounds were seized by police).

Though the court record indicated that even as recently as 1969 physicians had been given special exemption from the federal cyclamate ban to prescribe it to diabetic patients for whom the medical benefits outweighed the risks, the ban in 1970 revoked any such exception. Atkins's defense argued that his prescription of cyclamates may have been immoral, but, since he had only written (rather than filled) the prescription, his actions failed to violate the letter of the health code. The judge responded in kind, writing "The defense['s] position is as deficient in substance as cyclamate is lacking in nutritional value."[150] Damningly, Atkins had included recipes calling for cyclamates in his 1972 book, which baldly acknowledged the substance's illegality. For their actions, both he and Cumberland were fined.

After Atkins republished his *New Diet Revolution* in 1992, the events of 1974 seemed to play out all over again. In 1996, Atkins was sued by another patient, Gerry Ballinger, for advocating the use of artificial sweeteners that had damaged his health. Ballinger alleged that after beginning the Atkins diet in 1994, he had ingested large quantities of artificial sweeteners—in this case aspartame, sold under the NutraSweet label—in accordance with Atkins's program. He subsequently experienced "tachycardia, dizziness, anxiety, panic attacks, blurred vision, inability to concentrate, loss of memory, and shooting pains in his left arm."[151] To support his claim to injury, Ballinger requested the testimony of his personal physician, James Brodsky, and, bizarrely, Barry Sears, the diet guru behind The Zone. Both his witnesses were ultimately barred from testifying because Brodsky could not testify to Ballinger's injury with a reasonable degree of certainty and Sears had no special relevance to the case or expertise in medicine.[152] The case was dismissed.

Challenges for Complementary Medicine

Lawsuits did not stop Atkins from becoming a major agitator for American complementary medicine. It was during his time as a board member of the National Health Federation that the organization successfully lobbied to keep vitamins and other nutritional supplements beyond the reach of FDA regulation in the 1990s (see entremets III). He was also a founding member of the Foundation for the Advancement of Innovative Medicine (FAIM), which began in 1986 "as a voice for innovative medicine's professionals, physicians, patients, and suppliers."[153] FAIM members were especially motivated to insulate themselves against charges of malpractice because several high-ranking members, including Atkins, were shaken by what they perceived to be an unfair prosecution of an important fellow healer, Dr. Warren Levin.

Levin was a board-certified family practitioner who, in 1976, became one of the first in New York City to turn his medical practice to complementary medicine and clinical ecology: a contested medical discipline that investigates the cumulative health effects of low-level environmental toxins, which many physicians dismiss as akin to quackery.[154] Though Levin was dogged by litigation that many of his peers deemed unfair through the 1980s, the case in 1991 sent the biggest chill through the alternative healing community. One of Levin's patients, Glen Gersten, a twenty-nine-year-old man said to have been diagnosed with paranoid schizophrenia, died by apparent suicide. Levin allegedly exacerbated the man's paranoia by diagnosing him as a "universal reactor" and advising him to remain in a "pure" environment.[155] Career quack-buster Stephen Barrett claimed Levin said "drugs would aggravate [Gersten's] condition or kill him," implying that Levin had advised the man to stop taking his medication; further, he suggested Levin had even advised the man to "remove his furniture, seal his apartment with tape, and turn off his tap water in order to avoid toxins and pollutants."[156] When the verdict came down, Levin lost his medical license and was fined over $900,000 in the subsequent malpractice suit.[157]

Levin's loss became the subject of a dramatic novelization called *Prime Example* in which the author credits Levin's and Atkins's impassioned defense thereof with actually *saving* alternative medicine in NYC.[158] Atkins (alongside Nobel laureate and megavitamin promoter Linus Pauling) testified on Levin's behalf at trial that their own complementary practices included nearly identical procedures as his, including supplement cocktails, ozone therapy, hair analysis, chelation, and megavitamin injections. Atkins further spoke to the underrated value of experiential medicine, especially in a medical research environment that he saw as valuing pharmaceutical solutions over any alternatives: "I think . . . there are economic interests supporting the use of a pharmaceutical medicine. So a competing therapeutic which is non-pharmaceutical is not going to receive the financial support . . . and it does take financial backing to reach physicians. Physicians are reached mostly through medical journals which accept advertising mainly from pharmaceutical clients, and a position contrary to theirs is not likely to be accepted."[159] Atkins then offered a personal anecdote about a journal editor asking him to delete a phrase from an article he submitted for publication so as not to offend a pharmaceutical sponsor. When he was pressed at trial about what his supplements were for, he replied curtly, "Managing nutritional deficiencies."[160]

Although Levin lost his trial, it was such a shock to the complementary medical community that in 1994 they rallied to secure what initially seemed to be a huge victory in the Alternative Medicine Practice Act in New York City, which explicitly permitted any alternative medical practices deemed "effective," without requiring proof of efficacy. The act further mandated that at least two of the eighteen city board of medicine members be practitioners of nonconventional therapy and encouraged those board members to serve on hearing boards for disciplinary cases involving alternative practitioners.[161] Levin's loss had another silver lining in the form of personal vindication against a notorious anti-quackery activist, Victor Herbert (1927–2002). Herbert—who went on to call the Atkins diet "bullshit," and explained that the only reason people lost weight was out of boredom from eating "so much steak and eggs"—was the sole expert witness for the prosecution against Levin.[162] He was a hematologist at Mt. Sinai School of Medicine, former president of the American Society for Clinical Nutrition, and something of a career witness in cases involving accusations of health fraud. Herbert was also a close ally and occasional coauthor with retired physician Stephen Barrett, the most apparent heir of Fred Stare's midcentury anti-quackery crusade.[163] At a 1991 hearing for Levin's case, Herbert's neutrality as an expert witness was challenged because he had personally sued Levin several years prior and had called out his practice by name before Congress at Rep. Claude Pepper's (D-Florida) 1985 subcommittee hearing on health fraud and the elderly.[164] Herbert was subsequently barred from testifying to Levin and Atkins's great amusement.

Because Levin's case is so similar to situations in which Atkins found himself throughout his career, it is worth revisiting the narrative that opened this chapter—Vivian Coy's ozone injections and the subsequent suspension of Atkin's medical license—from Atkins's (and Coy's) perspective. After Coy was taken to the hospital and an embolism was diagnosed, her attending physician, Paul Gennis, requested her medical records from Atkins's office. Atkins refused to release them. His failure to comply with this request sparked a larger investigation, which led to Atkins's medical license being revoked in 1993. The dispute ended up in front of the New York Supreme Court, where a battle over Coy's subpoenaed medical records ensued.[165]

Notably, after her September 14 hospitalization, Coy returned to Atkins's office to continue her ozone treatments. During the trial, it was revealed that it was actually Coy who had asked Atkins to keep her records private, lest the suspension of his license imperil her therapy. In an affidavit she wrote to the court, Coy persuasively defended her right to choose Atkins's unconventional therapy over traditional chemotherapy and justified the withholding of her medical records from the state's case against him:

> I know that despite the miracles of modern science, conventional medicine is limited in its ability to control or cure various cancers including breast cancer. . . . Thanks to Dr. Atkins's therapy, I feel great today. CAT scans, bone scans, liver scans, mammograms, barium scans and other tests have all been negative. As an intelligent, autonomous woman, I have exercised my legal rights in choosing Dr. Atkins's therapy. I am particularly concerned that my ozone therapy not be discontinued. Accordingly, I request the Court enforce my legal right, and prevent the State from obtaining my patient records, or otherwise attempting to use me in its investigation of my primary care physician.[166]

The court was sympathetic to Coy's defense, and subsequently restored Atkins's license, ruling that "the state health commissioner acted unfairly when he suspended it last week."[167] Given what Atkins had seen happen to

Levin just two years prior, throughout his own trial he insisted that the plaintiff's motivation was "purely political" and that he felt unfairly targeted by the establishment over his support for alternative medicine.[168]

Many of Atkins's patients were happy to follow his unconventional recommendations and to try out experimental treatment because, like every other guru in this book, Atkins took his patients' holistic concerns to heart. A profile in *New York Magazine* described his appeal to patients as follows: "He understood the consumers on a more personal level . . . and they returned the favor, treating him like a savior. . . . Entire families came to him. Many sought him out as a last resort. They formed a loyal following and, sometimes, called his detractors 'pharisees.'"[169] Another of Atkins's patients, Diane Pinto, reported a positive experience with Atkins's therapies for her multiple sclerosis (MS). "Like a cruel joke," a journalist for *Allure* wrote, Pinto had gone "numb from the waist down on her honeymoon," and orthodox medicine, the article suggested, had offered Pinto only steroids as well as unhelpful advice to not get pregnant. With few other options available to her, Pinto sought help beyond medical orthodoxy, which landed her in Atkins's office. Fortunately, Atkins had an experimental treatment for MS: he had recently imported a controversial therapy involving an infusion of mineral-salts known as calcium ethylamino-phosphate (calcium EAP) from Germany. After seeing "tremendous improvement in her symptoms and energy" from her first injection in 1980, Pinto continued the therapy for eight more years. "It gave me hope again and I wasn't getting that anywhere else. You have to get to a point where you're so desperate that you say, What's the worst thing that could happen to me? Nothing."[170]

The same article in *Allure*, however, warned that trusting patient testimonies could be naive. Another of Atkins's patients suffering from MS, Edith Furman, underwent identical calcium EAP injections as had Pinto in 1987. Like Pinto, upon receiving a diagnosis of MS, Furman expressed her desperation: "I tried everything. . . . I was a desperate person. I wasn't going to wait for the MS Society to find a cure." Yet after receiving a few injections Furman went into cardiac arrest. She was taken to a hospital where she went into a coma for two weeks, after which she required a month of physical therapy to fully recover. Furman eventually sued Atkins for malpractice, and the case was apparently settled out of court for a "substantial sum," as Atkins wanted to protect his reputation and to continue to use calcium EAP.[171]

These cases did nothing to discourage Atkins from his work. As a pioneer of experiential medicine, Atkins's healing philosophy *assumed* therapies worked differently for different people—hence his skepticism of randomized, controlled trials. Because his style of practice was less insulated by government protections and institutional norms than orthodox medicine, he understood legal disputes like this to be an unfortunate but inevitable part of the process.

Atkins's Arteries

The famed diet guru passed away in 2003 at seventy-two years old. According to his death certificate, he "fell from an upright position," medical code that he had slipped on a patch of ice outside his Midtown office and cracked his skull, resulting in an epidural hematoma.[172] He died nine days later in the hospital after his wife took him off of life support. Many of his critics were quick to cast aspersions on the official circumstances of his death and demanded proof that the doctor had died as the papers and his relatives had claimed. Some of his more extreme opponents called for a detailed investigation of exactly how "healthy" Atkins was at the time of his death. As Atkins had promoted himself as a cardiologist, special attention was trained on the postmortem status of his heart. If Atkins's blasphemous dietary claims had been accurate, the reasoning goes, his heart should have been clear of obstructions. We will never know because Atkins's family, unlike Pritikin's, refused an autopsy, so there was no report (public or private) to deliver the much-awaited verdict on the state of Atkins's arteries.

As a controversial public figure, long before his death Atkins had been subject to intense scrutiny of both his practice and his person. That he masterminded this massively popular weight-loss regime as a visibly overweight man led dozens of commentators to openly deride his appearance and weight as hypocritical. One feature writer encapsulated this spirit when she wrote, "Atkins is 63 and, to put the gentlest spin possible on it, not exactly a walking advertisement for his diet. And most people want their stockbroker to be rich, their hairdresser to have a great cut, and their diet doctor to be a sylph—an issue that occurs to Atkins's patients from time to time."[173] *New York Magazine* reported that "he disguised his weight under layers of clothing."[174] Another article gossiped, "When a photographer arrived to photograph him for *The Observer*, Atkins insisted on standing. When he's photographed sitting down, he explains, it makes him look paunchy."[175] Even fellow low-carb guru Irwin Stillman joined in, saying, "Look, I'm not a diet doctor like Atkins. Incidentally, do you notice [Atkins is] always a little overweight?"[176] Though he never intended to be a living billboard for his ideology, that was the standard he was held to by his followers and critics alike.

An ablest, sizeist perspective animated Atkins and his patients, all of whom feared disabling changes to their bodies. Yet ableism and sizeism ironically fueled criticism of the Atkins diet as well. In life and in death, speculations that circulated about Atkins's personal health almost always used weight as a stand-in for general healthiness.

Shortly after he died, a startling batch of documents surfaced that appeared to betray the late Atkins's legacy. When he was first admitted to the hospital after his fall, Atkins's family had provided forms that listed his height, weight, and notes on his medical history. These documents were then illegally—albeit accidentally—released to a Nebraska cardiologist, Richard Fleming (an ironic turn of events given the contest over Coy's medical records). Fleming was a member of the medical activist group, the Physicians Committee for Responsible Medicine (PCRM), who had requested the documents as part of a sting operation to undermine Atkins's credibility. The PCRM was an organization of over 5,000 physicians, founded to advance the agenda of low-fat, plant-based diets from within the medical community. When Fleming received the report from the hospital despite not being Atkins's physician, he immediately leaked it to the media where it ignited a public frenzy.[177]

The documents contained two damning pieces of evidence that undermined the official narrative of Atkins's demise. First, Atkins's weight was listed at nearly 260 pounds at the time of death, giving him a body mass index of about 34, enough for him to be declared clinically obese. Second, on his medical history chart were notes referring to a history of myocardial infarction, congestive heart failure, and hypertension.[178] Years before his death, Atkins endured a cardiac event that nearly killed him at a restaurant, and a colleague successfully revived him with cardiopulmonary resuscitation. At the time, his family vehemently argued that Atkins's heart attack was the result of a viral infection that had critically weakened the musculature of his heart. Critics, however, interpreted his obesity and history of heart disease as evidence of profound deception: that he had profited from a system that he obviously knew to be mistaken and was endangering people's lives.

Atkins's family was rightly outraged that the doctor's private medical records had made their way into the public eye, but their fury almost lent credibility to the increasingly popular notion that there was something in Atkins's heart worth hiding. Neal Barnard, the president of the PCRM, which

had illegally obtained and released Atkins's records, said he was not interested in proving Atkins's hypocrisy per se, but rather that he was "concerned
about the Atkins machine trying to play the card that Atkins was healthy
and thin into old age."[179] Another PCRM member, Pritikin's long-time friend
John McDougall, said of Atkins, "I knew the man. . . . He was grossly overweight. I thought he was 40 to 60 pounds overweight when I saw him, and
I'm being kind."[180] Though the Whole Foods Plant-Based diet the PCRM pro-
motes is not explicitly oriented toward weight loss, the specter of the bad,
fat body haunts them still. Nor was this sentiment that Atkins had been a
hypocrite limited to his dietary opponents: none other than New York City
Mayor Michael Bloomberg was caught on tape making profanity-laced jokes
about Atkins's death, implying that Atkins's weight (and the fat-friendly nature of his diet) were responsible for his death.[181]

Those closest to Atkins responded to his naysayers with venom. Of
the PCRM, Veronica Atkins contended, "They're like the Taliban. They're the
vegetarian Taliban. . . . They're nasty."[182] Her sentiments were echoed by
Atkins's personal physician, colleague, and successor, Dr. Stuart Trager, who
said, "Here's a group of people who compare eating cheese to heroin, feeding children meat to child abuse. They don't think anyone should eat animal products. And it's clear they'll go to any extreme, any extreme, including
giving out records, breaking ethical violations to try to convince people."[183]
As for Mayor Bloomberg, Veronica Atkins demanded that he apologize, a
request Bloomberg initially ignored but to which he later relented.[184]

Despite the wave of popular skepticism targeting the late guru, Atkins's
staunchest supporters maintained that his medical records were misleading. Eventually, Veronica Atkins, exhausted from defending her husband's
honor with words alone, released his hospital admission record, which listed
his weight as 195 (still overweight but not clinically obese).[185] As his primary
spokesperson, Trager maintained that Atkins's cardiomyopathy was caused
by a virus, and that he had gained sixty-three pounds from fluid retention
during his hospital stay after his accident. This was supported by Atkins's
attending cardiologist, Dr. Fratellone, who said, somewhat cryptically,
"When we did his angiogram, I mean, the doctor who performed it, said it's
pristine for someone that eats his kind of diet. . . . Pristine, meaning these
are very clean arteries. I didn't want people to think that his diet caused
his heart muscle—it was definitely a documented viral infection."[186] For
low-carb hopefuls, the evidence that Atkins had suffered from a viral heart
infection at once redeemed his embattled dietary program and forgave the
"sin" of his weight. So long as his heart condition could be explained by

something other than a high-fat diet, Atkins could remain the renegade authority on heart health after his death (and his product empire could continue to profit accordingly). Critics of Atkins, however, rebuffed Trager's virus explanation, maintaining that such a rapid gain of sixty-three pounds from fluid retention was itself evidence of latent heart disease. It is ironic that the meaning of Atkins's death relied so heavily on the same kinds of up-for-interpretation medical measurements he had warned against his entire career.

Conclusion

Grain aversion was but one piece of Atkins's larger mission to ameliorate the glaring defects he saw in scientific medicine. Atkins was motivated above all by his patients and the work in his clinic. To serve what he understood as their needs, he became a leader for complementary medicine in New York City, helping to transform his adoptive city into a heterodox healing haven. That this key feature of Atkins's mission has been passed over despite the spotlight he once commanded signals the need to reconsider the place of dieting with respect to the American health care system. Diet gurus' cultural value has often been and continues to be reduced to the quality, veracity, or implications of their narrow nutritional claims. This way of thinking misses the greater cultural meaning of diet programs and their raison d'être.

Atkins's low-carb diet was explicitly grounded in his sweeping theory of chronic disease etiology. Yet everyone—from the hordes of casual dieters who tried his program and the columnists who advertised it to the critics who eviscerated it and the scholars who sifted through its ashes—focused exclusively on his diet's weight-loss promises. When it suited him, Atkins was happy to oblige such attention because it sold books and raised his public profile, but it also locked him in a tricky double-bind. Atkins's credibility as a weight-loss guru—his only real claim to fame—hinged on his public identity as a practicing cardiologist even though he had not, in actuality, practiced cardiology since shortly after opening his private practice. Yet his cardiological background, ironically, stunted the public reception of Atkins as a practitioner of complementary medicine. It was Atkins's complementary perspective that he most longed to spread because it was the linchpin to the hypoglycemia theory that laid at the heart of his ideology, around which he structured the treatments at his clinic and which fueled his attacks on the medical establishment, but his own success eclipsed his dream.

Atkins served as the major inspiration for contemporary low-carb movements, most notably the Paleolithic and ketogenic trends. His diet revolution is the clear predecessor of both movements—the contents (both consumable and rhetorical) of keto and Paleo reflect traditional ideals of masculinity and Americanness; they draw explicitly from Atkins's articulations of the underlying science of ketosis, his uncritical celebration of animal protein, and the legendary carnivory of exotic or prehistoric tribes; and, as benefactors of Atkins's low-carb popularity, each has been understood as a weight-loss program above all. Importantly, while these dietary movements are Atkins-esque in substance (unlimited portion sizes, rapid weight-loss philosophy, rebellious masculine spirit), they neglect Atkins's broader vision of health freedom. Focusing too intently on Atkins's low-carb structure obscures the diet's roots in medical disillusionment.

Although Atkins's commitment to complementary medicine perhaps bore less fruit than his low-carb program, it was his most cherished endeavor. After Atkins's death, several of his disciples, all physicians Atkins employed at his Center for Complementary Medicine, waged war against one another in a bid to claim this essential piece of his legacy for themselves. Critically, their competition was not centered on taking the low-carb, crash diet crown that made Atkins famous but rather on continuing his emphasis on complementary medicine and his "vital quality to provide a frisson for sophisticated urbanites."[187] Perhaps the best-known spin-off in that regard was Dr. Fred Pescatore's Hamptons diet—a program that rivaled Atkins's in decadence, replete with expensive, monounsaturated macadamia nut oil.[188] Pescatore was Atkins's longest friend; he said his program was faithful to the direction Atkins would have gone had he lived longer—as evident in Atkins's last true diet publication *Atkins for Life* (2003), which showcased that Atkins indeed understood that diets had to be lifelong regimens to offer sustainable health benefits.[189] The Hamptons diet had a worthy adversary in Dr. Keith Berkowitz, Atkins's "heir-apparent," who became the business director of Atkins's clinic after his death and who poached over 200 of former Atkins patients for his own Center for Balanced Health. Pescatore and another Atkins acolyte, Dr. Len Lipson, tried to undermine Berkowitz by opening their own clinic, Partners in Integrative Medicine, on Madison Avenue. As the chairman of the Atkins Physicians Council and the medical director of Atkins Nutritionals, Stuart Trager also sought Atkins's mantle for himself; he kept the Atkins-branded product empire afloat and even continued to publish posthumous diet books in Atkins's name.[190] And Atkins's personal physician and the chief of medicine and director of cardiology at his Manhattan clinic, Patrick Fratellone, spun off yet another clinic in Atkins's image, an integrative cardiology clinic called Fratellone Medical Associates.

We might take a note from those closest to Atkins who understood that the battle over his low-carb diet was a distraction from the grave circumstances facing patients who had been stripped of all hope and therapeutic opportunity. For them, Atkins's wider mission was questioning the standards of evidence by which scientific medicine justified negligence toward dying patients. In Atkins's mind, health was more than just a physical state. Like the National Health Federation, Atkins believed that physical health was only possible through (and thus entailed) a specific legal and political vision of medical freedom. But his holistic idealizations of health did not matter to the medical orthodoxy or his diet rivals, both of whom were only too eager to see Atkins's reputation tarnished so their own pet theories could reign again.

Atkins's friends and family understood that the quixotism of his central mission amounted more or less to his tilting at windmills. His misunderstood yet stalwart defiance of orthodox medicine was appropriately reflected at his memorial service, where the theme was "To Dream the Impossible Dream."[191]

Conclusion

Life, Death, and the Future of Dieting

••

In my own regular daily life, I have never consciously followed any specific nutritional protocols or the recommendations of any diet gurus. Still, I recognize that my life has nevertheless been profoundly shaped by their decades of work. As someone whose vegetarianism was more or less inherited, I have never felt the same zeal or sense of spiritual awakening reported by many of the figures in this book (let alone my parents). But I would still describe my dietary commitments as quasi-religious in nature: comforting and ritualistic.

My plant-forward habitus provides me with a source of subtle community. When I travel abroad, I always go out of my way to seek out meatless establishments, preferably the kind that veg-ify their native cuisines. It pushes me to go places I expect the average tourist does not venture in search of those increasingly globalized markers of like-mindedness, of intercultural acceptedness. People on the veg spectrum experience a special kind of social discrimination; the meat-eating world often turns a cold shoulder to those who, it assumes, think themselves ethically superior. Though I never try to coax others to my way of eating (even when I teach food politics to students), I fully expect to raise my child(ren) according to vegetarian principles. Yet, on the scale of dietary religiosity, I would not consider myself devout—I do not go to church, and I do not pray—but I still claim the secular identity and the attendant cultural practices because it gives my life unique meaning and flavor.

It is ironic though that while finishing this book about the social and cultural dimensions of dietary restrictions, I was made to endure a very different kind of dietary restriction while recovering from major (voluntary) jaw surgery that required my mouth to be wired shut for a month. During that time, I could consume only liquids that had been so thoroughly blended and carefully strained that they could be shot into my cheeks with a syringe or squeeze bottle, then sucked vigorously through my tightly interlocking molars (and around the cumbersome machinery holding them together). Like so many patients in this book, the dietary support I received from the medical orthodoxy to help me through this rather involved recovery process was pitifully inadequate. Whenever I pressed my otherwise competent oral surgeon about what I should do to sustain myself through this ordeal, he directed me to simply stock up on protein drinks like Ensure or Muscle Milk and to expect to lose between twenty-five and forty pounds (a ludicrous amount of weight for my frame) on this feeble regimen.

At the hospital, too, the food I was given was almost laughably inappropriate, as though the staff did not understand the basics of my condition. The kitchen gave me Jell-O that—while a staple of the kind of clear liquid diet I was assigned—was not of a consistency I could physically consume. I was also given zero-calorie (and thus entirely unhelpful) chicken broth powder, which I was apparently supposed to mix in hot water for myself, despite it not being vegetarian and at a time when I could barely manipulate the pen I needed to communicate nonverbally with my nurses. In short, the nutritional care to which I was subjected barely met the definition of either nutrition or care. My experience was not unique: though a select number of hospitals have made substantive efforts to revamp their food service of late, the industry standard still seems to be kitchens caught in a heartless and unimaginative fiscal race to the bottom of food quality.[1]

Thankfully, because of my heterodox upbringing and research interests, I have a higher-than-average nutritional literacy. That, along with the excellent caregiving of my partner, the *New York Times* Cooking app, a powerful blender on its last legs, several variety packs of unexpectedly delicious Soylent, and the recommendations of other "wired-shuts" on social media, we managed to cobble together a homespun routine on which I lost a mere seven pounds. As a fairly young, childless, overeducated white male with no chronic physical ailments, my pre-existing health circumstances and self-empowerment as a patient were about as close to ideal as possible. If this recovery was tough for me to navigate (and it was!), I can only imagine and shudder at the experience of others with multiple magnitudes of greater difficulty. My surgery was—by all accounts—a great success, and after months of recovery I had no major complications and bear no physical scars. However harrowing it felt to me, it is clear that my surgical experience only reflects a tiny kernel of a much more pervasive problem with the care system as the patients in this book repeatedly attested.

The inadequacy of American medical care presents a conundrum with respect to the public perception of the integrity of science writ large. Clearly, the patients in this book were not satisfied with state medicine limiting itself to playing the role of a public-interfacing, for-profit scientific industry that exacts bodily repair only in situations of acute crisis. Consequently, millions of Americans went looking for—and found in diet communities—a richer, humanistic experience where practitioners maintained a more holistic, politically salient yet optimistic vision of human well-being. It is important to recognize that these patients were not necessarily put off by individual orthodox practitioners; many continued to trust their primary care physicians and kept them apprised of their heterodox self-experimentation. Rather, patients were largely driven away by the failures of the system in its totality.

Their experiences remind us that in a public health or preventive medical context where the entire population ostensibly plays the patient, it is imperative to consider the emotional impact of the entire medical system as we might scrutinize an individual practitioner's bedside manner. And, unfortunately, many patients' experiences of the US health care system are still defined more by cold bureaucracy and malevolent financing than by care. Small wonder then that so many Americans have sought to care for themselves with the tools of the market, however inadequate they may be. We seem to know that the system fails regularly and at scale, but still there is a reflex to blame patients for their failures and to deflect the problem away from science and onto allegedly "irrational" human behavior.

The fact that millions of people still follow diet advice from tabloids and social media rather than their physicians signals the persistence of a tremendous rift between the provision of nutritional information and medical services on the one hand and patient expectations on the other. The dieters in this book were unified in their longing for expert advice in nutrition, a void many hoped would be filled by the health care system. By systematically neglecting this essential component of human health maintenance, organized allopathic medicine essentially fueled the public need for the very gurus they decried. And though it can be tempting to write off diet gurus and others who traffic in alternative facts and epistemologies—or those who maintain and live within separate information ecosystems—as dangerously misguided scientific heretics, this kind of public shaming typically only deepens the alienation that vulnerable groups feel toward medicine. As we know from COVID-19, many of medicine's harshest critics are people in dire need of health care, if not for themselves, then for their neighbors.

Assuming—as representatives of the scientific establishment often do— that those inclined toward heterodox ideas are merely bereft of the capacity to understand science or math (and shrieking "Science Is Real!" at them with our yard signs) misses the larger political and cultural underpinnings of medical hesitancy. The fact that during the pandemic we saw nurses, physicians, and pharmaceutical chemists—people who worked inside the system with enough mastery of medical science to have been hired in the first place—quit their jobs over mask and vaccine mandates should blare loudly that science, technology, engineering, and mathematics (STEM) education is not the problem. The specific content of a community's antiscience beliefs is irrelevant—mere window dressing—to the larger sociocultural concerns at the heart of their shared complaints and distrust.

To reckon with the root cause of contemporary medical hesitancy, we need to learn how to better listen to and empathize with the system's deepest skeptics—not to discern the logic of their specific healing beliefs so as to dismantle their closely held theories, nor to compromise scientific or medical values. We should want the public to have a healthy skepticism toward science and power, but to also know when it is appropriate to trust, not just in science but in governments, institutions, and credentialed experts generally. Educating the public in STEM fields will not inoculate against the sociopolitical barriers that underpin most patient skepticism. The wiser choice would be a robust *humanistic* approach that prioritizes patient empowerment through information literacy and an attention to positionality. In this, we can take a page from the guru's playbook.

The Guru's Playbook

How do heterodox healers like diet gurus find such success in a world replete with technological marvels and unceasing scientific innovation? It cannot be as simple as uttering platitudes to the gullible because not every charismatic heretical voice attracts a devoted following. The most successful gurus walk a delicate tightrope between radicalism and orthodoxy. Their ideas must have a certain degree of internal coherence; they must solve a pressing need that people cannot solve on their own and make sense of the world that creates such needs; and they must insist, convincingly, on their own righteousness. To be successful, gurus themselves must hold fast as medical experts loudly impugn their ideas and character and launch powerful legal assaults to counter their every effort at healing. Many do this with no formal training, no infrastructure to guide or safeguard their careers, no robust community of peers, no financial security, and no guarantee of success. Facing long odds, diet gurus must also grapple with the question of how to best prove their credibility and how to demonstrate the efficacy of their programs to their target audiences.

If the patient narratives in this book teach us anything, it is that people who shy away from orthodox medicine are often trying to save themselves and their loved ones from the realization of a specific fear. Alvenia Moody Fulton's community feared medical negligence and racism; George Ohsawa's followers saw looming danger in nuclear war and environmental devastation; a disproportionate number of Pritikinites fretted about the social isolation of physical immobility; Robert Atkins and his patients dreaded the intrusion of governmental regulation into experimental therapies. In a similar vein, underlying contemporary vaccine hesitancy we can see parents who are scared to have children with autism in a country where mental health is stigmatized and where social support for neurodiverse children varies wildly by community. During peak COVID, antimaskers demonstrated a phobia of partisan government control and a felt loss in personal autonomy and liberty. Though their theories or beliefs may not have aligned with science or greater society, health radicals throughout history have demonstrated that they are not necessarily interested in (or capable of) describing or creating a full-fledged and logically consistent alternative medical cosmology. Most just want to solve their immediate concerns.

While identifying problems in US health care is easy, filling gaps in public trust is not. Crafting adequate, actionable, preventive nutritional messaging for the public has been difficult, in large part due to the sheer complexity of nutrition science and the relatively low quality of data from which the major conclusions of nutrition science are derived. The lack of unambiguous experimental evidence has made it hard to craft simple recommendations to prevent chronic disease. Beyond that, the federal government's historical inability to extricate its recommendations—exemplified today by the MyPlate program—from the interests of high-powered lobbying groups has resulted in US Department of Agriculture standards that are simultaneously weak, culturally biased, and difficult to implement.[2] Such impotence erodes trust. Ideally, federal dietary recommendations would reflect the best available scientific evidence, but nutrition studies have had mostly weak, correlative evidence and frequently contradict each other. Scientific uncertainty, corporate lobbying, and sensational reporting have, together, produced bafflingly frequent tectonic shifts in public-facing nutrition advice. The resulting confusion has damaged the credibility of credentialed experts everywhere.[3] And although there have been several attempts at making clearer graphics, more nuanced recommendations, and more accessible guidelines for government programs, these newer messages are nonetheless infused with the same scientific dispassion, corporate corruption, and sense of walking bureaucratic tightropes as those that came before. The dieters featured in this book were largely unmoved and unsupported by such programs, signaling that efforts to induce widespread public behavioral change are likely to be wasted if they rely on well-explained scientific facts alone.

What would happen if we conceptualized science as just one of many ways of knowing through which we can approach the dilemmas of public health, rather than the only or even the most important way? Obviously scientific gatekeeping protects the integrity of its knowledge, but such gatekeeping also erects counterproductive barriers to limit the influence of other potentially valuable forms of expertise. Diet gurus constructed their theories using the same general scientific foundation as orthodox medicine, even though they sometimes interpreted (especially recent) information differently than the scientific community. But gurus were not trying to usurp the production of medical knowledge; they were not creating new diagnoses, identifying new diseases, or in any other way trying to revise medical concepts (again, with the ironic exception of Dr. Atkins). Instead, gurus blended that shared scientific foundation with other time-worn alternative medical techniques and personal experiences to construct actionable programs for the public. And gurus had the distinct advantage of not being bound to the same kinds of institutional disinterestedness as were scientists. Nutrition scientists' claims to objectivity lent them an air of detachment, which in some ways fundamentally limited the warmth, reception, and social utility of scientific knowledge in the public. Perfect is the enemy of good after all.

For the dieters in this book who rightfully mistrusted medical science, diet gurus and other unconventional healers offered a beacon of hope and provided a rich community that better fulfilled their perceived needs as patients. If orthodox medicine sought to outcompete these fringe ideologies, it would need to become a beacon of similar—if not superior—quality. Critically considering what diet gurus offered patients that orthodox medicine did not reveals a number of potential sites for change. Gurus prioritized a preventative approach to health, providing detailed models of affordable (relative to medical care) lifestyle change aimed at preempting, postponing, or even reversing chronic disease. Though it will not immediately boost insurance, pharmaceutical, or hospital profits, prevention rooted in robust public health infrastructure and sustained lifestyle changes remains one of the most humane and cost-effective medical interventions. After all, lessening the patient demand for medical services (especially as the population ages) would relieve some of the strain on the health care system. For the gurus in this book, particularly Fulton, prevention was never about securing perfect patient adherence to a proven diet plan. Their goal was instead encouragement: helping their patients see possibilities for their futures and deepening their patients' dedication to the pursuit of their own health. There's an admittedly fine line between empowering people to take control of their lives, recognizing that the capitalistic system in which such advice is situated is beyond our control, and directly stoking the flames of the neoliberal machine, but it is an important attitudinal difference even if the outcomes are the same.

Beyond making themselves relatable and their ideologies accessible, the gurus I have covered listened closely and carefully to the repeated frustrations their patients voiced about the medical system, and they designed programs that attended to their patients' specific needs and concerns. Yet comparing the followers from different dietary programs illuminates the uniqueness of each guru's audience. The simultaneous success of these four distinct (even contradictory) diet programs demonstrates clearly that even Americans united by medical disillusionment have never been homogeneous in their social or political attitudes—different patient populations respond to different appeals and tactics. These various patient groups did not speak clearly with one voice; many of their demands conflicted. It is unsurprising then that when government scientists privileged a one-size-fits-all model (even a powerful statistical one), it was necessarily unsuitable to the nutritional needs of all Americans.

The tactics that diet gurus have so successfully deployed to motivate preemptive dietary change remain underutilized by orthodox medicine. The entire ideology of scientific medicine rests on the assumption that all human bodies are fundamentally the same and that no matter what patients may say about their subjective experiences, the physical signs of illness inscribed in their bodies represent the objective Truth. These assumptions laid the groundwork for most of the important scientific advances in medicine from the past century and a half. Scientific medicine has equipped physicians with diagnostic equipment so powerful they can interrogate a sick body in complete disregard of patients' self-reported experiences, reducing patients' overall role and power in medical encounters.[4] But medicine's independence from patient voices has strayed too far, creating environments where certain classes of patients cannot be believed, cannot be understood, and cannot be comforted. Patients' individual, subjective experiences of holistic or heterodox care are dismissed with eyerolls as mere placebos—misinformed opinions to be overruled, not exceptions to be accrued and collectively analyzed. Even using the word "mere" to describe the effect of alleged placebos ignores the possibility that physiological mechanisms worthy of medical investigation might underpin this well-established experimental phenomenon in which states of belief apparently influence patient health outcomes. Perhaps this effect could even be harnessed—ethically, of course—by a more compassionate medical science.

The stories of the gurus in this book demonstrate the importance of recognizing that whether patients are inside or outside of medical contexts, they are always embedded in complex cultural environments. Each of these gurus connected with their followers around sets of common cultural values and fought alongside them in the trenches of cultural warfare, in some cases helping to structure the battlegrounds themselves. Their diet programs did not focus solely on the science or economies of eating but embraced the entire experience (and the embedded politics) of procuring, preparing, sharing, and communicating about food. Crucially, these diet gurus did not merely pay lip service to social movements: Fulton and Dick Gregory agitated for civil rights and taught students how to use their bodies in protest; macrobiotics provided the tools for hippies to resist the Cold War and to live in greater harmony with the natural environment; the Pritikin program reinvigorated senior citizens who had been encouraged to give up on their lives; Atkins created spaces where men constrained by gendered expectations of their behavior could feel comfortable performing lifestyle changes perceived to be effeminate. The gurus' attunement to the cultural values and forces at the heart of their patients' experiences was the backbone of their programs, and their tangible contributions to their respective social movements made them all the more persuasive.

The Guru's Journey

In each of the four dietary movements featured in this book, the guru's journey opens with a personal health crisis. For Fulton, it was ulcers and complications from fibroid tumors; for Gregory and Atkins, it was their weight (and the insufferable hunger that accompanied weight loss). Ohsawa contracted tuberculosis and watched helplessly as his entire family was swept away. Nathan Pritikin caught the early warning signs of severe heart disease and later leukemia. When orthodox medical care proved inadequate (or, as with Pritikin's leukemia, created the disease itself), each guru took it upon themselves to conduct independent research. Fulton found enlightenment in the Chicago health lecture circuit, then Gregory found it at Ful-tonia. Ohsawa stumbled across Sagen Ishizuka's dietary manual. Pritikin stole his way into medical conferences and accessed classified military data, then he and Atkins read copiously in medical literature. As they found the answers they sought, each experimented on themselves and found recov-ery in dietary change. In most cases, these figures understood their lives to be at stake, which endowed them with a wellspring of resilience.

Despite the fact that none of the gurus had formal credentials in nutri-tion (recall that Atkins's medical training was in cardiology), they all funded or participated in nutritional studies when given the chance. Gregory sub-mitted himself for study at the Flint-Goodridge Hospital in Louisiana (while Fulton supervised), and he also helped run trials to determine the suitabil-ity of his Formula 4X as a transition food for starving children in Africa. Both Pritikin and Michio Kushi hired their credentialed health worker sons to run studies with and for them. Pritikin and Atkins—unable to secure out-side funding, federal or otherwise—even used their own money to support trials (though Atkins only began funding such trials in the early 2000s).

None of these gurus could claim to have pioneered outright the diets they promoted—they had all clearly borrowed inspiration and ideas from their predecessors. Yet, because these gurus staked their claims to credibility on their personal experiences and self-mastery, the gurus' bodies were made uniquely to stand in as representative of the public body, exemplars onto which innumerable meanings were inscribed. Unlike regular physicians, diet gurus regularly shared intimate, personal medical details and invited their audiences to project concerns with their own bodies onto the gurus' body. Each guru's origin story served as a marker of their dual identity, blurring the distinctions between their public and private life, between their authority as a healer and their commonality as a patient, and be-tween their subjecthood and objecthood.

Because diet gurus occupied this special niche as both authority and pa-tient, they were granted more and different powers than traditional physi-cians. They were also held to different standards of evidence. In the public arena, gurus could resemble celebrities or other public figures in being sub-jected to greater than usual public scrutiny into their habits, their bodies, their self-contradictions, and their lives.[5] Their diets appeared in the same magazines where the idyllic bodies of celebrities were ritually worshiped and dissected, and they became, through a sort of osmosis, celebrities unto themselves. Though none of these gurus posed oily and scantily clad in the pages of the magazines where their work was featured, they were nevertheless judged by their appearance and health. When coverage was positive, it could provide special evidence of the potential healthfulness of their programs. For instance, when images of Dick Gregory's fluctuating weight loss and weight gain appeared in the Black press, it proved a powerful and visible testimonial to the power of Fulton's program. When the coverage was less positive—Atkins's apparent body consciousness in professional photography and on television—media encounters could put substantial pressure on those gurus whose appearance was deemed unfit.

Gurus themselves sometimes perpetuated this social pressure by hurling damaging bodily critiques at one another. During their televised debate, despite being fourteen years older than Atkins, Pritikin insisted to a national audience that he was by far the more handsome and appealing specimen. Pritikin then unabashedly extended his critique to anyone in ketosis, skewering their acetone breath and implying heavy-handedly that they were doomed to die.[6] Pritikin's followers—after seeing his encounter with Atkins—appealed to his vanity; one wrote flatteringly, "I just want you to know that you look a lot better than Dr. Atkins! (That's not saying much because of his fat Humma-Hummas. However, considering he is 20 years younger, it needs to be communicated.)"[7] Such ire was not reserved just for competitors either. Ohsawa launched critiques at public figures whose bodies were misaligned with the principles of macrobiotics; he habitually diagnosed various celebrities and world leaders with being *sanpaku* before making public predictions that they were nearing death.

Beyond their media appearances, gurus were scrutinized especially intensely regarding matters of their personal health and causes of death, a cultural trend that placed a public premium on their medical records. For Fulton, who lived to age ninety-two, and Dick Gregory, eighty-four, this might have been a boon for their credibility—both Fulton and Gregory had lived well beyond the peak of their careers, and their long lives served their followers as proof of the efficacy of their lifestyles. Fulton, who worked at Fultonia until her dying day, bragged about her health relative to her detractors in 1990 (she was then eighty-three) saying, "They all criticized me. . . . They're not now. Either they're in a wheelchair or in a nursing home or walking with a walker. They're not like I am anymore."[8]

For untimely or otherwise suspicious or premature deaths, including those of Ohsawa (seventy-two), Pritikin (sixty-nine), and Atkins (seventy-three), there was a need to protect the guru's and their program's integrity from posthumous claims of fraud or hypocrisy. Ohsawa's heart attack was explained away by his followers as the culmination of his penchant for smoking and the lingering effects of a parasitic infection he had allegedly acquired in Gabon on his trip to meet Albert Schweitzer. Pritikin's suspicious hospital pseudonym and suicide (after it became apparent his leukemia treatment was failing) were forgiven in light of his autopsy, showcasing his immaculate arteries. Longevity was not enough to insulate Michio Kushi from criticism. Despite living to age eighty-eight, Kushi died from pancreatic cancer, for which he—in open contradiction with the core premise of his program—had used orthodox medical treatment.[9] The practice of assessing dietary programs by the quality of the health and life of the leader is not new to this generation of gurus. Organic farming champion Jerome Rodale's reputation took a massive hit when he claimed, during a taping of the *Dick Cavett Show*, that he would live to be 100 years old before suddenly—during that very taping—suffering a fatal heart attack at seventy-two.[10] The same tragic irony also befell the pioneer of America's running culture, Jim Fixx, who suffered a fatal heart attack while jogging at age fifty-two.[11]

Unlike diet gurus, nutrition scientists were much more rarely judged for their bodies, their manners of death, or their life spans. Of course, they were much slower to incorporate their own biographies or their own medical narratives into their nutritional advice, too. Perhaps if they had been more willing to put themselves forward as lifestyle gurus, they would have made effective role models in a similar vein: Fred Stare died at age ninety-two, Bill Darby at eighty-two, and Stare's Harvard colleague Mark Hegsted at ninety-five. Physiologist Ancel Keys, who became somewhat of a guru himself, lived to be 100. It likely never occurred to them to showcase their bodies so openly because to them the technique smacked of quackery; however, their refusal to feature themselves as exemplars certainly made no inroads toward their missions of reinforcing public faith in the industrial food system or decoupling diet and disease risk. Regardless, the fact that diet gurus were judged harshly for their bodies and medical outcomes while nutrition scientists were not speaks to how each group donned the mantle of expertise and to what ends.

Without their figureheads, many of these dietary movements came apart. Macrobiotics still has roots in communities scattered all over the world but has no clear contemporary leadership. The Pritikin Longevity Center and Spa in Miami, Florida, is still operational and covered by Medicare, but it is not well known.[12] Fultonia is gone, but there have been varying attempts, including by an artist group in her West Englewood neighborhood in Chicago, to resurrect and honor her legacy.[13] The Atkins Foundation still purports to educate the public about Atkins's ideas, yet almost immediately after his death they retreated from Atkins's firebrand-esque defense of un-limited meat consumption to emphasize lean cuts instead.[14] Although these activities hardly capture the original energy or intent of their creators, as I signaled at the end of each chapter, the programs' true spirits live on in the other, allied movements they helped inspire.

Dieting in the Digital World

The gurus featured in this book were, in some ways, the first and last of their kind. They were situated at a unique historical juncture between World War II and the end of the millennium, a period of scientific and technologi-cal abundance but not yet oversaturation. As with many other facets of con-temporary life in the new millennium, diets have since spread online where their mythologies are supported by innumerable passionate dieters, bloggers, vloggers, social media influencers, and start-up brands. Atkins was among the first diet gurus with his own website in 1996 (it was little more than a landing page that sold his signature energy bars), but the internet has changed dramatically since then, and the dietary landscape followed suit. The number of new would-be gurus exploded with the accessibility of the internet. The most influential of these live and breathe Twitter (X), Tik-Tok, YouTube, and Instagram.

The older generation of traditional diet gurus tried to adapt their tech-niques to meet the challenges of the Digital Age, too. Though several, like Pritikin-inspired Dr. Michael Greger, have seen breakout success online, countless others have yielded power to their grassroots social networks. It is rarer now for a diet to have a singular leader. Members of the new digital class of "microgurus" instead function as nodes in a broader decentralized network of shared dietary thought and expertise. Like vegetarianism, mi-crogurus in the Paleo, Keto, Whole30, or Whole Foods Plant-Based (WFPB) sects piggyback on one another and promote the same general dietary in-terests. They form community through comments, shout outs, keywords, hashtags, and backlinks. They share each other's advice, make each other's recipes, use the same fonts and color schemes, and use the same styles of food photography. Digital diet communities even go to war together. Ad-herents of the Paleo and WFPB diets, for instance, often skirmish in the com-ment sections of each others' YouTube videos and on Twitter (X). Like Pritikin and Atkins, they are locked in an eternal struggle over which studies to be-lieve, which chemical pathways to emphasize, and who is generally health-ier, fitter, more attractive, or more ethical. Though the formative imprints of the gurus in this book can be clearly seen in these emergent diet cultures, the contemporary dietary landscape has shifted so drastically that to excavate its twenty-first century history would require a rather different methodology than what I have employed here.

Much of the dietary innovation from the past two decades has been driven by the architecture of the digital platforms on which new diet trends are emerging. Not by coincidence, Silicon Valley (and the financial culture that has grown to support it) is a hotbed of bizarre nutritional theories and trends. When Soylent—an unassuming (if gruesomely named) line of meal replacement shakes—first reached the market, it was heralded as "the end of food."[15] Founded on the premise that the problem of human nutrition could be "hacked" (part of the larger trend of "lifehacking" or "biohacking"), Soylent combined crowd-sourced data with the principles of bioengineering to eliminate such inefficiencies of modern life as shopping, cooking, and eating. Unlike other meal replacement shakes, Soylent was initially crowd-funded and later attracted the attention of venture capitalists, who have since helped the company develop an international supply chain.[16] Venture capitalists have also been pouring money into biotech firms to produce such culinary marvels as laboratory-grown meat and the Impossible Burger—the now-ubiquitous faux meat product that duplicates the taste and texture of ground beef and even "bleeds." Not entirely by coincidence, technology icons themselves have developed some unusual dietary predilections. Apple Inc.'s cofounder Steve Jobs was an avid fruitarian (some have even speculated his diet underlaid the fruity namesake of the company); Dave Asprey went from the vice president of cloud security at the cybersecurity firm Trend Micro to the lifestyle guru behind the Bulletproof diet; several early Bitcoin developers were responsible for pioneering the Atkins-esque movement variously called "Zero-Carb," "ZC," or the carnivore diet.[17] Importantly, these developments are not simply a product of technological progression or innovation; rather, they are reflective of the changing value systems driving the adoption of new lifestyles. In the case of Silicon Valley, it seems its peculiar hybrid of environmentalism and hypermasculine productivity culture has driven much of its thinking (and anxiety) about the future of meat eating.

Despite incredible changes in the delivery and propagation of dietary advice, the overlap between alternative medicine and diet in particular is as strong as ever. Even online, diet advice and all manner of heterodox medical therapies still comingle throughout the rising wellness industry via social media and in the blogosphere, picking up radicals from throughout the political spectrum. Diet trends are also still closely allied with exercise trends, as elite athletes and the devotees of the new gym cults, including yoga, rock climbing, CrossFit, and indoor cycling, eagerly share targeted diet tips among themselves. While the twentieth-century-style diet guru may no longer exist at the center of the American dietary ecosystem, budding young diet movements are nevertheless finding new ways to interrogate and renegotiate the meanings, boundaries, and behaviors of the healthy, consuming body.

Acknowledgments

There are many people to whom I owe a debt of gratitude for their support of my work. Foremost among these is my incredible wife Kathleen—there's no thanking you enough for your dedication or support. It is impossible to overstate how critical you were to me and my general sanity, let alone to the actual project. All the hours you spent reading drafts, spreading outlines all over our floors, bailing me out in the archive, and writing in the trenches right alongside me for years on end—I could never ever have done it without you (and Turdle, too).

Thank you next to my parents—for letting me write their story in my own words and for living the perfectionistic lifestyle that inspired this entire project in the first place. Thanks for always supporting my education and pushing me to follow my ideas as far as they can go. If the research material I built my dissertation around hadn't been so personal to me, I don't know if I could have mustered the conviction I needed to finish the damn thing—let alone this book.

I certainly couldn't have done justice to the figures (or "dieteers" as they were almost called) in this book, nor to their quirkiness without the guidance, enthusiasm, encouragement, and general inspiration of my graduate advisor and dissertation supervisor, Sue Lederer. On top of all the academic, logistical, and material support you've given me throughout this project, thank you most of all for teaching me how to find joy in academic writing by digging up all the colorful little details that make for a compelling narrative.

Thank you to all my other academic mentors, advisors, and committee members: Sarah Tracy, Nicole Nelson, Luc Richert, Nan Enstad, Lydia Zepeda, Sally Dwyer-McNulty, and Sandy Gliboff. Thanks to all the faculty and office staff in History of Medicine & Bioethics and History of Science, Medicine and Technology at the University of Wisconsin–Madison. Thanks also to my history of nutrition conference crew and dissertation group members: Emily Hutcheson, Emer Lucey, Molly Laas, Emily Contois, and Andrew Ruis. Thank you to all the patient and talented people who assisted me in finding source material at the various archives and libraries I visited: the California Historical Society, the San Francisco Public Library, the University of California–Los Angeles Special Collections, the University of California–San Francisco Special Collections, the American Medical Association, the Chicago History Museum, the Harold Washington Library, the University of Chicago Special Collections, the Carter Woodson Regional Library, the National Museum of American History, the Countway Library of Medicine Special Collections at Harvard University, the Vanderbilt Special Collections, the Wisconsin Historical Society, and the Brooklyn Historical Society. I especially appreciate the librarians and student aids at the University of Wisconsin–Madison and Marist library systems who assisted me in innumerable ways throughout this project.

The writing and research for this book project was funded by several Vilas Student Research Travel Grants, several conference travel grants from the Associated Students of Madison and the History of Science Society, the Maurice L. Richardson Fellowship, and the University Fellowship at the University of Wisconsin–Madison. Parts of this work were presented at the annual meetings for the American Association for the History of Medicine, the History of Science Society, the Association for the Study of Food and Society, the Graduate Association for Food Studies, and the Midwest Junto for the History of Science where I received invaluable feedback and encouragement. I also presented parts of this work at the Cermes3 Workshop "Health Sciences and the Social" in Paris, France; the Cambridge Body and Food Histories Group Virtual Conference "The Ideal Body"; the Dietary Innovation and Disease conference in Venice, Italy; and at the Aaron and June Gillespie Forum at Marist College. An earlier draft of my chapter on Alvenia Fulton received an honorable mention for the Shryock Medal from the American Association for the History of Medicine. A later version was published in the *Journal of the History of Medicine and Allied Sciences* and received honorable mentions for both the Warren Belasco Prize for Scholarly Excellence from the Association for the Study of Food and Society and the Nursing Clio Prize for Best Journal Article. Thank you to everyone involved.

Last but not least, I owe a steep debt of gratitude to my editor Lucas Church for being so chill and buying into my project right away, to my anonymous reviewers for *JHMAS* and the University of North Carolina Press, who really brought so much clarity and focus to the book, and to Tom Bedenbaugh and the rest of the University of North Carolina Press team. Thank you all.

Notes

Introduction

1. Bernard Jensen and Sylvia Bell, *Tissue Cleansing through Bowel Management* (Escondido, CA: Bernard Jensen Enterprises, 1981).

2. John Alan Schwartz, dir., *Faces of Death*, written by John Alan Schwartz, featuring Michael Carr (n.p., Gorgon Video, 1978), videocassette (VHS), 105 min.

3. Michel Poulain, Anne Herm, and Gianni Pes, "The Blue Zones: areas of exceptional longevity around the world," *Vienna Yearbook of Population Research* 11 (2013): 87–108.

4. Peter N. Stearns, *Fat History: Bodies and Beauty in the Modern West* (New York: New York University Press, 1997); Amy Erdman Farrell, *Fat Shame: Stigma and the Fat Body in American Culture* (New York: New York University Press, 2011).

5. Georges Vigarello, *The Metamorphoses of Fat: A History of Obesity*, trans. C. Jon Delogu (New York: Columbia University Press, 2013); Christopher Forth, *Fat: A Cultural History of the Stuff of Life* (London: Reaktion, 2019); Joan Jacobs Brumberg, *Fasting Girls: The History of Anorexia Nervosa* (New York: Vintage, 2000).

6. Emma McDonnell, "Nutrition Politics in the Quinoa Boom: Connecting Consumer and Producer Nutrition in the Commercialization of Traditional Foods," *International Journal of Food and Nutritional Science* 4, no. 1 (2016): 1–7, https://doi.org/10.15436/2377-0619.16.1212.

7. Harvey Levenstein, *Revolution at the Table: Transformation of the American Diet* (Oxford: Oxford University Press, 1988); Warren Belasco, *Appetite for Change: How the Counterculture Took on the Food Industry* (Ithaca, NY: Cornell University Press, 2007).

8. Data taken from Google N-Gram; Jean-Baptiste Michel et al., "Quantitative Analysis of Culture Using Millions of Digitized Books," *Science* 331, no. 6014 (2010): 176–82.

9. Colleen Derkatch, *Why Wellness Sells: Natural Health in a Pharmaceutical Culture* (Baltimore: Johns Hopkins University Press, 2022), 3.

10. The honorific "guru" has a controversial, if slightly pejorative, history in the United States. The term rose to prominence first in the 1960s with the mass importation of Indian philosophy and lifestyles to the West; the title has been used dismissively, especially by scientists and the intelligentsia, to ridicule Eastern thought. In alternative health circles, however, the term guru is not considered derogatory— "quack" or "faddist" were the terms the alternative health community found offensive. Moreover, "diet guru" is the specific title most commonly deployed by the consumers of diet literature, intended to describe not just a teacher but an

experienced long-term role model who helps motivate and shape lifestyle values as much as impart specific nutritional knowledge. The word guru is still endearingly applied to wellness and fitness experts by their followers, the media, and the experts themselves today. Mariana Caplan, "'Guru' as a Four-Letter Word: Criticisms of Spiritual Teachers, and the Nature of Spiritual Scandals," in *The Guru Question: The Perils and Rewards of Choosing a Spiritual Teacher* (Boulder, CO: Sounds True, 2011), 31–47.

11. George Weisz, *Chronic Disease in the 20th Century: A History* (Baltimore: Johns Hopkins University Press, 2014), 102.

12. Weisz, *Chronic Disease.*

13. Chris Feudtner, *Bittersweet: Diabetes, Insulin, and the Transformation of Illness* (Chapel Hill: The University of North Carolina Press, 2003).

14. Emily K. Abel, *Sick and Tired: An Intimate History of Fatigue* (Chapel Hill: The University of North Carolina Press, 2021), 2.

15. One of Keys's earliest critics was, notably, the Harvard nutrition scientist Fred Stare, who will recur throughout the book. Harry M. Marks, *The Progress of Experiment: Science and Therapeutic Reform in the United States, 1900–1990* (Cambridge: Cambridge University Press, 1997), 183.

16. US Senate Select Committee on Nutrition and Human Needs, *Dietary Goals for the United States* (Washington, DC: US Government Printing Office, February 1977), also known as the McGovern Report.

17. Helen Zoe Veit, *Modern Food, Moral Food: Self-Control, Science, and the Rise of Modern American Eating in the Early Twentieth Century* (Chapel Hill: The University of North Carolina Press, 2013); Nick Cullather, "The Foreign Policy of the Calorie," *American Historical Review* 112, no. 2 (2007) 337–64.

18. For a recent example of this attitude from medical professionals, see Rebecca M. Marton et al., "Science, Advocacy, and Quackery in Nutritional Books: An Analysis of Conflicting Advice and Purported Claims of Nutritional Best-sellers," *Palgrave Communications* 6, no. 43 (2020): 43, https://doi.org/10.1057/s41599-020-0415-6.

19. There has been much attention to personalization in medicine in the past few decades. Within the context of this project, when I use the term *personalization* I do not mean to invoke the contemporary push for data-driven or precision medicine. Instead, I am referring to the ways in which diet gurus harkened back to the kind of tailored approach to healing that was long employed by Hippocratic practitioners and, more recently, other sorts of alternative healers.

20. Even where records have been faithfully preserved, animosity toward alternative healing groups maintains a presence in the archive itself. For example, the American Medical Association maintains one of the only major collections on quackery, which is, suspiciously, their only publicly available collection. The documents housed there were also clearly collected by hostile actors with intent to prosecute rather than preserve. Similarly, when I was conducting research for this project, an archivist at the National Museum of American History, which houses the Michio and Aveline Kushi Collection on macrobiotics, bent down and whispered in my ear, "It's a cult!"

21. By alternative medicine, I do not necessarily mean to imply organized alternative medical sects like naturopathy or homeopathy. Instead, I mean to label those practices beyond the purview of orthodox medicine that could also be labeled popular or vernacular medicine.

22. William Mayo to Morris Fishbein, November 3, 1932, Fishbein, Morris, papers, box 99, folder 9, Hanna Holborn Gray Special Collections Research Center, University of Chicago Library.

Chapter 1

Epigraph: Althea Smith, "A Farewell to Chitterlings: Vegetarianism Is on the Rise among Diet Conscious Blacks," *Ebony*, September 1974, 104–112, 104.

1. This chapter draws from material published previously as Travis A. Weisse, "Alone in a Sea of Rib-Tips": Alvenia Fulton, Natural Health, and the Politics of Soul Food," *Journal of the History of Medicine and Allied Sciences* 74, no. 3 (2019): 292–315, https://doi.org/10.1093/jhmas/jrz028.

2. Clyde Haberman, "Dick Gregory, 84, Dies; Found Humor in the Civil Rights Struggle," *New York Times*, August 19, 2017, www.nytimes.com/2017/08/19/arts/dick -gregory-dies-at-84.html.

3. "Comedians: They Have Overcome," *Time*, February 5, 1965, 100, https:// content.time.com/time/subscriber/article/0,33009,839260,00.html.

4. Adrian Miller, *Soul Food: The Surprising Story of an American Cuisine, One Plate at a Time* (Chapel Hill: The University of North Carolina Press, 2013), 32.

5. Alvenia Fulton, *Radiant Health through Nutrition* (Chicago: Life Line, 1980), 11.

6. Fulton, *Radiant Health*, 11.

7. Sharla M. Fett, *Working Cures: Healing, Health, and Power on Southern Slave Plantations* (Chapel Hill: The University of North Carolina Press, 2002), 63.

8. Wonda L. Fontenot, *Secret Doctors: Ethnomedicine of African Americans* (Westport, CT: Greenwood, 1994), 131.

9. Fulton, *Radiant Health*, 16.

10. Earl Calloway, "Actors Inquire about Healthful Diets from Nutritionist," *Chicago Defender*, December 26, 1974, 16; "County WCTU Meeting Set," *Marion Star* (Ohio), September 23, 1948, 14.

11. Harold M. Mayer and Richard C. Wade, *Chicago: Growth of a Metropolis* (Chicago: University of Chicago Press, 1969), 402.

12. Mayer and Wade, *Chicago*, 406.

13. Jessica B. Harris, *High on the Hog: A Culinary Journey from Africa to America* (London: Bloomsbury, 2012), 202.

14. Laura Miller, *Building Nature's Market: The Business and Politics of Natural Foods* (Chicago: University of Chicago Press, 2017), 91–92.

15. Fulton, *Radiant Health*, 15. Fulton also cited as influential the lectures of Thomas Gains, Howard Inches, Florence McCullum, V. Earl Irons, Lelord Kordel, Victor Lindlahr, Christopher Gurais-Cursio, Henry Shelton, and Joseph Liss.

16. Garnett Cheney, "Rapid Healing of Peptic Ulcers in Patients Receiving Fresh Cabbage Juice," *California Medicine* 70, no. 1 (1949): 10–15; Garnett Cheney, Samuel H.

Waxler, and Ivan J. Miller, "Vitamin U Therapy of Peptic Ulcer: Experience at San Quentin Prison," *California Medicine* 84, no. 1 (1956): 39–42. Vitamin U was the name given to *S*-methylmethionine, which was later discovered not to fit the narrow technical definition of a vitamin.

17. Toni Anthony, "Illness Turns Lady to Field of Nutrition, Health Foods," *Chicago Daily Defender*, November 3, 1969, 4.

18. Fulton, *Radiant Health*, 15.

19. Anthony, "Illness Turns Lady to Field," 4.

20. Dorothea Drew, "Weekly Review of the News," *Chicago Metro News*, January 10, 1976; "Dr. Fulton Opens New Health Store," *Chicago Metro News*, February 12, 1977; Alvenia Fulton, "Notice," advertisement, *Chicago Metro News*, February 5, 1977, 4.

21. Smith, "A Farewell to Chitterlings," 112.

22. "Open House for Health Food Unit," *Chicago Defender*, May 7, 1966, 3; "Health Food Center Sponsors Open House," *Chicago Defender*, June 4, 1966, 21.

23. Robert B. McKersie, *A Decisive Decade: An Insider's View of the Chicago Civil Rights Movement during the 1960s* (Carbondale: Southern Illinois University Press, 2013), 108; Dick Gregory, *Callus on My Soul: A Memoir* (Atlanta: Longstreet, 2000), 121.

24. Gregory, *Callus on my Soul*, 121.

25. After completing the fast, Gregory fasted two more weeks. Dave Potter, "Gregory Starts Eating Again after 54 Days," *Chicago Daily Defender*, January 10, 1968, 3.

26. Gregory, *Callus on My Soul*, 124.

27. Fruitarianism is a diet of mostly fruit. Gregory also speaks admiringly of breatharianism—the alleged ability to live on sunlight—in Dick Gregory, *Dick Gregory's Natural Diet for Folks Who Eat: Cookin' with Mother Nature* (New York: Harper & Row, 1973), 5.

28. Clovis Semmes, "Entrepreneur of Health: Dick Gregory, Black Consciousness, and the Human Potential Movement," *Journal of African American Studies* 16, no. 3 (2012): 537–49, https://doi.org/10.1007/s12111-011-9208-8.

29. "Dick Gregory Ill, but Refuses to Break Fast," *Jet*, July 18, 1968, 6; "Dick Gregory Vows to Fast until All Prisoners Freed," *Jet*, February 22, 1973, 5; "Dick Gregory Endures 40-Day Fast in Support of Michael Jackson," *Jet*, January 26, 2004, 36; "Dick Gregory Prays, Fasts 167 Days to Lose 68 Lbs., Dramatize World Hunger," *Jet*, September 3, 1984, 12.

30. Doris Witt, *Black Hunger: Soul Food and America* (Minneapolis: University of Minnesota Press, 2004), 149.

31. Smith, "Farewell to Chitterlings," 112.

32. Each celebrity's name appears in at least one article about Fulton. Calloway, "Actors Inquire about Healthful Diets"; "Meet Diet Columnist," *Chicago Daily Defender*, May 1, 1971, 24; "Authors on Eating and Health Featured on 'That's Your Opinion,'" *Chicago Metro News*, May 10, 1986, 6; Fultonia Health and Fasting Institute, advertisement, *Chicago Metro News*, June 2, 1984, 2; "Dr. Fulton Conducts 'Health-A-Rama' Seminar," *Chicago Metro News*, June 11, 1983, 1.

33. Anthony, "Illness Turns Lady to Field," 4.

34. Potter, "Gregory Starts Eating Again," 3.

35. Smith, "Farewell to Chitterlings," 110. Adjusted for inflation, the price of such a shot would be equivalent to just over $1,000 in 2024.

36. Calloway, "Actors Inquire about Healthful Diets," 16.

37. Alvenia Fulton, "Eating for Health . . . and Strength," *Chicago Daily Defender*, May 18, 1972, 29; Alvenia Fulton, *The Fasting Primer: The Book That Tells You What You Always Wanted to Know about Fasting* (Chicago: B.C.A. Publishing, 1978), 1.

38. "Why Pet Milk Should Cultivate the Negro Market through the Pages of Ebony Magazine," Johnson Publishing marketing report, February 1962, box 18, folder 2, Ben Burns Collection, Vivian G. Harsh Research Collection, Carter Woodson Regional Library, Chicago, 12.

39. Her main radio show, *The Joy of Living*, broadcast on stations as far away as Los Angeles. Her views on nutrition were featured in major national publications: *Newsweek, Ebony, Cosmopolitan*, the *Chicago Tribune* and the *Chicago Sun Times. Joy of Living* Radio Talk Show, advertisement, *Chicago Metro News*, November 13, 1982, 1; *Joy of Living* Radio Talk Show, advertisement, *Chicago Metro News*, June 16, 1984, 10; "Appreciation Day for Dr. Fulton," *Chicago Metro News*, April 3, 1976, 1.

40. Fulton had interviews around the country on NBC, ABC, and CBS on *Morning Express Cleveland, Sunday Live Baltimore, Alive and Well, Los Angeles*, the *Lu Palmer Show*, and the *Today Show*. Douglas G. Griswold, "Dr. A. Fulton Strives for Nutritional Harmony," *Chicago Defender*, February 22, 1982.

41. In the mid-1970s, Fulton self-published four books, *The Nutrition Bible, Vegetarianism Fact or Myth: Eating to Live, Radiant Health through Nutrition*, and *The Fasting Primer*, and coauthored a book with Dick Gregory, *Dick Gregory's Natural Diet for Folks Who Eat: Cookin' with Mother Nature*.

42. "Local Nutritionist on Tour," *Chicago Defender*, September 11, 1975, 26.

43. "International Women's Year Honors Two Chicago Women," *Chicago Defender*, March 22, 1975, 12; "Howalton Luncheon to Recognize Civic Contributors," *Chicago Defender*, May 26, 1973, 14; Toni Anthony, "Liaison Committee Show Helps Needy Families," *Chicago Daily Defender*, November 29, 1969, 25; "Windy Citians Give a 'Special Valentine' to Dr. Jenkins," *Chicago Defender*, February 27, 1960, 14. The quoted phrase has been the tagline of the *Chicago Metro News* since 1972.

44. "Dr. Fulton Opens New Health Store," *Chicago Metro News*, February 12, 1977, 11; Alvenia Fulton, "Notice," advertisement, *Chicago Metro News*, February 5, 1977, 4.

45. Smith, "Farewell to Chitterlings," 110.

46. Richard Gillum and Kuo Chang Liu, "Coronary Heart Disease Mortality in United States Blacks, 1940–1978: Trends and Unanswered Questions," *American Heart Journal* 108, no. 3 (September 1984): 728–32, https://doi.org/10.1016/0002 -8703(84)90665-3.

47. "Heart Disease Leads in Cause of Death," *Chicago Daily Defender*, October 24, 1960, A6.

48. Gillum and Liu, "Coronary Heart Disease." This apparent absence of women's heart disease has recently been challenged, too. See Cara Kiernan Fallon, "Husbands' Hearts and Women's Health: Gender, Age, and Heart Disease in Twentieth-Century

America," *Bulletin of the History of Medicine* 93, no. 4 (2019): 577–609, https://doi.org/10.1353/bhm.2019.0073.

49. "The Negro and Heart Disease" *Ebony*, December 1962, 125–30, 125.

50. Anne Pollock, *Medicating Race: Heart Disease and Durable Preoccupations with Difference* (Durham, NC: Duke University Press, 2012), 86.

51. Elianne Riska, *Masculinity and Men's Health: Coronary Heart Disease in Medical and Public Discourse* (Lanham, MD: Rowman & Littlefield, 2004), 75.

52. Richard Gillum, "The Epidemiology of Coronary Heart Disease in Blacks," *Journal of the National Medical Association* 77, no. 4 (1985): 282, www.ncbi.nlm.nih.gov/pmc/articles/PMC2561855/.

53. Riska, *Masculinity and Men's Health*, 75.

54. Riska, *Masculinity and Men's Health*, 75.

55. John Hoberman, *Black and Blue: The Origins and Consequences of Medical Racism* (Berkeley: University of California Press, 2012), 101.

56. "The Negro and Heart Disease," 129.

57. Alondra Nelson, *Body and Soul: The Black Panther Party and the Fight against Medical Discrimination* (Minneapolis: University of Minnesota Press, 2011), 9.

58. Pollock, *Medicating Race*, 89.

59. Alvenia Fulton, "The Black Male Drain," *Black X-Press*, June 30, 1973, 15.

60. Audrey T. Weaver, "Faulty Diet Blamed for High Death Rate among Blacks," *The Chicago Courier*, December 17, 1977, 8.

61. Alvenia Fulton, "An Open Letter to Black Women from Dr. Alvenia M. Fulton, Nutritionist," *Word Chatham/South Shore* (Chicago), November 1976.

62. Harvey Levenstein, *Revolution at the Table: Transformation of the American Diet* (Oxford: Oxford University Press, 1988), 178.

63. Ancel Keys and Margaret Keys, *Eat Well and Stay Well* (Garden City, NY: Doubleday, 1959). See also Todd M. Olszewski, "The Causal Conundrum: The Diet-Heart Debates and the Management of Uncertainty in American Medicine," *Journal of the History of Medicine and Allied Sciences*, 70, no. 2 (2015): 218–49; and Ann F. La Berge, "How the Ideology of Low-Fat Conquered America," *Journal of the History of Medicine and Allied Sciences*, 63, no. 2 (2008): 139–77.

64. "The Good Life May Be Killing Us," *Chicago Daily Defender*, January 20, 1968, 20.

65. Miller, *Soul Food*, 41; Tracy N. Poe, "The Origins of Soul Food in Black Urban Identity: Chicago, 1915–1947," *American Studies International* 37, no. 1 (1999): 10, www.jstor.org/stable/41279638.

66. Miller, *Soul Food*, 36.

67. Poe, "Origins of Soul Food," 8.

68. Komozi Woodard, *A Nation within a Nation: Amiri Baraka (LeRoi Jones) and Black Power Politics* (Chapel Hill: University of North Carolina Press, 1999), 32.

69. Elaine Bowen, *Old School Adventures from Englewood—South Side of Chicago* (Chicago: Lulu Publishing Services, 2014), 21. Bowen recalled gatherings at local soul food restaurants on Fulton's block to discuss politics and vote.

70. Fulton, *Radiant Health*, 11.

71. Alvenia Fulton, "Eating for Health . . . and Strength," *Chicago Daily Defender*, June 24, 1971, 28.

72. Miller, *Soul Food*, 46.

73. Janet Shim, *Heart-Sick: The Politics of Risk, Inequality, and Heart Disease* (New York: New York University Press, 2014), 94.

74. Amie Breeze-Harper, "Going Beyond the Normative White 'Post-Racial' Vegan Epistemology," in *Taking Food Public: Redefining Foodways in a Changing World*, ed. Psyche Williams-Forson and Carole Counihan, 155–74 (New York: Routledge, 2012), 166.

75. Frederick Douglass Opie, *Hog and Hominy: Soul Food from Africa to America* (New York: Columbia University Press, 2008), 172.

76. Miller, *Soul Food*, 17.

77. Miller, *Soul Food*, 45.

78. Toni Tipton-Martin, *The Jemima Code: Two Centuries of African American Cookbooks* (Austin: University of Texas Press, 2015), 3.

79. Rebecca Sharpless, *Cooking in Other Women's Kitchens: Domestic Workers in the South, 1865–1960* (Chapel Hill: The University of North Carolina Press, 2010), 31.

80. Tipton-Martin, *Jemima Code*, 2.

81. Opie, *Hog and Hominy*, xi.

82. Frederick Douglass Opie, *Southern Food and Civil Rights: Feeding the Revolution* (Charleston, SC: American Palate, 2017), 89.

83. Sheryl Fitzgerald, "Creating a New American Diet Is Essential," *Chicago Daily News*, December 5, 1977.

84. John T. Edge, *The Potlikker Papers: A Food History of the Modern South* (New York: Penguin, 2017), 72; Doris Witt, "From Fiction to Foodways: Working at the Intersections of African American Literary and Culinary Studies," in *African American Foodways: Explorations of History and Culture*, edited by Anne L. Bower, 101–25 (Urbana: University of Illinois Press, 2007), 115.

85. Alvenia Fulton, "Eating for Health . . . and Strength" *Chicago Daily Defender*, June 24, 1971, 28.

86. L. F. Palmer Jr., "Soul Food with a Mission," *Chicago Daily News*, 1969.

87. Opie, *Hog and Hominy*, 155. Some scholars have subsumed Fulton and Gregory's health reform efforts under other food rebels, many of whom were Fulton's competitors as much as her peers. Religious studies scholar R. Marie Griffith argues Dick Gregory's enthusiasm for fasting and natural foods were derived from the fasting and dietary restrictions set forth by Elijah Muhammad. R. Marie Griffith, *Born Again Bodies: Flesh and Spirit in American Christianity* (Berkeley: University of California Press, 2004), 157. Likewise, literary scholar Doris Witt notes that Fulton regularly ran ads in *Muhammad Speaks*, suggesting Fulton owed an unarticulated intellectual debt to Muhammad as well. Witt, *Black Hunger*, 134. Conversely, an article in the *Defender* suggested that "[Dick Gregory] is just one of the thousands of persons who have benefited from [Fulton's] nutrition regimens. The late Hon. Elijah Muhammed [*sic*] was another." Joy Darrow, "Putting Some of the Myths to

Sleep," *Chicago Defender*, July 29, 1975, 9. Ideologically, though Fulton shared much with other food rebels—especially her reasoning for rejecting soul food and elements of the dietary lifestyle she submitted as a replacement—their actions and attitudes should not be conflated.

88. Opie, *Hog and Hominy*, 159.

89. Elijah Muhammad, *How to Eat to Live* (Atlanta: Elijah Muhammad Propagation Society, 1967); *How to Eat to Live, Book Two* (Chicago: Muhammad's Temple of Islam No. 2, 1972).

90. Elijah Muhammad, "How to Eat to Live: The Deliberate Poisoning of Good Food and Good Drinks by the Avowed Enemy," *Muhammad Speaks*, April 5, 1968.

91. Opie, *Southern Food and Civil Rights*, 143; Mary Potorti, "Eat to Live: Culinary Nationalism and Black Capitalism in Elijah Muhammad's Nation of Islam," in *New Perspectives on the Nation of Islam*, ed. Dawn Marie Gibson and Herbert Berg, 68–94 (New York: Routledge, 2017).

92. Edward E. Curtis IV, *Black Muslim Religion in the Nation of Islam, 1960–1975* (Chapel Hill: The University of North Carolina Press, 2006), 191.

93. Margarite Fernández Olmos and Lisabeth Paravisini-Gebert, *Creole Religions of the Caribbean: An Introduction from Vodou and Santeria to Obeah and Espiritismo* (New York: New York University Press, 2011), 197.

94. Tonde Lumumba, oral history interview conducted by Monica Parfait et al., March 22, 2010, Crown Heights History Project, 2010.020, Brooklyn Historical Society. Also see Randy Kandel et al., "Diet and Acculturation: The Case of Black-American Immigrants," in *Nutritional Anthropology*, ed. Norge W. Jerome, Gretel H. Pelto, and Randy F. Kandel, 275–324 (New York: Redgrave, 1979).

95. Harris, *High on the Hog*, 214. Vertamae Smart-Grosvenor, *Vibration Cooking, or, the Travel Notes of a Geechee Girl* (1970; repr., Athens, GA: University of Georgia Press, 2001); Helen Mendes, *The African Heritage Cookbook* (New York: Macmillan, 1971).

96. William L. Van Deburg, *New Day in Babylon: The Black Power Movement and American Culture, 1965–1975* (Chicago: University of Chicago Press, 1992), 168.

97. Dave Hoekstra, *The People's Place: Soul Food Restaurants and Reminiscences from the Civil Rights Era to Today* (Chicago: Chicago Review Press, 2015), 206–7.

98. Opie, *Hog and Hominy*, 170.

99. Black studies scholar Clovis Semmes locates Fulton's program (via Dick Gregory) within the broader Human Potential Movement, which he argues strove to raise Black consciousness about the power of the body as revealed through natural healing and self-discipline. Semmes, "Entrepreneur of Health."

100. Miller, *Building Nature's Market*, 16–17.

101. Potter, "Gregory Starts Eating Again," 3.

102. "Meet Diet Columnist," 24.

103. Fulton, *Radiant Health*, 15–24; Anthony, "Illness Turns Lady to Field," 4. An ND is a doctor of naturopathy, which was a formally recognized degree in several US states until the 1950s. Fulton may not have actually been the first African Amer-

ican with an ND. See Susan Cayleff, *Nature's Path: A History of Naturopathic Healing in America* (Baltimore: Johns Hopkins University Press, 2016), 362.

104. "Dr. Fulton to Keynote Health Fed. Dinner," *Chicago Metro News*, May 31, 1980, 1; Lee Paige, "World Reknown Nutritionist Speaks Out," *Chicago Metro News*, February 9, 1980, 1.

105. Cayleff, *Nature's Path*, 223.

106. Cayleff, *Nature's Path*, 249.

107. Roxane Arnold, "Vitamin King: To Critics, He's a Quack, but Kurt Donsbach Has Built a Multimillion-Dollar Empire Pushing Value of Nutrition," *Los Angeles Times*, July 12, 1982, B3.

108. Stephen Barrett and William T. Jarvis, eds., *The Health Robbers: A Close Look at Quackery in America* (Buffalo, NY: Prometheus, 1993).

109. Katherine Bouton, "Wrapped in Data and Diplomas, It's Still Snake Oil," *New York Times*, November 2, 2010, D4, www.nytimes.com/2010/11/02/science/02scibks .html.

110. Weaver, "Faulty Diet Blamed," 8.

111. For two late examples of Fulton's innovation, including super blue-green algae and computerized nutrition assessments, see "Is Super Algae the Food for '90s?" *Janesville Gazette*, March 13, 1990, 2C; and Fultonia Health and Fasting Institute, advertisement, *Chicago Metro News*, May 17, 1980, 12.

112. Illinois General Assembly, House Resolution 130, *House Journal, House of Representatives*, Ninety-First General Assembly, 27th Legislative Day, Tuesday, March 16, 1999.

113. "Nutritionist Fulton Featured at Ritz Carlton," *Chicago Metro News*, April 12, 1980, 1; "Dr. Fulton to Keynote Health Fed. Dinner."

114. Griffith, *Born Again Bodies*, 117; Catherine Carstairs, "The Granola High: Eating Differently in the Late 1960s and 1970s," in *Edible Histories, Cultural Politics: Towards a Canadian Food History*, ed. Franca Iacovetta, Valerie J. Korinek, and Marlene Epp, 305–25 (Toronto: University of Toronto Press, 2012).

115. Melanie DuPuis, *Dangerous Digestion: The Politics of American Dietary Advice* (Oakland: University of California Press, 2015); Helen Zoe Veit, *Modern Food, Moral Food: Self-Control, Science, and the Rise of Modern American Eating in the Early Twentieth Century* (Chapel Hill: The University of North Carolina Press, 2013); Charlotte Biltekoff, *Eating Right in America: The Cultural Politics of Food and Health* (Durham, NC: Duke University Press, 2013).

116. Fulton, *Radiant Health*, 15.

117. Fulton, *Radiant Health*, 31.

118. See Gregory, *Dick Gregory's Natural Diet*; Gregory, *Callus on My Soul*; Dick Gregory, *Nigger: An Autobiography by Dick Gregory with Robert Lipsyte* (New York: E. P. Dutton, 1964). It is difficult to know whether it is intentional or coincidental that Formula 4X mimics the scheme by which members of the Nation of Islam adopted new names after their conversion.

119. Victoria Mucie, ". . . But by Prayer and Fasting," *Chicago Metro News*, January 31, 1976.

120. "An Option to Consider," editorial, *Wichita Eagle* (Kansas), May 29, 1976.

121. Gregory, *Callus on My Soul*, 187–91.

122. Notably, Habte also later served as the first president of the Ethiopian Academy of Sciences.

123. "Ethiopia Calls for Widespread Use of Gregory's Nutritional Formula to Restore Malnourished Youth," press release, April 21, 1985, series III, box 1, folder 6, William Jefferson Darby Papers, Eskind Biomedical Library Manuscripts Collection, Vanderbilt University (hereafter cited as Darby Papers); "Dick Gregory Delivers His Nutritional Formula to Starving Ethiopians," *Jet*, May 13, 1985, 11; "Dick Gregory's Formula to Be Used All Over Ethiopia Following Successful Tests," *Jet*, May 27, 1985, 13.

124. Berhane Deressa to Dick Gregory, April 15, 1985, series III, box 1, folder 6, Darby Papers.

125. Gregory, *Callus on My Soul*, 153.

126. Jeannine Stein, "Through Thick and Thin: Dick Gregory Has a Weight-Loss Plan That's Highly Controversial, but His Faithful Clients See It as a Last, Best Hope," *Los Angeles Times*, February 17, 1989, 1.

127. Semmes, "Entrepreneur of Health," 546; James Carter to William Jefferson Darby, June 20, 1985, series III, box 1, folder 6, Darby Papers. Cernitin was a subsidiary of the Swedish health food company A. B. Cernelle, which was founded in the 1950s and run by Dr. David Allen. A. B. Cernelle was best known for selling bee pollen supplements for prostate health. A. B. Cernelle was run by (principal medical and research advisor) Olov Lindahl, a professor of orthopedic surgery and founder of the *Swedish Journal of Biological Medicine*.

128. Gregory, *Callus on My Soul*, 224.

129. Gregory tried to offer Correction Connection to Marvin Gaye to help with his drug problem, but Gaye reportedly refused his help.

130. Before this grand empire even began, Gregory's business partners and he had a falling out. In 1988, Gregory's cofounders Larry Depte and Sandra Henderson sued him for control of the company. Gregory eventually prevailed in court three years later, but this was too late: Gregory lost his house, and the company's potential had already run dry. The formula was never sold again. "Dick Gregory Finds Business Dispute No Laughing Matter," *United Press International*, October 18, 1988, www.upi.com/Archives/1988/10/18/Dick-Gregory-finds-business-dispute-no-laughing-matter/7710593150400/; "Gregory Regains Control of Diet Formula Business," *Buffalo News* (New York), October 27, 1991, https://buffalonews.com/1991/10/27/gregory-regains-control-of-diet-formula-business/.

131. Semmes, "Entrepreneur of Health," 546.

132. Around the same time, Gregory also reportedly tried to buy a cruise ship to serve as a floating weight loss resort.

133. Marjorie Williams, "Gregory's Gathering," *Washington Post*, June 23, 1988, www.washingtonpost.com/archive/lifestyle/1988/06/23/gregorys-gathering/ed2907e1-7cf4-4f8c-b38d-2deb2dc04d3d/.

134. "Gregory Diet Center Unsafe, Report Says," *United Press International*, July 25, 1989, www.upi.com/Archives/1989/07/25/Gregory-diet-center-unsafe-report -says/5125617342400/.

135. Stein, "Through Thick and Thin," 1.

136. Stein, "Through Thick and Thin," 1.

137. Stein, "Through Thick and Thin," 1.

138. Luis C. Rodrigues, "White Normativity, Animal Advocacy, and PETA's Campaigns," *Ethnicities* 20, no. 1 (2019): 71–92; Breeze-Harper, "Going Beyond the Normative," 157.

139. Cass R. Sunstein, "The Rights of Animals," *University of Chicago Law Review* 70, no. 1 (2003): 387–401, https://chicagounbound.uchicago.edu/uclrev/vol70/iss1 /25; Brycchan Carey, "Abolishing Cruelty: The Concurrent Growth of Anti-Slavery and Animal Welfare Sentiment in British and Colonial Literature," *Journal for Eighteenth-Century Studies* 43 (2020): 203–20, https://doi.org/10.1111/1754-0208.12686.

140. Ellen Bring, "Moving Toward Coexistence: An Interview with Alice Walker," *Animals' Agenda* 8, no. 3 (1988): 6–9; Jon Hochschartner, "Vegan Angela Davis Connects Human and Animal Liberation," *Counterpunch*, January 24, 2014, www .counterpunch.org/2014/01/24/vegan-angela-davis-connects-human-and-animal -liberation/; Wesleyan University, "The Legacy of and Memorial to Dr. King," *Wesleyan University*, www.wesleyan.edu/mlk/posters/legacy.html.

141. Breeze-Harper, "Going Beyond the Normative"; Tracye McQuirter, "This Civil Rights Activist Is the Reason I've Been Vegan for 30 Years" *Bon Appetit*, September 1, 2017, www.bonappetit.com/story/dick-gregory-vegan-civil-rights; Tracye Lynn McQuirter, *By Any Greens Necessary: A Revolutionary Guide for Black Women Who Want to Eat Great, Get Healthy, Lose Weight, and Look Phat* (Chicago: Lawrence Hill, 2017); Queen Afua, *Sacred Woman: A Guide to Healing the Feminine Body, Mind, and Spirit* (New York: Random House, 2000).

142. Laura Reiley, "The Fastest-Growing Vegan Demographic Is African Americans. Wu-tang Clan and Other Hip-Hop Acts Paved the Way," *Washington Post*, January 24, 2020, www.washingtonpost.com/business/2020/01/24/fastest-growing -vegan-demographic-is-african-americans-wu-tang-clan-other-hip-hop-acts-paved -way/.

143. Opie, *Hog and Hominy*, 137.

144. Alvenia Fulton, "Eating for Health . . . and Strength," *Chicago Defender*, June 17, 1971, 24; Alvenia Fulton, "Eating for Health . . . and Strength," *Chicago Defender*, July 1, 1971, 24; Alvenia Fulton, "Eating for Health . . . and Strength," *Chicago Defender*, June 3, 1971, 24; Alvenia Fulton, "Eating for Health . . . and Strength," *Chicago Defender*, October 28, 1971, 32.

Entremets I

1. Nick Cullather, "American Pie: The Imperialism of the Calorie," *History Today* 57, no. 2 (February 2007): 34–40, www.historytoday.com/archive/american-pie -imperialism-calorie.

2. As part of American war propaganda, civilians were urged to ration wheat (so it could be sent to starving and war-torn Europe) and to plant victory gardens (so they could eat more to keep strong, patriotic bodies while not parasitizing the food system).

3. Lulu Hunt Peters, *Diet and Health with Key to the Calories* (Chicago: Reilly and Lee, 1918), 110.

4. Chin Jou, "The Progressive Era Body Project: Calorie-Counting and 'Disciplining the Stomach' in 1920s America," *Journal of the Gilded Age and Progressive Era* 18, no. 4 (2019): 422–40, 423, https://doi.org/0.1017/S1537781418000348.

5. Perhaps the best evidence of nutrition scientists maintaining focus on issues of hunger and malnutrition rather than the chronic disease and obesity more characteristic of late-twentieth century America is the trajectory of the Senate Select Committee on Nutrition and Human Needs. The committee, chaired by George McGovern (D-South Dakota), was assembled in 1968 to investigate the problem of malnutrition and hunger in the United States, having been spurred into action by the shocking May 21, 1968, CBS exposé, "CBS Reports: Hunger in America" ("Hunger in America: The 1968 CBS Documentary That Shocked America," May 21, 2018, https://www.cbsnews.com/video/hunger-in-america-the-1968-cbs-documentary -that-shocked-america/). After several years of investigation into American hunger, McGovern's subcommittee performed an about-face to investigate the problems with false nutritional advice, overnutrition, obesity, and chronic disease instead. After five more years of testimony from 1973–77, the Senate Select Subcommittee published what came to be known as the McGovern Report, the first federal document to proclaim a relationship between diet and disease. United States Senate Select Committee on Nutrition and Human Needs, Dietary Goals for the United States (Washington, DC: US Government Printing Office, February 1977).

6. Andrew N. Case, "Looking for Organic America: J. I. Rodale, the Rodale Press, and the Popular Culture of Environmentalism in the Postwar United States" (PhD diss., University of Wisconsin–Madison, 2012), ProQuest books and Theses Global (3509898).

7. Lynn K. Nyhart, "Home Economists in the Hospital, 1900–1930," in *Rethinking Home Economics: Women and the History of a Profession*, ed. Sarah Stage and Virginia B. Vincenti, 125–44 (New York: Cornell University Press, 1997).

8. This tradition dates back to Sylvester Graham himself who warned against the dangers of industrial food production on the devitalization of essential foods.

Chapter 2

Epigraph: Robert Christgau, "Beth Ann and Macrobioticism," *New York Herald Tribune,* January 23, 1966, 10–15.

1. Paul Sherlock and Edmund O. Rothschild, "Scurvy Produced by a Zen Macrobiotic Diet," *Journal of the American Medical Association* 199, no. 11 (1967): 794–98, https://doi.org/10.1001/jama.1967.03120110066009.

2. Karlyn Crowley, "'Gender on a Plate': The Calibration of Identity in American Macrobiotics," *Gastronomica* 2, no. 3 (Summer 2002): 37–48, https://doi.org/10.1525

/gfc.2002.2.3.37; William Shurtleff and Akiko Aoyagi, *History of Tofu and Tofu Products (965 C.E. to 2013)* (Lafayette, CA: Soyinfo Center, 2013), 3266.

3. William Shurtleff and Akiko Aoyagi, *History of Macrobiotics (1715–2017)* (Lafayette, CA: Soyinfo Center, 2017), 9. Georges Ohsawa, *Zen Macrobiotics: The Art of Rejuvenation and Longevity*, rev. ed., ed. Lou Oles (Los Angeles: Ohsawa Foundation, 1965); and *The Book of Judgment: Philosophy of Macrobiotics*, 5th ed. (Los Angeles: Ohsawa Foundation, 1966).

4. Herman Aihara, *Basic Macrobiotics* (Oroville, CA: George Ohsawa Macrobiotic Foundation, 1998), 29.

5. George Alexander, "Brown Rice as a Way of Life," *New York Times*, March 12, 1972, 87, www.nytimes.com/1972/03/12/archives/brown-rice-as-a-way-of-life-brown-rice.html.

6. Ohsawa, *Zen Macrobiotics*. The original 1960 edition only existed in mimeographed form and is difficult to locate.

7. Fred Stare, "The Zen Macrobiotic Diet," p. 2, statement prepared for Harvard University Health Services, n.d., box 17, folder 3, Mark Hegsted Papers, Center for the History of Medicine Repository, Francis A. Countway Library of Medicine, Harvard University (hereafter cited as Hegsted Papers).

8. FDA Press Release, June 2, 1966, box 17, folder 3, Hegsted Papers.

9. Alexander, "Brown Rice," 87.

10. FDA Press Release; Walter Alvarez, "Zen Diet Termed Health Risk," *Los Angeles Times*, February 8, 1973, J8.

11. FDA Press Release.

12. William Shurtleff and Akiko Aoyagi, *History of Soybeans and Soyfoods in Southeast Asia (13th Century to 2010)* (Lafayette, CA: Soyinfo Center, 2010), 645. Some macrobiotic loyalists also blamed Ohsawa's death on the filarial parasites he apparently contracted during his stay with Albert Schweitzer in Lambarene, Gabon, in the mid-1950s.

13. Susan E. Lederer, "Darkened by the Shadow of the Atom: Burn Research in 1950s America," in *Man, Medicine, and the State: The Human Body as an Object of Government Sponsored Medical Research in the 20th Century*, ed. Wolfgang Uwe Eckart, 263–78 (Stuttgart: Franz Steiner Verlag, 2006).

14. George (or Georges) Ohsawa's Japanese name was sometimes reported as Yukikazu Sakurazawa, Sakurazawa Jyoichi, Nyoiti or Nyoichi Sakurazawa, and Musagendo Sakurazawa.

15. Shurtleff and Aoyagi, *History of Macrobiotics*, 9. The term "macrobiotics" actually had some scattered earlier uses in the West, but while the term generally denoted the same "long life" concept and perhaps captured some superficial similarities, the way it was used by these Western predecessors did not signal an attention to *shoku-yo* philosophy per se.

16. Ishizuka's next text, *Shokumotsu Yojoho: Ichimei Kagakuteki Shoku-yo Taishin-ron* (A Method of Nourishing Life through Food: A Unique Chemical Food Nourishment Theory of Body and Mind), was a practical guide to his earlier work and gained widespread distribution in Japan, going through twenty-three editions. Ronald Ernst Kotzsch, "Georges Ohsawa and the Japanese Religious Tradition" (PhD

diss., Harvard University, 1981) ProQuest Dissertations and Theses Global (0354664), 50.

17. Ronald Kotzsch, "Understanding Macrobiotics," *Vegetarian Times*, April 1986, 15–18; Kotzsch, "Georges Ohsawa," 47.

18. Despite his insistence on brown rice, there is no evidence that Ishizuka understood the connection between rice husks and beriberi. Ishizuka's challenge to the historical self-conception of the Japanese, however, has been supported by more recent scholarship. See Emiko Ohnuki-Tierney, *Rice as Self: Japanese Identities through Time* (Princeton, NJ: Princeton University Press, 2001).

19. Ishizuka's insistence that people from a given region could only attain optimal health by eating foods specific to that region presents a strong parallel to the humoralist tradition in the West. See Rebecca Earle, *The Body of the Conquistador: Food, Race and the Colonial Experience in Spanish America, 1492–1700* (Cambridge: Cambridge University Press, 2012); Trudy Eden, "Food, Assimilation and the Malleability of the Human Body in Early Virginia," in *A Center of Wonders: The Body in Early America*, ed. Janet Lindman and Michele Tarter, 29–42 (Ithaca, NY: Cornell University Press, 2001).

20. Kotzsch, "Georges Ohsawa," 54.

21. Kotzsch, "Georges Ohsawa," 63.

22. Ishizuka's 3:7 sodium/potassium ratio is strikingly similar to Ohsawa's recommended 5:1 ratio between yin and yang foods because Ohsawa appropriated Ishizuka's mineral ratio to describe his own yin/yang dichotomy when formulating macrobiotics. In Ohsawa's system, potassium was yin, and sodium was yang. The ratios were not identical, however, because potassium and sodium were not the only factors to consider when determining a food's relative yin or yang value.

23. Kotzsch, "Georges Ohsawa," 11.

24. Kotzsch, "Georges Ohsawa," 47.

25. Shurtleff and Aoyagi, *History of Macrobiotics*, 412.

26. Ronald E. Kotzsch, *Macrobiotics: Yesterday and Today* (New York: Japan Publications, 1985), 106.

27. It was as ambassadors to the World Federalist Movement/World Government Association that Michio and his soon-to-be wife, Aveline (born Tomoko Yokoyama), met as Ohsawa's students. Printed copy of "About Us" page from Kushi Institute website, June 16, 2006, box 60, folder 1, Michio and Aveline Kushi Macrobiotics Collection, Archives Center, National Museum of American History (hereafter cited as Kushi Collection).

28. William Shurtleff and Akiko Aoyagi, *History of Erewhon: Natural Foods Pioneer in the United States (1966–2011)* (Lafayette, CA: Soyinfo Center, 2011), pp. 22, 144, 194.

29. Kotzsch, *Macrobiotics*, 107.

30. Michael K. Masatsugu, "'Bonded by Reverence toward the Buddha': Asian Decolonization, Japanese Americans, and the Making of the Buddhist World, 1947–1965," *Journal of Global History* 8 (2013): 142–64, 153, https://doi.org/10.1017/S174002 2813000089.

31. Kotzsch, "Georges Ohsawa," 238.

32. Kotzsch, *Macrobiotics*, 166.

33. Kotzsch, *Macrobiotics*, 166.

34. Sawako Hiraga, "How I Survived the Atomic Bomb," trans. Herman Aihara, *Macrobiotics Today*, June 1986, 7.

35. Jonathan Kauffman, *Hippie Food: How Back-to-the-Landers, Longhairs, and Revolutionaries Changed the Way We Eat* (New York: William Morrow, 2018), 58–59.

36. Kotzsch, *Macrobiotics*, 167.

37. Warren Belasco, *Appetite for Change: How the Counterculture Took on the Food Industry* (Ithaca, NY: Cornell University Press, 2007), 56.

38. Alexander, "Brown Rice," 87.

39. Alexander, "Brown Rice," 87, Crowley, "Gender on a Plate," 37–48.

40. Mary Daniels, "A Loaf of Whole-Grain Bread, a Jug of Bancha and Thou," *Chicago Tribune*, August 1, 1971, F18.

41. Carl Ferre, "From Tragedy to Happiness: The Origins of West Coast Macrobiotics, Part 3," *Macrobiotics Today*, November–December 2011, 25–28. One man reportedly even used LSD to derive key macrobiotic principles independently; he tasted brown rice while tripping and suddenly concluded that it was the best food possible.

42. Daniels, "Loaf of Whole-Grain Bread," F18.

43. Jane Iwamura, *Virtual Orientalism: Asian Religions and American Popular Culture* (Oxford: Oxford University Press, 2011), 5.

44. Michael K. Masatsugu, "'Beyond This World of Transiency and Impermanence': Japanese Americans, Dharma Bums, and the Making of American Buddhism during the Early Cold War Years," *Pacific Historical Review* 77, no. 3 (2008): 423–51, 438, https://doi.org/10.1525/phr.2008.77.3.423.

45. Masatsugu, "Beyond This World," 440.

46. Mark Lewis Taylor, "Oriental Monk as Popular Icon: On the Power of U.S. Orientalism," *Journal of the American Academy of Religion* 79, no. 3 (2011): 735–46, https://doi.org/10.1093/jaarel/lfr014.

47. Iwamura, *Virtual Orientalism*, 19.

48. Tom Monte, *The Way of Hope: Michio Kushi's Anti-AIDS Program* (New York: Grand Central Publishing, 1990), 61.

49. Fred Stare, "The Zen Macrobiotic Diet," statement prepared for Harvard University Health Services, n.d., p. 2, box 17, folder 3, Hegsted Papers.

50. Stare, "Zen Macrobiotic Diet," Hegsted Papers.

51. Alvarez, "Zen Diet Termed Health Risk," J8.

52. Stare, "The Zen Macrobiotic Diet," Hegsted Papers.

53. Daniels, "Loaf of Whole-Grain Bread,," F18; Ronald Kotzsch, "Macrobiotics: Yesterday and Today," *MacroMuse*, October 1985, 28.

54. Eugen Herrigel, *Zen and the Art of Archery*, trans. Richard F. C. Hull (London: Routledge & Kegan Paul, 1953), first published in German in 1948. Herrigel's book eventually spurred dozens of copycats, including Robert Pirsig's 1974 classic *Zen and the Art of Motorcycle Maintenance: An Inquiry into Values* (New York: William Morrow).

55. Stare, "Zen Macrobiotic Diet," Hegsted Papers.

56. Patricia Wells, "Diet Is More Than Brown Rice," *Chicago Tribune*, July 25, 1978, A1.

57. Julian Wasser, "Modern Living: The Kosher of the Counterculture," *Time*, November 16, 1970, https://content.time.com/time/magazine/article/0,9171,904481,00.html; Alexander, "Brown Rice," 87.

58. Christgau, "Beth Ann and Macrobioticism," 10–15. Among the drugs they used were "hashish, cocaine, heroin, amphetamine, LSD and DMT."

59. Sakurazawa Nyoiti [George Ohsawa], *You Are All Sanpaku*, trans. William Dufty (Hyde Park, NY: University Books, 1965).

60. Alexander, "Brown Rice," 87. The term *sanpaku* had been featured in mass media before the *New York Times* picked it up, though its spread was limited. Other demises predicted by or ascribed to the sanpaku principle included those of Marilyn Monroe, Abraham Lincoln, Julius Caesar, Adolf Hitler, and Princess Diana. See Don Bell, "Ohsawa and the Yin and Yang of Health," *Chicago Tribune*, August 1, 1971, F23; Jane Trahey, "The Grain to Sanpaku," *Harper's Bazaar*, August 1966, 61–62.

61. Other celebrity followers included musicians John Lennon, Yoko Ono, and John Denver, actors Dirk Benedict, Peter Fonda, and Rod Serling, celebrity promoter Earl Blackwell, and theatrical producer Michael Butler. Daniels, "Loaf of Whole-Grain Bread," F18; John David Mann, "Myths of Macrobiotics," *Solstice*, Summer 1989, pp. 20–35, box 80, folder 11, Kushi Collection.

62. Annemarie Colbin, "Interview with Irma Paule: February 9, 2002," *Macrobiotics Today*, March/April 2003, 10–13.

63. Colbin, "Interview with Irma Paule," 10–13.

64. Christgau, "Beth Ann and Macrobioticism," 10–15.

65. Christgau, "Beth Ann and Macrobioticism," 10–15.

66. Though Paule had been an important early figure for Ohsawa's transition into the American market, her role was significantly diminished after he passed away. When her office was raided, Paule reported having been largely abandoned by the other macrobiotics' leaders and devotees, who kept their heads down—a move she credited with her eventual disenchantment with the movement. Colbin, "Interview with Irma Paule," 10–13.

67. Monte, *Way of Hope*, 59.

68. Shurtleff and Aoyagi, *History of Macrobiotics*, 599. R.H. stood for Resurrection of Humanity.

69. Gloria Emerson, "Japanese Specialty Store to Open on Fifth Avenue," *New York Times*, June 27, 1958, 22, www.nytimes.com/1958/06/27/archives/japanese-specialty-store-to-open-on-fifth-avenue.html.

70. Lawrence Kushi et al., "The Macrobiotic Diet in Cancer," *Journal of Nutrition*, 131, no. 11 (2001): 3056S–3064S, https://doi.org/10.1093/jn/131.11.3056S.

71. For more information regarding macrobiotics' domination of the health food industry, see Belasco, *Appetite for Change*; Laura J. Miller, *Building Nature's Market: The Business and Politics of Natural Foods* (Chicago: University of Chicago Press, 2017); Kauffman, *Hippie Food*.

72. The company took the name from Ohsawa's favorite book, the Samuel Butler novel of the same name. The word itself is an anagram of the word "nowhere," spelled (almost) backward.

73. Monte, *Way of Hope*, 66. Monte says Erewhon was eventually passed off to the Kushis' students, before going bankrupt in 1983. Chico-San was eventually bought by Heinz.

74. Anthony J. Sattilaro and Tom Monte, *Recalled by Life* (New York: Avon, 1982), 180.

75. Jack Raso, "Vitalistic Gurus and Their Legacies," in *The Health Robbers: A Close Look at Quackery in America*, ed. Stephen Barrett and William T. Jarvis, 236–40 (Buffalo, NY: Prometheus, 1993), 227.

76. Alvarez, "Zen Diet Termed Health Risk," J8.

77. Kotzsch, "Macrobiotics Yesterday and Today," 28.

78. Hiraga, "How I Survived the Atomic Bomb," 7; Michio Kushi and Robert S. Mendelsohn, *Cancer and Heart Disease: The Macrobiotic Approach to Degenerative Disorders*, ed. Edward Esko (Tokyo: Japan Publications, 1982), 192.

79. Yuki Miyamoto, "Unbearable Light/ness of the Bombing: Normalizing Violence and Banalizing the Horror of the Atomic Bomb Experiences," *Critical Military Studies* 1, no. 2 (2015): 116–30, https://doi.org/10.1080/23337486.2015.1050268.

80. Tatsuichiro Akizuki, *Nagasaki 1945: The First Full-length Eyewitness Account of the Atomic Bomb Attack on Nagasaki*, ed. Gordon Honeycombe, trans. Keiichi Nagata (New York: Quartet, 1981). Akizuki was also the author of *Health Condition and Diet/Constitution and Food: A/The Way to Health*, trans. Hiroko Furo, August 29, 2009, https://yufoundation.org/pdfs/akizuki.pdf.

81. Susan Southard, *Nagasaki: Life After Nuclear War* (New York: Viking 2015).

82. Lorenz K. Schaller, review of *Nagasaki: Life After Nuclear War* by Susan Southard, in Shurtleff and Aoyagi, *History of Macrobiotics*, 1118–20.

83. Alexandra Dundas Todd, *Double Vision: An East-West Collaboration for Coping with Cancer* (Hanover, NH: University Press of New England, 1994); Michio Kushi and Alex Jack, *The Cancer Prevention Diet: Michio Kushi's Macrobiotic Blueprint for the Prevention and Relief of Disease* (New York: St. Martin's Griffin, 1993), 333; Sara Shannon, *Diet for the Atomic Age* (Wayne, NJ: Avery, 1987); Steve Schrecter, "Radiation: What You Can Do," *Vegetarian Times*, December 1981, 39–45.

84. Tatsuichiro Akizuki, "How We Survived Nagasaki," *East-West Journal*, December 10, 1980, 12–13.

85. Alex Jack, "Soviets Embrace Macrobiotics: Special Report from Moscow and Leningrad," *One Peaceful World* 6, no. 1 (Autumn/Winter 1990): 7–10; L. M. Iakushina et al., "The Effect of Vitamin- and Beta-Carotene-Enriched Products on the Vitamin A Allowance and the Concentration of Different Carotenoids of the Blood Serum in Victims of the Accident at the Chernobyl Atomic Electric Power Station" (article in Russian), *Voprosy Pitaniia* 1 (1996): 12–15.

86. For examples, see S. C. Skoryna, T. M. Paul, and D. W. Edward, "Studies on Inhibition of Intestinal Absorption of Radioactive Strontium. I. Prevention of

Absorption from Ligated Intestinal Segments," *Canadian Medical Association Journal* 91, no. 6 (1964): 285–88; Y. Tanaka, D. Waldron-Edward, and S. C. Skoryna, "Studies on Inhibition of Intestinal Absorption of Radioactive Strontium. VII. Relationship of Biological Activity to Chemical Composition of Alginates Obtained from North American Seaweeds," *Canadian Medical Association Journal* 99, no. 4 (1968): 169–75; Hiromitsu Watanabe, "Beneficial Biological Effects of Miso with Reference to Radiation Injury, Cancer, and Hypertension," *Journal of Toxicologic Pathology* 26, no. 2 (2013): 91–103, https://doi.org/10.1293/tox.26.91; Hiromitsu Watanabe et al., "A Miso (Japanese Soybean Paste) Diet Conferred Greater Protection against Hypertension than a Sodium Chloride Diet in Dahl Salt-Sensitive Rats," *Hypertension Research* 29 (2006): 731–38, https://doi.org/10.1291/hypres.29.731; M. Ohara et al., "Radioprotective Effects of Miso (Fermented Soy Bean Paste) against Radiation in B6c3f1 Mice: Increased Small Intestinal Crypt Survival, Crypt Lengths and Prolongation of Average Time to Death," *Hiroshima Journal of Medical Sciences* 50, no. 4 (2001): 83–86.

87. Shurtleff and Aoyagi, *History of Macrobiotics*. Kushi especially took the idea seriously that macrobiotics had antiradiation properties, going so far as to teach himself new scientific techniques such as spectroscopy to classify radioactive materials into Ohsawa's yin/yang system. Under his model, for example, products of nuclear fallout such as strontium-90 were determined to be too yin based on the blue pattern that emerged as a result of its spectroscopic analysis.

88. Raso, "Vitalistic Gurus," 231.

89. Aihara, *Basic Macrobiotics*, 9.

90. Angela N. H. Creager, *Life Atomic: A History of Radioisotopes in Science and Medicine* (Chicago: University of Chicago Press, 2013), 150.

91. Ellen Leopold, *Under the Radar: Cancer and the Cold War* (New Brunswick, NJ: Rutgers University Press, 2009), 78.

92. Also see M. Susan Lindee, *Suffering Made Real: American Science and the Survivors at Hiroshima* (Chicago: University of Chicago Press, 1994).

93. Gerald Kutcher, *Contested Medicine: Cancer Research and the Military* (Chicago: University of Chicago Press, 2009), 193.

94. Aihara, *Basic Macrobiotics*, 82; Fumimasa Yanagisawa, *A New Theory on Longevity, Medical Studies on Calcium and Magnesium Metabolism* (Tokyo: Toyo Keisai Shinposha, 1962).

95. Kushi, et al., "Macrobiotic Diet in Cancer," 3056S–3064S. Notably, Kushi's son Lawrence became a physician. He served on the board of the American Cancer Society, held a chair in nutrition at Columbia University, and currently serves as the director of science policy for Kaiser Permanente in northern California. At least one of his studies on macrobiotics was conducted with funding from the National Institutes of Health Office of Alternative Medicine from 2001; when the funds ran out, the study was canceled, leaving the results inconclusive.

96. Mann, "Myths of Macrobiotics," 21.

97. For examples, see Michio Kushi and the East-West Foundation, *The Macrobiotic Approach to Cancer: Toward Preventing and Controlling Cancer with Diet and Lifestyle* (Wayne, NJ: Avery, 1982); Michio Kushi and Alex Jack, *The Cancer Preven-*

tion Diet: Michio Kushi's Macrobiotic Blueprint for the Prevention and Relief of Disease (New York: St. Martin's Press, 1983); Aveline Kushi and Wendy Esko, The Macrobiotic Cancer Prevention Cookbook (Garden City Park, NY: Avery, 1988); Georges Ohsawa, Cancer and the Philosophy of the Far East (Binghamton, NY: Swan House, 1971); Jean Charles Kohler and Mary Alice Kohler, Healing Miracles from Macrobiotics: A Diet for All Diseases (West Nyack, NY: Parker, 1979); Virgina Brown and Susan Stayman, Macrobiotic Miracle: How a Vermont Family Overcame Cancer (New York: Japan Publications, 1984); Hugh Faulkner, Physician, Heal Thyself: A Doctor's Dietary Recovery from Incurable Cancer (Becket, MA: One Peaceful World, 1992); Elaine Nussbaum, Recovery: From Cancer to Health through Macrobiotics (New York: Japan Publications, 1986); and Ann Fawcett and Cynthia Smith, Cancer-Free: 30 Who Triumphed Over Cancer Naturally (New York: Japan Publications, 1991).

98. Mann, "Myths of Macrobiotics," 21.

99. Sattilaro and Monte, Recalled by Life, 54. It should be noted that Tom Monte is a macrobiotically trained natural health guru in his own right.

100. Monte, Way of Hope, 40; Anthony Sattilaro and Tom Monte, "Physician, Heal Thyself: A Doctor Believes a Macrobiotic Diet Cured His Cancer," Life, August 1982; Sattilaro and Monte, Recalled by Life.

101. Mann, "Myths of Macrobiotics," 21.

102. Nussbaum, Recovery; Brown and Stayman, Macrobiotic Miracle; Dirk Benedict, Confessions of a Kamikaze Cowboy: A True Story of Discovery, Acting, Health, Illness, Recovery, and Life (Garden City Park, NY: Square One, 2013).

103. J. P. Carter et al., "Hypothesis: Dietary Management May Improve Survival from Nutritionally Linked Cancers Based on Analysis of Representative Cases," Journal of the American College of Nutrition 12, no. 3 (1993): 209–26, https://doi.org/10.1080/07315724.1993.10718303; B. B. Bowman et al., "Macrobiotic Diets for Cancer Treatment and Prevention," Journal of Clinical Oncology 2, no. 6 (1984): 702–11, https://doi.org/10.1200/JCO.1984.2.6.702; Joellyn Horowitz and Mitsuo Tomita, "The Macrobiotic Diet as Treatment for Cancer: Review of the Evidence," Permanente Journal 6, no. 4 (2002): 34–37; Andrew J. Vickers and Barrie R. Cassileth, "Unconventional Therapies for Cancer and Cancer-related Symptoms," Lancet Oncology 2, no. 4 (2001): 226–32, https://doi.org/10.1016/S1470-2045(00)00293-X; "Unproven Methods of Cancer Management: Macrobiotic Diets," CA: A Cancer Journal for Clinicians, 34, no. 1 (1984): 60–63, https://doi.org/10.3322/canjclin.22.6.372; J. Dwyer, "The Macrobiotic Diet: No Cancer Cure," Nutrition Forum 7, no. 2 (1990): 9–11; Canlas Meritess, Shayne Small, and Megan Waltz-Hill, "Alternative Nutrition Therapies in Cancer Patients," Seminars in Oncology Nursing 21, no. 3 (2005): 173–76, https://doi.org/10.1016/j.soncn.2005.04.005; Ernst Edzard and Barrie Cassileth, "Cancer Diets: Fads and Facts," Cancer Prevention International 2, no. 3–4 (1996): 181–87, https://doi.org/10.3727/108399896792195419; Yogeshwer Shukla and Sanjoy Kumar Pal, "Dietary Cancer Chemoprevention: An Overview," International Journal of Human Genetics 4, no. 4 (2004): 265–76, https://doi.org/10.1080/09723757.2004.11885905; and Sheila Weitzman, "Alternative Nutritional Cancer Therapies," International Journal of Cancer 78, no. S11 (1999): 69–72, https://doi.org/10.1002/(SICI)1097-0215(1998)78:11+<69::AID-IJC20>3.0.CO;2-7.

104. Aihara, *Basic Macrobiotics*, 9.

105. Sattilaro and Monte, *Recalled by Life*, 171–72.

106. For more detailed discussions of alternative cancer therapies, see David Cantor, "Cancer, Quackery and the Vernacular Meanings of Hope in 1950s America," *Journal of the History of Medicine and Allied Sciences* 61, no. 3 (2006): 324–68, https://doi.org/10.1093/jhmas/jrj048; James Harvey Young and Richard E. McFadyen, "The Koch Cancer Treatment," *Journal of the History of Medicine and Allied Sciences* 53, no. 3 (1998): 254–84, https://doi.org/10.1093/jhmas/53.3.254; Eveleen Richards, *Vitamin C and Cancer: Medicine or Politics?* (London: Macmillan, 1991); and David J. Hess, *Can Bacteria Cause Cancer?: Alternative Medicine Confronts Big Science* (New York: New York University Press, 1997).

107. James S. Olson, *Bathsheba's Breast: Women, Cancer, and History* (Baltimore: Johns Hopkins University Press, 2005), 152.

108. Don Bell, "Ohsawa and the Yin and Yang of Health," *Chicago Tribune*, August 1, 1971, F23.

109. Michio Kushi, foreword to Jean Charles Kohler and Mary Alice Kohler, *Healing Miracles from Macrobiotics: A Diet for All Diseases* (West Nyack, NY: Parker, 1979).

110. See box 60, folder 8, Kushi Collection.

111. "Aveline Kushi; Leader in Macrobiotic Diet," *Los Angeles Times*, July 6, 2001, https://www.latimes.com/archives/la-xpm-2001-jul-06-me-19319-story.html; congressman and presidential candidate Dennis Kucinich gave a eulogy at Michio Kushi's funeral. Shurtleff and Aoyagi, *History of Macrobiotics*, 1097.

112. Stephen Barrett, "'Alternative' Cancer Treatment: Doublespeak That Can Kill You," in *The Health Robbers: A Close Look at Quackery in America*, ed. Stephen Barrett and William T. Jarvis, 83–100 (Buffalo, NY: Prometheus Books, 1993), 99.

113. Anthony J. Sattilaro and Tom Monte, *Living Well Naturally* (Boston: Houghton Mifflin, 1985); Len Lear, "Local Doctor with Stage 4 Cancer Found Lifesaving Diet," *Chestnut Hill Local* (Pennsylvania), September 4, 2015, https://www.chestnuthilllocal.com/2015/09/04/local-doctor-with-stage-4-cancer-found-life-saving-diet/.

114. Quote in subtitle from Ronald Kotzsch, "AIDS: Putting an Alternative to the Test," *East-West Journal*, September 1986, p. 66, box 21, folder 24, Kushi Collection.

115. For more on how Kaposi's sarcoma became the hallmark of the disease, see Sally Smith Hughes, "The Kaposi's Sarcoma Clinic at the University of California, San Francisco: An Early Response to the AIDS Epidemic," *Bulletin of the History of Medicine* 71, no. 4 (1997): 651–88, https://doi.org/10.1353/bhm.1997.0179.

116. "Letters from AIDS Friends Supporting the Studies on the Macrobiotic Dietary Approach to AIDS," May 15, 1984, box 21, folder 21, Kushi Collection.

117. Monte, *Way of Hope*, 38.

118. Steven Epstein, "The Construction of Lay Expertise: AIDS Activism and the Forging of Credibility in the Reform of Clinical Trials," *Science, Technology, and Human Values* 20, no. 4 (1995): 408–37, https://doi.org/10.1177/016224399502000402; Patrick Wallis, "Debating a Duty to Treat: AIDS and the Professional Ethics of Amer-

ican Medicine," *Bulletin of the History of Medicine* 85, no. 4 (2011): 620–49, https://doi.org/10.1353/bhm.2011.0092.

119. "Letters from AIDS Friends Supporting the Studies on the Macrobiotic Dietary Approach to AIDS," May 15, 1984, box 21, folder 21, Kushi Collection.

120. "Letters from AIDS Friends."

121. Kotzsch, "AIDS," 66.

122. Kotzsch, "AIDS," 67.

123. "Message from Michio Kushi for 'Wipe Out AIDS' Friends," January 11, 1984, box 21, folder 17, Kushi Collection.

124. Karlyn Crowley, "When Spirits Take Over: Gender and American New Age Culture" (PhD diss., University of Virginia, 2002); Randy F. Kandel, "Rice, Ice Cream, and the Guru: Decision-Making and Innovation in a Macrobiotic Community" (PhD diss., City University of New York, 1975); Belasco, *Appetite for Change*.

125. Kotzsch, "AIDS," 67.

126. "Message from Michio Kushi."

127. "Influence of Diet on Immune Status of People with AIDS," May 16, 1984, research proposal, p. 4, box 20, folder 19, Kushi Collection.

128. Kotzsch, "AIDS," 67.

129. Monte, *Way of Hope*, 66.

130. "Influence of Diet on Immune Status," 4.

131. Elinor M. Levy, Martha C. Cottrell, and Paul H. Black, "Psychological and Immunological Associations in Men with AIDS Pursuing a Macrobiotic Regimen as an Alternative Therapy: A Pilot Study," *Brain, Behavior, and Immunity* 3, no. 2 (1989): 175–82, https://doi.org/10.1016/0889-1591(89)90018-4.

132. Elinor Levy to Michio Kushi, June 28, 1985, box 21, folder 17, Kushi Collection.

133. Elinor Levy et al., "Patients with Kaposi Sarcoma Who Opt for No Treatment," *Lancet* 326, no. 8448 (1985): P223, https://doi.org/10.1016/S0140-6736(85)91542-9.

134. Kotzsch, "AIDS," 67.

135. Mann, "Myths of Macrobiotics," 21.

136. Mann, "Myths of Macrobiotics," 23.

137. Belasco, *Appetite for Change*, 56.

138. Dundar Kaya Buharli to Jim Sleeper, January 22, 1992, box 60, folder 8, Kushi Collection; Jim Sleeper to Dundar Kaya Buharli, January 23, 1992, box 60, folder 8, Kushi Collection; Jim Sleeper to Dundar Kaya Buharli, February 6, 1992, box 60, folder 8, Kushi Collection; Dundar Kaya Buharli to Jim Sleeper, February 7, 1992, box 60, folder 8, Kushi Collection; Jim Sleeper to Dundar Kaya Buharli, February 20, 1992, box 60, folder 8, Kushi Collection. Kushi apparently maintained this kind of medical correspondence with a significant number of people (mostly cancer patients outside the United States). Kushi's advice to them usually included minor dietary and other behavioral changes along with slight modifications of their regular medical treatment program.

139. Kimberly J. Lau, *New Age Capitalism: Making Money East of Eden* (Philadelphia: University of Pennsylvania Press, 2000), 78.

140. Mann, "Myths of Macrobiotics," 25.

141. Wells, "Diet Is More Than Brown Rice," A1.

142. Mann, "Myths of Macrobiotics," 25.

143. In June 1989, Jack Raso, a registered dietitian, attended a "five-day Michio Kushi Seminar for Medical Professionals" as an opposition researcher. In his description of Kushi's program, his writing was dripping with condescension and scare quotes, and he even blamed his difficulty understanding the macrobiotic system on Kushi's ethnic heritage, stating "[Kushi's] broken English often made him unintelligible." Raso, "Vitalistic Gurus," 231.

144. Mann, "Myths of Macrobiotics," 25.

145. Enid Nemy, "For the Nine O'Clocks, Time Is Rolled Back to Paris of the 1920's," *New York Times*, December 2, 1971, 62, www.nytimes.com/1971/12/02 /archives/for-the-nine-oclocks-time-is-rolled-back-to-paris-of-the-1920s.html.

146. Mann, "Myths of Macrobiotics," 26.

147. Mary Virginia Orna, Marco Fontani, and Mariagrazia Costa, *The Lost Elements: The Periodic Table's Shadow Side* (New York: Oxford University Press, 2015), 540.

148. Michio Kushi, "Message to the Government AIDS Symposium in Brazzaville, Peoples Republic of the Congo Africa," December 1, 1987, box 13, folder 9, Kushi Collection.

149. Kushi's actions contain echoes of the power dynamics and assumptions of colonialism. However, he inverts the classical power structure by arguing that a macrobiotic Congo could "demonstrate to so-called developed countries in Europe, North America, and the Far East the more healthy way of living because these developed countries are facing serious physical, mental, and social degeneration primarily as a direct result of improper dietary and nutritional practices." Kushi, "Message to the Government AIDS Symposium."

150. Kushi, "Message to the Government AIDS Symposium."

151. There are still hundreds of macrobiotics outposts around the globe, but their recognition in broader culture seems to have waned significantly.

Entremets II

1. "The Truth about This Man, Fred J. Hart," n.d., carton 2, folder 7, Margaret Hart Surbeck Papers, UCSF Library and Center for Knowledge Management, Archives and Special Collections, University of California, San Francisco.

2. Roxane Arnold, "Vitamin King: To Critics, He's a Quack, but Kurt Donsbach Has Built a Multimillion-Dollar Empire Pushing Value of Nutrition," *Los Angeles Times*, July 12, 1982, B3.

3. Eric W. Boyle, *Quack Medicine: A History of Combating Health Fraud in Twentieth-Century America* (Santa Barbara, CA: Praeger, 2013), 136.

4. When a member of the NHF, Clinton Miller, asked the AMA to justify their estimate, they could not. In a private memo, AMA member Robert Throckmorton essentially admitted Miller had caught them with their pants down. Clinton R. Miller

to American Medical Association, February 24, 1964, box 529, folder 6, Historical Health Fraud and Alternative Medicine Collection, American Medical Association Archive (hereafter cited as HHF Collection); Robert B. Throckmorton to Oliver Field, memorandum, March 2, 1964, box 529, folder 6, HHF Collection.

5. Laura J. Miller has been one of the few scholars to recognize the magnitude of this estimate and its consequences for the natural health food movement. Laura J. Miller, *Building Nature's Market: The Business and Politics of Natural Foods* (Chicago: University of Chicago Press, 2017), 145.

6. Aaron Bobrow-Strain, *White Bread: A Social History of the Store-Bought Loaf* (Boston: Beacon, 2013).

7. Upton Sinclair, *The Jungle* (New York: Doubleday, Page & Co, 1906).

8. Deborah Blum, *The Poison Squad: One Chemist's Single-Minded Crusade for Food Safety at the Turn of the Twentieth Century* (New York: Penguin, 2018).

9. Jean Mayer, "Nutritional Quackery," *Consultant*, February 1963.

10. Proceedings, National Congress on Medical Quackery, October 6–7, 1961, p. 67, box 100, folder 1, Morris Fishbein papers, Special Collections Research Center, University of Chicago.

11. D. Mark Hegsted, "Frederick John Stare (1910–2002)," *Journal of Nutrition* 134, no. 5 (2004): 1007–9.

12. Hunger was the major focus of elite, anti-quackery nutrition scientists through the 1970s. Vanderbilt nutrition scientist William J. Darby, who was Stare's ally and corporate fundraiser extraordinaire, built his career on iron deficiency anemia. Likewise, Stare's Harvard colleague Jean Mayer founded the National Council on Hunger and Malnutrition and helped create the food stamps and school lunch programs.

13. "AMA Seeks to Kill Competition: Sponsors Shocking 'Quackery' Congress," box 529, folder 4, HHF Collection.

14. "Washington Week," *Sponsor*, October 16, 1961, 55.

Chapter 3

Epigraph: Harry Oliphant to Nathan Pritikin, October 22, 1981, box 23, folder "Creative Tributes," Nathan Pritikin Papers, Library Special Collections, Charles E. Young Research Library, University of California, Los Angeles (hereafter cited as Pritikin Papers).

1. Joseph N. Bell, "The Woman Who Refused to Give Up" (repr. *Today's Health* magazine), in *Hearings before the Select Committee on Nutrition and Human Needs of the United States Senate, Diet Related to Killer Diseases II*, 95th Cong. 124 (February 1–2, 1977), pp. 124–8 (enclosure to a letter from Nathan Pritikin to Hon. Robert L. Leggett), https://www.google.com/books/edition/Diet_Related_to_Killer _Diseases/NuOLAyu5DigC.

2. Bell, "Woman Who Refused to Give Up."

3. Rose Dosti, "Senior Olympic Athletes: Don't Look Now, but That's Grandma Out on the Track," *Los Angeles Times*, May 1, 1975, H1.

4. Marian Burros, "Longevity: Is Diet the Answer?" *Washington Post*, April 7, 1977; Tom Monte, *Unexpected Recoveries: Seven Steps to Healing Body, Mind, and Soul When Serious Illness Strikes* (New York: St. Martin's Griffin, 2005), 183.

5. Bell, "Woman Who Refused to Give Up."

6. Monte, *Unexpected Recoveries*, 183.

7. Bell, "Woman Who Refused to Give Up."

8. Shelly McKenzie, *Getting Physical: The Rise of Fitness Culture in America* (Lawrence: University Press of Kansas, 2013), 109.

9. Bell, "Woman Who Refused to Give Up."

10. Patrick McGrady, "A Diet-Exercise Program That Could Add Years to Your Life," *Woman's Day*, November 1976, 88.

11. Carol Lawson, "Behind the Best Sellers," *New York Times*, July 1, 1979, 5, www.nytimes.com/1979/07/01/archives/behind-the-best-sellers-nathan-pritikin.html.

12. Burros, "Longevity," 183.

13. Monte, *Unexpected Recoveries*, 183.

14. Bell, "Woman Who Refused to Give Up."

15. Bell, "Woman Who Refused to Give Up."

16. Judith Willis, "Sorting Out and Understanding Today's Fad Diets," *Chicago Tribune*, July 1, 1982, S_B11.

17. Gyorgi Scrinis, *Nutritionism: The Science and Politics of Dietary Advice* (New York: Columbia University Press, 2015). Notably, while Scrinis pioneered the concept, it was popularized by Michael Pollan.

18. Chris Feudtner, *Bittersweet: Diabetes, Insulin, and the Transformation of Illness* (Chapel Hill: The University of North Carolina Press, 2003); Jeremy Greene, *Prescribing by Numbers: Drugs and the Definition of Disease* (Baltimore: Johns Hopkins University Press, 2007); Joseph Dumit, *Drugs for Life: How Pharmaceutical Companies Define Our Health* (Durham, NC: Duke University Press, 2012).

19. Tim Jahns, "The Crusader: A Profile of Nathan Pritikin," [unpublished article], n.d., p. 10, box 1, folder "Biographical Article (Never Published) by Tim Jahns, 1979," pp. 1–17, Pritikin Papers.

20. See Thomas Cole, *The Journey of Life: A Cultural History of Aging in America* (Cambridge: Cambridge University Press, 1992); Mike Featherstone and Andrew Wernick, eds., *Images of Aging: Cultural Representations of Later Life* (London: Routledge, 1995); Pat Thane, ed., *The Long History of Old Age* (London: Thames and Hudson, 2005); Steven Katz, *Disciplining Old Age: The Formation of Gerontological Knowledge: Disciplinary and Beyond* (Charlottesville: University Press of Virginia, 1996).

21. See Margaret Morganroth Gullete, *Declining to Decline: Cultural Combat and the Politics of the Midlife* (Charlottesville: University Press of Virginia, 2004); Lawrence R. Samuel, *Aging in America: A Cultural History* (Philadelphia: University of Pennsylvania Press, 2017); Louise Aronson, *Elderhood: Redefining Aging, Transforming Medicine, Reimagining Life* (New York: Bloomsbury, 2019).

22. Aimee Medeiros and Elizabeth Siegel Watkins, "Live Longer Better: The Historical Roots of Human Growth Hormone as Anti-Aging Medicine" *Journal of the History of Medicine and Allied Sciences* 73, no. 3 (2018): 333–59, https://doi.org/10.1093/jhmas/jry001.

23. Tom Monte, *Pritikin: The Man Who Healed America's Heart* (Emmaus, PA: Rodale Press, 1988), 7.

24. Monte, *Pritikin*, 32.

25. Harry M. Marks, *The Progress of Experiment: Science and Therapeutic Reform in the United States, 1900–1990* (Cambridge: Cambridge University Press, 1997), 167.

26. Monte, *Pritikin*, 25; Nathan Pritikin and John McDougall, "Nathan Pritikin: A Casual Conversation with Dr. John McDougall," originally aired on PBS Hawaii, October 1982, and posted by Dr. McDougall Health & Medical Center, February 7, 2013, YouTube video, 56:04, www.youtube.com/watch?v=qOj4rzSkqok.

27. Barbara Newborg and Florence Nash, *Walter Kempner and the Rice Diet: Challenging Conventional Wisdom* (Durham, NC: Carolina Academic Press, 2011). Newborg and Nash say Pritikin tried to paint himself as an ally of Kempner, but Kempner refused to be associated with him.

28. Monte, *Pritikin*, 38.

29. Burt A. Folkart, "Lester Morrison; Pioneer in Diet, Health," *Los Angeles Times*, May 28, 1991, www.latimes.com/archives/la-xpm-1991-05-28-mn-2586-story.html.

30. For histories covering other early developments connecting heart disease and diet, see Nicholas Rasmussen, "Group Weight Loss and Multiple Screening: A Tale of Two Heart Disease Programs in Postwar American Public Health," *Bulletin of the History of Medicine* 92, no. 3 (2018): 474–505, https://doi.org/10.1353/bhm.2018 .0056; Todd M. Olszewski, "The Causal Conundrum: The Diet-Heart Debates and the Management of Uncertainty in American Medicine," *Journal of the History of Medicine and Allied Sciences* 70, no. 2 (2015): 218–49, https://doi.org/10.1093/jhmas /jru001; Robert Aronowitz, "The Framingham Heart Study and the Emergence of the Risk Factor Approach to Coronary Heart Disease, 1947–1970," *Revue d'Histoire des Sciences* 54, no. 2 (July–December 2011): 263–95, https://doi.org/10.3917/rhs.642 .0263; and Maiko Spiess, "Food and Diet as Risk: The Role of the Framingham Study," in *Proteins, Pathologies, and Politics: Dietary Innovation and Disease from the Nineteenth Century*, ed. D. Gentilcore and M. Smith, 81–94 (London: Bloomsbury, 2018).

31. Folkart, "Lester Morrison."

32. "Health Autobiography of N.P.," box 4, folder "Health Biography N.P.," Pritikin Papers.

33. "Health Autobiography of N.P."

34. Monte, *Pritikin*, 41. Pritikin's radiation dosages were well-above the 50 rem (roentgen equivalent man) threshold needed to detect proto-cancerous blood changes. For comparison, according to the FDA, a standard X-ray dose now is 0.02 mSv (millisieverts), or 1/500 rem, even a modern computed tomography scan is only 16 mSv, or 1.6 rem. Using these figures, therefore, I estimate Pritikin received the equivalent of 110,000 chest X-rays—a lot of radiation.

35. His archival materials offer further evidence of his meticulous record keeping as he went even so far as to request the submission of his own blood slides into the archive.

36. Neal D. Barnard, "The Pritikin Legacy," *Vegetarian Times*, May 1991, 69.

37. "The Pritikin Regimen for a Long, Healthy Life," *Chicago Tribune*, September 2, 1979, J3.

38. Barnard, "Pritikin Legacy," 67.

39. Jon N. Leonard to Nathan Pritikin, August 11, 1972, box 5, folder "Longevity Foundation. Nathan's Influence Re: Direction of Activities," Pritikin Papers.

40. Jon N. Leonard, Jack L. Hofer, and Nathan Pritikin, *Live Longer Now: The First One Hundred Years of Your Life—the 2100 Program* (New York: Grosset & Dunlap,1974); Mary Knoblauch, "Giving Up the Sweet Life for a Good Life," *Chicago Tribune*, December 1, 1974, F11.

41. Barnard, "Pritikin Legacy," 67. Explaining Pritikin's justification for lying in the book, Robert Pritikin said, "My father thought that if he didn't make up this fiction, and it all came from a guy without any degrees, who'd believe it?"

42. Knoblauch, "Giving Up the Sweet Life," F11.

43. Nathan Pritikin and Patrick M. McGrady Jr., *The Pritikin Program for Diet and Exercise* (New York: Grosset & Dunlap, 1979); Jack Jones, "Nathan Pritikin, Crusader for Fitness, Kills Himself," *Los Angeles Times*, February 23, 1985, A1, www .latimes.com/archives/la-xpm-1985-02-23-mn-1021-story.html.

44. According to Pritikin's son Robert, when Pritikin presented at the American Academy of Medical Preventives, most of the other speakers emphasized prostheses, wheelchairs, and other kinds of technical aids to help people cope with age-related disabilities. Pritikin felt like the black sheep for preaching disease reversal instead.

45. John Kern to Nathan Pritikin, July 27, 1974, box 6, folder "VA Hospital Investigation: Kern's Correspondence in Investigator's File," Pritikin Papers; transcript from deposition of Nathan Pritikin, p. 551, box 6, Folder "V.A. Hospital Investigation. Deposition of Nathan Pritikin," Pritikin Papers.

46. Jahns, "The Crusader," 10–11.

47. Transcript from deposition of Nathan Pritikin, p. 551.

48. Nathan Pritikin et al., "Diet and Exercise as a Total Therapeutic Regime for the Rehabilitation of Patients with Severe Peripheral Vascular Disease," *Archives of Physical Medicine and Rehabilitation* 56, no. 558 (1975).

49. The name of this organization has changed several times over the years. For example, it was once known as the American Academy of Physical Medicine and Rehabilitation.

50. Jahns, "The Crusader," 10–11.

51. Pritikin and McDougall, "Nathan Pritikin: A Casual Conversation."

52. Barnard, "Pritikin Legacy," 68.

53. Jahns, "The Crusader," 10–11.

54. Barnard, "Pritikin Legacy," 69.

55. Jones, "Nathan Pritikin, Crusader for Fitness, Kills Himself," A1.

56. Jahns, "The Crusader," 11.

57. Jahns, "The Crusader," 12.

58. Elaine Markoutsas, "Nutrition Guru Is No Ordinary Health Nut," *Chicago Tribune*, May 8, 1979, A1.

59. By 1985, the costs of attendance had dropped slightly (adjusting for inflation) to $5,800 for couples and $4,700 for individuals. "Nutritionist Pritikin, Ill with Leukemia, Kills Self," *Los Angeles Times*, February 22, 1985, A1, www.latimes

.com/archives/la-xpm-1985-02-22-mn-598-story.html; Elaine Louie, "The Boom in Health Clubs," *New York Times Magazine*, October 7, 1979, SM20, www.nytimes .com/1979/10/07/archives/the-boom-in-health-clubs.html; Judy Klemesrud, "At the Spas: Shedding Holiday Excesses," *New York Times*, May 10, 1984, A20, www .nytimes.com/1985/01/20/style/at-the-spas-shedding-holiday-excesses.html; Pamela Hollie, "Spas Thrive on Diet, Fitness Craze: Profits Mount for Owners," *New York Times*, November 6, 1978, 82, www.nytimes.com/1978/11/06/archives/spas -thrive-on-diet-fitness-craze-profits-mount-for-owners.html; and Marian Burros, "Toning Up at the Sleekest of Health Spas," *New York Times*, January 27, 1987, 19, www.nytimes.com/1987/01/25/travel/toning-up-at-the-sleekest-of-health-spas .html.

60. Stephen Randall, "Healthful Eating: Take it to Heart," *Women's Wear Daily*, April 8, 1977, 10–11.

61. Hillel Schwartz, *Never Satisfied: A Cultural History of Diets, Fantasies, and Fat* (New York: Free Press, 1986), 250.

62. Patrick McGrady, "A Diet-Exercise Program That Could Add Years to Your Life," *Woman's Day*, November 1976, 158.

63. Jahns, "The Crusader," 11.

64. Pritikin and McDougall, "Nathan Pritikin: A Casual Conversation."

65. Michael Balter, "Pritikin Son Carries on Crusade: A Firm Believer in Diet's Influence on Heart Health," *Los Angeles Times*, September 9, 1986, G1, www.latimes .com/archives/la-xpm-1986-09-09-vw-12738-story.html.

66. McGrady, "Diet-Exercise Program," 158. Patrick McGrady helped Pritikin write *The Pritikin Program for Diet and Exercise*; Stephen Barrett labels him a quack in his own right.

67. McGrady, "Diet-Exercise Program," 158.

68. Randall, "Healthful Eating," 10–11.

69. Some prime examples include Rebecca Weiner to Nathan Pritikin, August 7, 1980, box 23, folder "Birthday Book Replies 3," Pritikin Papers; Sylvia Siegle to Nathan Pritikin, August 23, 1980, box 23, folder "Birthday Book Replies 3," Pritikin Papers; Maury Leibovitz, "Ode to Nathan," box 23, folder "Creative Tributes." Pritikin Papers; William Hermanns, "O Francis," March 23, 1982, box 23, folder "Creative Tributes," Pritikin Papers.

70. Randall, "Healthful Eating," 10–11.

71. Lawson, "Behind the Best Sellers," 5.

72. Markoutsas, "Nutrition Guru," A1.

73. Pritikin and McDougall, "Nathan Pritikin: A Casual Conversation."

74. Harold Snow to Nathan Pritikin, August 5, 1980, box 25, folder "Hospital Plan: Using Pritikin Program," Pritikin Papers.

75. Keay Davidson, "Troubled Hospital Turns to Weight-Loss Plan," *Los Angeles Times*, April 5, 1983, SD_A1.

76. Davidson, "Troubled Hospital," SD_A1.

77. "Pritikin ICR: Pritikin Intensive Cardiac Rehab," Pritikin Longevity Center, accessed November 11, 2019, www.pritikin.com/your-health/health-benefits /reverse-heart-disease/pritikin-icr.html.

78. Studies conducted by Pritikin's Longevity Center staff include John A. Hall, Gerald H. Dixson, R. James Barnard, and Nathan Pritikin, "Effects of Diet and Exercise on Peripheral Vascular Disease," *Physician and Sports Medicine* 10, no. 5 (1982): 90–101, https://doi.org/10.1080/00913847.1982.11947226; Monroe B. Rosenthal, R. James Barnard, David P. Rose, Stephen Inkeles, John Hall, and Nathan Pritikin, "Effects of a High-Complex-Carbohydrate, Low-fat, Low Cholesterol Diet on Levels of Serum Lipids and Estradiol," *American Journal of Medicine* 78, no. 1 (1985): 23–27, https://doi.org/10.1016/0002-9343(85)90456-5; R. James Barnard, Manzoor R. Massey, Samuel Cherny, Lynne Trexler O'Brien, and Nathan Pritikin, "Long-term Use of a High-Complex-Carbohydrate, High-Fiber Diet and Exercise in the Treatment of NIDDM Patients," *Diabetes Care* 6, no. 3 (1983): 268–73, https://doi.org/10.2337/diacare.6.3.268; R. James Barnard, Peter M. Guzy, Jerry Rosenberg, and Lynne Trexler O'Brien, "Effects of an Intensive Exercise and Nutrition Program on Patients with Coronary Artery Disease: Five-Year Follow-up," *Journal of Cardiac Rehabilitation* 3, no. 3 (1983): 183–90; John A. Hall and R. James Barnard, "The Effects of an Intensive 26-Day Program of Diet and Exercise on Patients with Peripheral Vascular Disease," *Journal of Cardiac Rehabilitation* 2, no. 7 (1982): 569–74; Fran Weber, R. James Barnard, and Douglas Roy, "Effects of a High-Complex-Carbohydrate, Low-Fat Diet and Daily Exercise on Individuals 70 Years of Age and Older," *Journal of Gerontology* 38, no. 2 (1983): 155–61, https://doi.org/10.1093/geronj/38.2.155; R. James Barnard, Leza Lattimore, Robert G. Holly, Samuel Cherny, and Nathan Pritikin, "Response of Non-Insulin-Dependent Diabetic Patients to an Intensive Program of Diet and Exercise," *Diabetes Care* 5, no. 4 (1982): 370–74, https://doi.org/10.2337/diacare.5.4.370; R. James Barnard, John Hall, and Nathan Pritikin, "Effects of Diet and Exercise on Blood Pressure and Viscosity in Hypertensive Patients," *Journal of Cardiac Rehabilitation* 5, no. 4 (1985): 185–90; and R. James Barnard et al., "Effects of a High Complex-Carbohydrate Diet and Daily Walking on Blood Pressure and Medication Status of Hypertensive Patients," *Journal of Cardiac Rehabilitation* 3, no. 12 (1983): 839–50.

79. Monte, *Pritikin*.

80. US Senate Select Committee on Nutrition and Human Needs, *Dietary Goals for the United States* (Washington, DC: US Government Printing Office, February 1977), also known as the McGovern Report.

81. Marion Nestle, *Food Politics: How the Food Industry Influences Nutrition and Health* (Berkeley: University of California Press, 2013).

82. Ann F. La Berge, "How the Ideology of Low-Fat Conquered America," *Journal of the History of Medicine and Allied Sciences* 63, no. 2 (2008): 139–77, https://doi.org/10.1093/jhmas/jrn001; Gary Taubes, "What If It's All Been a Big Fat Lie?" *New York Times Magazine*, July 7, 2002, www.nytimes.com/2002/07/07/magazine/what-if-it-s-all-been-a-big-fat-lie.html. It was also the first report to use the term "complex carbohydrates."

83. Edward J. Boyer, "'Fellow Crusader' George McGovern at Rites: Pritikin Eulogized as a Bold Pioneer," *Los Angeles Times*, March 1, 1985, www.latimes.com/archives/la-xpm-1985-03-01-mn-23924-story.html. The exact date and circumstances of their meeting is unknown. The *Los Angeles Times* only reported that

McGovern first met Pritikin in the early 1970s, ambiguously placing Pritikin and McGovern's meeting around the time the senator's committee began to transition its focus away from hunger toward issues of overnutrition.

84. George McGovern, "Tribute to Nathan Pritikin," *The Center Post* (Longevity Center alumni newsletter), April 1986, box 1, folder "PRF Memorial Newsletter Center Post 'Tribute,'" Pritikin Papers.

85. Pritikin's testimony was supported by testimony from a British physician, Hugh Trowell, who served on the Longevity Research Institute's board and who likened the Pritikin program to the Kikuyu peasant diet he favored from his anthropological research in Kenya (he may also have joined the Pritikin program as a spy to report on his patients' candid responses to the program).

86. Transcript from deposition of John Kern, pp. 236–340, box 6, folder "V.A. Hospital Investigation Deposition of Dr. John Kern," Pritikin Papers.

87. Another crucial error in the study report that arose from the deposition was the fact that Pritikin was unable to secure the necessary funds and donations to cover the meal costs for the experimental group for nine months; he solicited a $2 fee from each patient to cover their meals, after which several of them dropped out of the study, a fact that was omitted from the publication itself. Transcript from deposition of John Kern, p. 283, box 6, folder "V.A. Hospital Investigation Deposition of Dr. John Kern," Pritikin Papers.

88. Transcript from deposition of John Kern, pp. 236–40, box 6, folder "V.A. Hospital Investigation Deposition of Dr. John Kern," Pritikin Papers.

89. Aside from the fact that it was housed in New York, I was unable to find any information about this funding agent. Pritikin merely said they paid Robert's salary.

90. John Kern to American Heart Association, March 6, 1976, box 6, folder "VA Hospital Investigation. Kern's Correspondence in Investigation File," Pritikin Papers.

91. Nathan Pritikin to John Kern, February 20, 1976, box 6, folder "VA Hospital Investigation. Kern's Correspondence in Investigation File," Pritikin Papers.

92. Pritikin et al., "Diet and Exercise as a Total Therapeutic Regime."

93. John Kern to Ralph Bodfish, February 11, 1976, box 6, folder "VA Hospital Investigation: Kern's Correspondence in Investigator's File," Pritikin Papers.

94. John Kern to Nathan Pritikin, February 11, 1976, box 6, folder "VA Hospital Investigation: Kern's Correspondence in Investigator's File," Pritikin Papers.

95. John Kern to American Heart Association, March 6, 1976, box 6, folder "VA Hospital Investigation: Kern's Correspondence in Investigator's File," Pritikin Papers; John Kern to Ralph E. Bodfish, February 11, 1976, box 6, folder "VA Hospital Investigation: Kern's Correspondence in Investigator's File," Pritikin Papers.

96. Transcript from deposition of John Kern, p. 254, box 6, folder "VA Hospital Investigation Deposition of Dr. John Kern," Pritikin Papers.

97. Transcript from deposition of Nathan Pritikin, p. 550, box 6, folder "VA Hospital Investigation Deposition of Nathan Pritikin," Pritikin Papers.

98. Markoutsas, "Nutrition Guru," A1.

99. Jahns, "The Crusader," 14.

100. Fred Stare and Elizabeth Hubbard, "Pritikin, Scarsdale Diets Not Recommended," *Tampa Tribune*, April 3, 1980, 72, www.newspapers.com/article/the-tampa-tribune-stare-on-pritikin-1980/37631833/.

101. Judith Willis, "Sorting Out and Understanding Today's Fad Diets," *Chicago Tribune*, July 1, 1982, S_B11; Andy Kroll and Jeremy Schulman, "Leaked Documents Reveal the Secret Finances of a Pro-Industry Science Group," *Mother Jones*, October 28, 2013, www.motherjones.com/politics/2013/10/american-council-science-health-leaked-documents-fundraising/.

102. Robert I. Levy to Robert L. Leggett, July 30, 1976, in *Hearings Before the Select Committee on Nutrition and Human Needs of the United States Senate—Diet Related to Killer Diseases II*, 95th Cong. 122–123 (February 1–2, 1977).

103. Randall, "Healthful Eating," 10–11. Also see Martha Smilgis, "Pritikin Will Eat No Fat, Atkins Will Eat No Grain—and That Feeds a Fierce Dispute over Diet," *People*, December 3, 1979, https://people.com/archive/pritikin-will-eat-no-fat-atkins-will-eat-no-grain-and-that-feeds-a-fierce-dispute-over-diet-vol-12-no-23/.

104. Al Martinez, "The Fun Part of Hog Fat," *Los Angeles Times*, October 15, 1988, H2.

105. Markoutsas, "Nutrition Guru," A1. Markoutsas reports that his followers called Pritikin a "medical messiah," and says his center was known as "the Lourdes of the West."

106. Markoutsas, "Nutrition Guru," A1.

107. Jon Van, "Pritikin's Diet Philosophy Is Main Course at Conference," *Chicago Tribune*, June 10, 1984, 4.

108. Pritikin and McDougall, "Nathan Pritikin: A Casual Conversation."

109. Pritikin and McDougall, "Nathan Pritikin: A Casual Conversation."

110. Markoutsas, "Nutrition Guru," A1.

111. Pritikin and McDougall, "Nathan Pritikin: A Casual Conversation."

112. Nathan Pritikin and Ilene Pritikin, *The Official Pritikin Guide to Restaurant Eating* (Indianapolis: Bobbs-Merrill, 1984).

113. Marilyn Schwartz, "Nathan Pritikin Gets Picky at a Mexican Restaurant," *Los Angeles Times*, February 9, 1984, S50.

114. Max Jacobson, "Pritikin Chinese? A Little 'Diet' Oil Goes a Long Way," *Los Angeles Times*, December 27, 1990, OC25, www.latimes.com/archives/la-xpm-1990-12-27-ol-9845-story.html; L. N. Halliburton, "Testing Low-Calorie Menu at Vito's," *Los Angeles Times*, November 7, 1986, 115, www.latimes.com/archives/la-xpm-1986-11-07-ca-15564-story.html; Rose Dosti, "Pastas: The 'Light' Food Movement Has Embraced a Culinary Heavy—Pasta," *Los Angeles Times*, April 5, 1990, H1, www.latimes.com/archives/la-xpm-1990-04-05-fo-600-story.html.

115. "Founder of Longevity Center Is Banquet Speaker," *The Gold Leaf* (newsletter published by the American Academy of Gold Foil Operators), August 1982, www.jopdentonline.org/userimages/ContentEditor/1399312603418/1982%20August.pdf.

116. Calvin Trillin, "Noble Experiment," *New Yorker*, January 12, 1981, 86–91, www.newyorker.com/magazine/1981/01/12/noble-experiment-3.

117. Captain R. W. Ware to Nathan Pritikin, December 7, 1982, box 34, folder "Diet Prepared by Pritikin Research Foundation for Voyage," Pritikin Papers.

118. Nathan and Ilene Pritikin to Members of the Pritikin "Family," September 21, 1981, box 25, folder "Pritikin Pantry," Pritikin Papers.

119. Richard Arnold to Nathan Pritikin, December 9, 1980, box 24, folder "United Airlines Diet," Pritikin Papers.

120. Nathan Pritikin to Richard Arnold, November 18, 1980; Nathan Pritikin to Richard Arnold, September 30, 1980; Nathan Pritikin to Richard Arnold, December 18, 1980; Nathan Pritikin to Richard Arnold, June 11, 1980; Nathan Pritikin to Richard Arnold, May 27, 1980; all in box 24, folder "United Airlines Diet," Pritikin Papers.

121. Nathan Pritikin to Richard Arnold, August 8, 1980; Nathan Pritikin to Richard Arnold, January 10, 1981; both in box 24, folder "United Airlines Diet," Pritikin Papers.

122. Richard Arnold to Nathan Pritikin, December 10, 1980, box 24, folder "United Airlines Diet," Pritikin Papers.

123. Richard Arnold to Nathan Pritikin, December 31, 1980, box 24, folder "United Airlines Diet," Pritikin Papers.

124. "North American Brief: Quaker Oats Co.," *Asian Wall Street Journal*, June 29, 1995, 22.

125. As is typical in testimonials of any sort, the quality of evidence here is necessarily problematic. The authors of these letters have likely employed embellished language in an attempt to praise and flatter Pritikin on his birthday. Regardless of whether they exaggerated their claims of success on the program, the call for testimonials in the first place creates a self-selecting crowd. Although it is possible that Ilene Pritikin cherry-picked the submissions that she let into the archive, she preserved a significant amount of criticism in other places of the archive.

126. Rebecca Weiner to Nathan Pritikin, August 7, 1980; Philip Philibosian, August 22, 1980; both in box 23, folder "Birthday Book Replies 3," Pritikin Papers.

127. Frieda E. London to Nathan Pritikin, August 29, 1980, box 23, folder "Birthday Book Replies 4," Pritikin Papers; Sam S. Becker to Nathan Pritikin, September 25, 1980, box 23, folder "Birthday Book Replies 3," Pritikin Papers.

128. Letters that call this quality out explicitly include Lauren T. Blount to Nathan Pritikin, August 19, 1980; Morris and Pearl Schaffer to Nathan Pritikin, August 3, 1980; Lester G. Abeloff to Nathan Pritikin, August 5, 1980; all in box 23, folder "Birthday Book Replies 3," Pritikin Papers.

129. H. Curtis Wood to Nathan Pritikin, August 14, 1980; Frances and Herman Benjamin, September 24, 1980; both in box 23, folder "Birthday Book Replies 3," Pritikin Papers.

130. Susan Yager, *The Hundred Year Diet: America's Voracious Appetite for Losing Weight* (New York: Rodale, 2010), 133.

131. Deborah Hastings, "Pritikin Suicide Linked to Scalpel Provided by Nurse," *Los Angeles Times*, March 11, 1985, OC3, www.latimes.com/archives/la-xpm-1985-03-11-me-34027-story.html.

132. Balter, "Pritikin Son Carries on Crusade," G1; Michael Balter, "The Continuation of the Pritikin Legacy," *Baltimore Sun*, March 11, 1985, 9.

133. J. D. Hubbard, S. Inkeles, and R. J. Barnard, "Nathan Pritikin's Heart," *New England Journal of Medicine* 313, no. 1 (1985): 52, https://doi.org/10.1056/nejm 198507043130119; "Pritikin: Vindication from the Grave?" *Medical World News*, August 13, 1985, box 4, folder "Autopsy Report," Pritikin Papers; Jones, "Nathan Pritikin, Crusader," A1; Hastings, "Suicide of Pritikin," OC3.

134. "McGovern Will Deliver Pritikin Eulogy," *Desert Sun* (California), February 25, 1985.

135. George McGovern, "Tribute to Nathan Pritikin," *The Center Post*, April 1986, box 1, folder "PRF Memorial Newsletter Center Post 'Tribute,'" Pritikin Papers.

136. Van, "Pritikin's Diet Philosophy," F1.

137. Boyer, "'Fellow Crusader' George McGovern."

138. John McDougall to Ilene Pritikin, July 1, 1985, box 19, folder "Physicians and Supporters II—John A. McDougall, M.D.," Pritikin Papers.

139. Michael Greger and Gene Stone, *How Not to Die: Discover the Foods Scientifically Proven to Prevent and Reverse Disease* (New York: Flatiron, 2015); Michael Greger, *How Not to Diet: The Groundbreaking Science of Healthy, Permanent Weight Loss* (New York: Pan Macmillan, 2021).

140. Michael Greger, "The Story of NutritionFacts.org," NutritionFacts.org, accessed April 12, 2020, https://nutritionfacts.org/video/the-story-of-nutritionfacts -org/.

141. La Berge, "How the Ideology of Low-Fat Conquered America," 139–77.

142. Daniel Goleman, "New Study Says Diet Can Heal Arteries," *New York Times*, November 15, 1988, 1, www.nytimes.com/1988/11/15/science/new-study-says-diet -can-heal-arteries.html.

143. Dean Ornish et al., "Can Lifestyle Changes Reverse Coronary Heart Disease? The Lifestyle Heart Trial," *Lancet* 336, no. 8708 (1990): 129–33, https://doi.org/10 .1016/0140-6736(90)91656-u.

144. "Heart Beat: Ornish, Pritikin Get Medicare Okay for Cardiac Rehab," *Harvard Health Publishing*, December, 2010, www.health.harvard.edu/newsletter _article/ornish-pritikin-get-medicare-okay-for-cardiac-rehab.

145. As of this writing, the American College of Lifestyle Medicine offers a certification in lifestyle medicine that serves as a complement to other formalized board certifications. Notably, the organization has conferred its highest honors on some of the key founders of the Whole Foods, Plant-Based (WFPB) movement. For instance, Dr. Neal Barnard won their 2016 Lifestyle Medicine Trailblazer Award and Dr. John McDougall won their 2018 Lifetime Achievement award.

146. Greger, "Story of NutritionFacts.org." Lifestyle medicine is similar in spirit and philosophy to modern osteopathy; many DOs consider themselves practitioners of lifestyle medicine. Pritikin received an honorary doctorate from Kirksville College of Osteopathic Medicine.

Entremets III

1. Cristin E. Kearns, Laura A. Schmidt, and Stanton A. Glantz, "Sugar Industry and Coronary Heart Disease Research: A Historical Analysis of Internal Industry

Documents," *JAMA Internal Medicine* 176, no. 11 (2016): 1680–85, https://doi.org/10.1001/jamainternmed.2016.5394.

2. David Merrit Johns and Gerald M. Oppenheimer, "Was There Ever Really a 'Sugar Conspiracy'?" *Science* 359, no. 6377 (2018): 747–50, https://doi.org/10.1126/science.aaq1618.

3. Hank Campbell, "Fred Stare Was Not in Cahoots with Big Sugar," *American Council on Science and Health (ACSH.org)*, September 22, 2016, www.acsh.org/news/2016/09/22/fred-stare-was-not-cahoots-big-sugar-10161.

4. Elizabeth M. Whelan and Fredrick John Stare, *Panic in the Pantry: Food Facts, Fads, and Fallacies* (New York: Atheneum, 1975); John L. Hess, "Harvard's Sugar-Pushing Nutritionist," *Saturday Review*, 1978, 10–14, www.unz.com/print/SaturdayRev-1978aug-00010.

5. Hess, "Harvard's Sugar-Pushing Nutritionist."

6. Hess, "Harvard's Sugar-Pushing Nutritionist."

7. Frederick J. Stare to Carlton Fredericks, March 10, 1960, series IIB, box 15, folder 28, William Jefferson Darby Papers, Eskind Biomedical Library Manuscripts Collection, Vanderbilt University (hereafter cited as Darby Papers). This idea has since been reproposed and attempted (unsuccessfully) on several occasions. Stare was once even sued for an article he wrote in *McCall's* magazine in which he defended white bread as healthful. A confused reader wrote to the magazine's editor asking Stare to clarify his position about the healthfulness of white flour. To her concerned letter, she fastened a newspaper clipping that condemned refined white flour as bereft of nutritional value. In response, Stare wrote, "These scare tactics are typical of the food-faddist organizations. . . . From a practical viewpoint in most American diets, dark flour and enriched white flour are the same in food value and they both make important contributions to our diet. To imply or suggest that enriched white flour can cause or contribute to [chronic disease] is a cruel and reckless fraud"; quoted in Ralph Lee Smith, "The Vitamin Healers," *The Reporter*, December 16, 1965, Earl R. Thayer Research Files, Division of Library, Archives, and Museum Collections, Wisconsin Historical Society.

8. Hess, "Harvard's Sugar-Pushing Nutritionist."

9. Darby's letters to Henry Sebrell show that he was aware that soft drinks were probably unhealthy, but rather than eliminate them or recommend their removal, he wanted to use them as a vehicle for nutritional betterment (i.e., enrich them with vitamins). For example, he alludes to having corresponded with officials at Coca-Cola about the high levels of vitamin C in Hi-C and wanted to start more projects like that. William Darby to W. Henry Sebrell, series I, box 19, folder 10, Darby Papers.

10. Jean Mayer, "Nutritional Quackery," *Consultant* 3, no. 2 (February 1963): 21.

11. Jean Mayer was on the board of Monsanto and Miles Laboratories (later Bayer). William H. White to Jean Mayer, March 6, 1972, box 9, folder 4, Jean Mayer Papers, Center for the History of Medicine Repository Francis A. Countway Library of Medicine, Harvard University (hereafter cited as Mayer Papers); Jean Mayer to Walter Compton, August 11, 1972, box 9, folder 21, Mayer Papers. Bill Darby's research was funded by the National Dairy Council, to whom he offered insider

information regarding the activities of the AMA's Council on Food and Nutrition and to tip them off early about future FDA regulations. Elwood W. Speckmann to William J. Darby, August 19, 1968, series 1, box 20, folder 14, Darby Papers. He had kept his relationship and substantial fundraising efforts with the Campbell Soup Company secret from his dean because of matters of a "personal nature." See William J. Darby to Don Knight, July 26, 1971, series I, box 5, folder 4; and Don Knight to William J. Darby, July 20, 1971, series I, box 5, folder 4, Darby Papers. Darby helped the Pillsbury Company weather an FTC investigation regarding false claims on product packaging. William J. Darby to Joel Burke, September 7, 1971, series I, box 5, folder 11, Darby Papers. He also did outside consulting work for General Foods, Carnation, and Heinz.

12. Hess, "Harvard's Sugar-Pushing Nutritionist."

13. For NHF leaders, the 1961 NCMQ was little more than a naked power grab. In the *National Health Federation Bulletin*'s report on the event, one NHF member wrote, "Never has the dressed up, modern propaganda for the medical apparatus more blatantly portrayed big business characteristics"; Harold Edwards, "Washington Office Report on Congress of Quackery," *National Health Federation Bulletin* 7, no. 11–12 (November–December 1961), p. 3, box 529, folder 4, Historical Health Fraud and Alternative Medicine Collection, American Medical Association Archive (hereafter cited as HHF Collection). Insofar as hegemonic medicine operated like a business, it became obvious to the NHF that the AMA's goal in hosting these national congresses was to claim complete dominion over the provision of health care to maximize its own profits and suffocate its competition. The NHF and its allies decided to troll their opponents by creating their own conference, the deliberately similar National Congress on Medical Monopoly (NCMM). The medical monopoly congresses attracted major figures. For instance, America's first diet guru with medical credentials, Adelle Davis, spoke at one of the conferences in 1966. Conference organizers for the NHF purposely scheduled the NCMM to be hosted in the same city and during the same dates as the NCMQ to confuse its participants. On several occasions, their dummy conference did apparently attract a few bewildered nurses and physicians, but it was not a winning strategy overall. "F-D-C Reports," October 28, 1963, p. 10, box 529 folder 5, HHF Collection.

14. "F-D-C Reports," 12.

15. Food Additives Amendment of 1958 to the Food, Drugs, and Cosmetic Act of 1938, Pub. L. No. 85-929, 52 Stat. 1041, 21 USC 321 (1958), www.govinfo.gov/content /pkg/STATUTE-72/pdf/STATUTE-72-Pg1784.pdf.

16. Harrison Wellford and Samuel Epstein, "The Conflict over the Delaney Clause," *New York Times*, January 13, 1973, 31, www.nytimes.com/1973/01/13 /archives/the-conflict-over-the-delaney-clause.html.

17. "F-D-C Reports," August 10, 1959, box 529, folder 4, pp. 7–8, HHF Collection.

18. Dietary Supplement Health and Education Act of 1994 Amendment to the Federal Food, Drug, and Cosmetic Act of 1938, Pub. L. No. 103-417, 108 Stat. 4325 (1994), www.govinfo.gov/content/pkg/STATUTE-108/pdf/STATUTE-108-Pg4325 .pdf.

19. Laura A. W. Khatcheressian, "Regulation of Dietary Supplements: Five Years of DSHEA," *Food and Drug Law Journal* 54 (1999): 623–44.

20. Although NHF leaders insisted they were not enemies of scientific medicine per se, they became avid opponents of many well-intentioned public health interventions under the banner of health freedom. They opposed mandatory public vaccination, for instance, advising their membership to reject the polio vaccine. In place of the vaccine, the NHF advised its members they could keep their children safe from polio by cutting sugar from their diets. The NHF later joined forces with Christian Scientists to fight the fluoridation of public water and promoted Hoxsey therapy, laetrile, Krebiozen, and several other infamous heterodox cancer remedies.

Chapter 4

1. Michael T. Kaufman, "The Maze of Alternative Medicine," *New York Times*, March 6, 1993, 26, www.nytimes.com/1993/03/06/nyregion/about-new-york-the-maze-of-alternative-medicine.html.

2. Aimee Lee Ball, "The Trials of a Famous Fat Doctor," *Allure*, April 1994, 178.

3. Ball, "Trials of a Famous Fat Doctor"; Rick Hampson, "Diet Doc's License Suspended over Unconventional 'Ozone' Cancer Therapy," *Associated Press*, August 12, 1993, https://apnews.com/cb368dbefa9115b60255d992f76 291d3.

4. Essiac is a compound of burdock root, slippery elm, Indian rhubarb, and sheep sorrel pioneered in the 1920s as an alternative cancer therapy.

5. Ball, "Trials of a Famous Fat Doctor," 178.

6. Hampson, "Diet Doc's License Suspended"; Steve Fishman, "The Diet Martyr," *New York Magazine*, March 5, 2004, https://nymag.com/nymetro/news/people/features/n_10035/.

7. Kaufman, "Maze of Alternative Medicine," 26.

8. Hampson, "Diet Doc's License Suspended"; Fishman, "Diet Martyr."

9. Verlyn Klinkenborg, "Sorting Out an Eating Plan in a Nation Filled with Dietary Confusion," *New York Times*, May 5, 2003, A22, www.nytimes.com/2003/05/05/opinion/editorial-observer-sorting-eating-plan-nation-filled-with-dietary-confusion.html. Quote in section subheading from Lisa Heldke, Kerri Mommer, and Cynthia Pineo, eds., *The Atkins Diet and Philosophy: Chewing the Fat with Kant and Nietzsche* (New York: Open Court, 2013), 232.

10. Robert C. Atkins and Ruth West Herwood, *Dr. Atkins' Diet Revolution: The High Calorie Way to Stay Thin Forever* (New York: David McKay, 1972).

11. Chin Jou, "The Progressive Era Body Project: Calorie-Counting and 'Disciplining the Stomach' in 1920s America," *Journal of the Gilded Age and Progressive Era* 18, no. 4 (2019): 422–40, https://doi.org/10.1017/S1537781418000348.

12. Daniel O'Connell, "Brillat-Savarin's Nineteenth-Century Proto-Atkins Diet: A Case Study in Inductive Inference," in *The Atkins Diet and Philosophy: Chewing the Fat with Kant and Nietzsche*, ed. Lisa Heldke, Kerri Mommer, and Cynthia Pineo, 57–68 (New York: Open Court, 2013).

13. Vilhjalmur Stefansson, *The Fat of the Land* (New York: MacMillan, 1946). Also see Agnes Arnold-Forster, "The Pre-History of the Paleo Diet: Cancer in the 19th C.,"

in *Proteins, Pathologies, and Politics: Dietary Innovation and Disease Since the Nineteenth Century*, eds. David Gentilcore and Matthew Smith, 15–24 (London: Bloomsbury, 2018).

14. Richard Mackarness, *Eat Fat and Grow Slim* (London: Harvill Press, 1958).

15. John Yudkin, *Pure, White, and Deadly: How Sugar Is Killing Us and What We Can Do to Stop It* (London: Davis-Poynter, 1972), published in the United States as *Sweet and Dangerous: The New Facts about Sugar You Eat as a Cause of Heart Disease, Diabetes, and Other Killers* (New York: Peter H. Wyden, 1972); John Yudkin, *This Slimming Business* (London: Macgibbon & Kee, 1960). Rachel Meach, "From John Yudkin to Jamie Oliver: A Short but Sweet History on the War against Sugar," in *Proteins, Pathologies, and Politics: Dietary Innovation and Disease Since the Nineteenth Century* ed. David Gentilcore and Matthew Smith, 95–108 (London: Bloomsbury, 2018).

16. Evelyn L. Fiore, ed., *The L-C Diet: The Low Carbohydrate Diet* (New York: Ridge Press, 1965); per the cover copy, "Widely known as the low carbohydrate Air Force diet."

17. Herman Taller, *Calories Don't Count* (New York: Simon and Schuster, 1961).

18. Clarence Petersen, "Living off the Fat—and Fads—of the Land with Million-Dollar Diet Doctors," *Chicago Tribune*, September 8, 1981, A1.

19. Petersen, "Living off the Fat," A1. Gardner Jameson [Robert Cameron], *The Drinking Man's Diet: Or How to Lose Weight with a Minimum of Will Power* (San Francisco: Cameron Books, 1964); Irwin Maxwell Stillman and Samm Sinclair Baker, *Doctor's Quick Weight Loss Diet* (Englewood Cliffs, NJ: Prentice-Hall, 1967).

20. Adrienne Rose Johnson, "The Paleo Diet and the American Weight Loss Utopia, 1975–2014," *Utopian Studies* 26, no. 1 (2015): 101–24, 104, https://doi.org/10.5325/utopianstudies.26.1.0101. Walter L. Voegtlin, *The Stone Age Diet: Based on In-depth Studies of Human Ecology and the Diet of Man* (New York: Vantage, 1975).

21. Herman Tarnower and Samm Sinclair Baker, *The Complete Scarsdale Medical Diet: Plus Dr. Tarnower's Lifetime Keep-Slim Program* (New York: Rawson, Wade, 1978).

22. Joel Stein, "The Low-Carb Diet Craze," *Time*, October 24, 1999, http://content.time.com/time/magazine/article/0,9171,33169,00.html. Mary Dan Eades and Michael R Eades, *Protein Power: The High-Protein/Low-Carbohydrate Way to Lose Weight, Feel Fit, and Boost Your Health—in Just Weeks!* (New York: Bantam, 1996); Ray Audette and Troy Gilchrist, *NeanderThin: Eat Like a Caveman to Achieve a Lean, Strong, Healthy Body* (New York: St. Martin's Press, 1999); Pierre Dukan, *The Dukan Diet: The French Medical Solution for Permanent Weight Loss* (London: Hodder & Stoughton, 2010), first published in French in 2000; Loren Cordain, *The Paleo Diet: Lose Weight and Get Healthy by Eating the Food You Were Designed to Eat* (Hoboken, NJ: John Wiley & Sons, 2002); H. Leighton Steward, Sam S. Andrews, Morrison C. Bethea, and Luis A. Balart, *Sugar Busters! Cut Sugar to Trim Fat* (New York: Ballantine, 2001); Arthur Agatston, *The South Beach Diet: The Delicious, Doctor-Designed, Foolproof Plan for Fast and Healthy Weight Loss* (New York: Random House, 2003); Dave Asprey, *The Bulletproof Diet: Lose up to a Pound a Day, Reclaim Your Energy and Focus, and Upgrade Your Life* (New York: Rodale, 2014). Atkins's influence

can also be seen on programs that are not explicitly low-carb, such as Barry Sears's *The Zone: A Dietary Roadmap* (Los Angeles: Regan Books, 1995), Jennie Brand Miller and Kaye Foster, *The Glucose Revolution: Your Heart the Top 100 Low Glycemic Foods* (New York: Marlowe & Company, 1998), and Jordan Rubin, *The Maker's Diet* (Lake Mary, FL: Siloam, 2004), to the Quick Weight Loss Center program (popularized in 2009 by Rush Limbaugh) and the 2017 Optavia Diet (formerly Medifast).

23. Jack Speer, "Atkins Nutritionals Files for Bankruptcy," *NPR*, August 1, 2005, www.npr.org/templates/story/story.php?storyId=4780891.

24. For other work on male dieting, see Sander Gilman, *Fat Boys: A Slim Book* (Lincoln: University of Nebraska Press, 2004); Fabio Parasecoli, "Feeding Hard Bodies: Food and Masculinities in Men's Fitness Magazines," *Food and Foodways* 13, no. 1–2 (2005): 17–37, https://doi.org/10.1080/07409710590915355; Emily Contois, "'Lose Like a Man': Gender and the Constraints of Self-Making in Weight Watchers Online," *Gastronomica* 17, no. 1 (2017): 33–43, https://doi.org/10.1525/gfc.2017.17.1.33.

25. Amy Bentley, "The Other Atkins Revolution: Atkins and the Shifting Culture of Dieting," *Gastronomica* 4, no. 3 (2004): 34–45, https://doi.org/10.1525/gfc.2004.4.3.34. For similar arguments on masculinity and modern diets, see Tanfer Emin Tunc, "The 'Mad Men' of Nutrition: *The Drinking Man's Diet* and Mid-Twentieth-Century American Masculinity," *Global Food History* 4, no. 2 (2018): 189–206, https://doi.org/10.1080/20549547.2018.1434353; Contois, "Lose Like a Man," 33–43; Jesse Berrett, "Feeding the Organization Man: Diet and Masculinity in Postwar America," *Journal of Social History* 30, no. 4 (1997): 805–25, 805, https://doi.org/10.1353/jsh/30.4.805. For an important exploration of masculinity and food restriction from an earlier time period, see R. Marie Griffith, *Born again Bodies: Flesh and Spirit in American Christianity* (Berkeley: University of California Press, 2004).

26. Bentley, "Other Atkins Revolution," 34–45.

27. D. L. Stewart, "Thin Memories: Author of Controversial Diet Has Dayton Roots, but His Heart's in NYC," *Dayton Daily News*, February 20, 2003, C1.

28. Stewart, "Thin Memories," C1.

29. Fishman, "The Diet Martyr."

30. Fishman, "The Diet Martyr."

31. Douglas Martin, "Dr. Robert C. Atkins, Author of Controversial but Best-Selling Diet Books, Is Dead at 72," *New York Times*, April 18, 2003, D9, www.nytimes.com/2003/04/18/nyregion/dr-robert-c-atkins-author-controversial-but-best-selling-diet-books-dead-72.html.

32. Stewart, "Thin Memories," C1.

33. Pamela Howard and Sandy Treadwell, "Dr. Atkins Says He's Sorry," *New York Weekly*, March 26, 1973, as cited in *Hearings Before the Select Committee on Nutrition and Human Needs of the United States Senate—Obesity and Fad Diets I*, 93rd Cong. 68 (April 12, 1973), enclosed in Item 3—Articles Pertinent to Hearing Pertaining to Dr. Atkins's "Diet."

34. The following papers were the basis of the Pennington or Dupont diet: Alfred W. Pennington, "A Reorientation on Obesity," *New England Journal of Medicine* 248, no. 23 (1953): 959–64, https://doi.org/10.1056/nejm195306042482301;

Alfred W. Pennington, "Treatment of Obesity: Developments of the Past 150 Years," *American Journal of Digestive Diseases* 21, no. 3 (1954): 65–69, https://doi.org/10.1007/bf02880976; Alfred W. Pennington, "An Alternate Approach to the Problem of Obesity," *American Journal of Clinical Nutrition* 1, no. 2 (1953): 100–106, https://doi.org/10.1093/ajcn/1.2.100; Alfred W. Pennington, "Treatment of Obesity with Calorically Unrestricted Diets," *American Journal of Clinical Nutrition* 1, no. 5 (1953): 343–48, https://doi.org/10.1093/ajcn/1.5.343; Alfred W. Pennington, "Obesity: Overnutrition or Disease of Metabolism," *American Journal of Digestive Diseases* 20, no. 9 (1953): 268–74, https://doi.org/10.1007/BF02881331.

35. For examples, see A. Kekwick and G.L.S. Pawan, "Calorie Intake in Relation to Body-weight Changes in the Obese," *Lancet* 268, no. 6935 (1956): 155–61, https://doi.org/10.1016/S0140-6736(56)91691-9; T. M. Chalmers, A. Kekwick, and G.L.S. Pawan, "On the Fat-Mobilising Activity of Human Urine," *Lancet* 271, no. 7026 (1958): 866–69, https://doi.org/10.1016/S0140-6736(58)91624-6; A. Kekwick and G.L.S. Pawan, "Metabolic Study in Human Obesity with Isocaloric Diets High in Fat, Protein or Carbohydrate," *Metabolism* 6, no. 5 (1957): 447–60.

36. Megan Rosenfeld, "Going against the Grain," *Washington Post*, October 12, 1999, C1, www.washingtonpost.com/wp-srv/health/nutrition/stories/diet101299.htm; Howard and Treadwell, "Dr. Atkins Says He's Sorry."

37. William Leith, "Robert Atkins: Diet Guru Who Grew Fat on the Proceeds of the Carbohydrate Revolution," *Guardian* (London), April 18, 2003, www.theguardian.com/news/2003/apr/19/guardianobituaries.williamleith.

38. Martin, "Dr. Robert C. Atkins," D9.

39. Martin, "Dr. Robert C. Atkins," D9; Stewart, "Thin Memories," C1.

40. Natalie Gittelson, "How to Lose Weight Without Hunger," *Harper's Bazaar*, January 1966, 130–31; Jean Pierson, "How to S-T-A-Y 10 Lbs. Thinner," *Vogue*, June 1970, 158–59.

41. Howard and Treadwell, "Dr. Atkins Says He's Sorry."

42. Howard and Treadwell, "Dr. Atkins Says He's Sorry"; Diane K. Shah, "Critics Choke over Dr. Atkins' Diet," both as cited in *Hearings Before the Select Committee on Nutrition and Human Needs of the United States Senate—Obesity and Fad Diets I*, 93rd Cong. 63 (April 12, 1973), included in Item 3—Articles Pertinent to Hearing, Pertaining to Dr. Atkins's "Diet."

43. Shah, "Critics Choke over Dr. Atkins' Diet."

44. Freda Aron, "Nutritionist Hits Fads—Advises 'Eat Less,'" *The Skokie*, February 1, 1973, as cited in *Hearings Before the Select Committee on Nutrition and Human Needs of the United States Senate—Obesity and Fad Diets I*, 93rd Cong. 61 (April 12, 1973), enclosed in Item 3—Articles Pertinent to Hearing Pertaining to Dr. Atkins's "Diet."

45. Howard and Treadwell, "Dr. Atkins Says He's Sorry."

46. Martin, "Dr. Robert C. Atkins," D9.

47. Howard and Treadwell, "Dr. Atkins Says He's Sorry." Dr. Irwin Maxwell Stillman was already quite well-known as a diet guru and public figure when Atkins entered the scene, having made regular appearances on talk shows since the late 1960s. Between 1970 and 1974, he appeared on *The Tonight Show with Johnny*

Carson thirty-one times, and another fourteen times on *The Mike Douglas Show* between 1968 and 1975.

48. *Hearings Before the Select Committee on Nutrition and Human Needs of the United States Senate—Obesity and Fad Diets I*, 93rd Cong. (April 12, 1973), vi; Howard and Treadwell, "Dr. Atkins Says He's Sorry"; Martin, "Dr. Robert C. Atkins," D9.

49. Howard and Treadwell, "Dr. Atkins Says He's Sorry."

50. Linda Lee, "The Man Who Took Their Bread Away," *New York Times*, April 20, 2003, ST2; Lisa Rogak, *Dr. Robert Atkins: The True Story of the Man behind the War on Carbohydrates* (New York: Chamberlain Bros., 2005), 67.

51. Rogak, *Dr. Robert Atkins*, 96.

52. Rogak, *Dr. Robert Atkins*, 97.

53. Rogak, *Dr. Robert Atkins*, 69.

54. Rogak, *Dr. Robert Atkins*, 67.

55. A version of the original warning was published several months later in "A Critique of Low-Carbohydrate Ketogenic Weight Reduction Regimens: A Review of Dr. Atkins' Diet Revolution," *Journal of the American Medical Association* 224, no. 10 (1973): 1415–19, https://doi.org/10.1001/jama.1973.03220240055018. For an earlier, albeit more indirect critique, see "Statement on Hypoglycemia," *Journal of the American Medical Association* 223, no. 6 (1973): 682, https://doi.org/10.1001/jama.1973.03220060056016. Direct quote from March 10 statement from "Atkins Issues Reply to A.M.A. Criticism," *New York Times*, March 10, 1973, 21, www.nytimes.com/1973/03/10/archives/atkins-issues-reply-to-ama-criticism.html.

56. "Diet Doctor Hits Back at AMA Charge," *Dallas Times Herald*, March 9, 1973, as cited in *Hearings Before the Select Committee on Nutrition and Human Needs of the United States Senate—Obesity and Fad Diets I*, 93rd Cong. 65 (April 12, 1973), enclosed in Item 3—Articles Pertinent to Hearing Pertaining to Dr. Atkins's "Diet"; "Atkins Issues Reply," 21; Jane E. Brody, "Atkins Diet: A 'Revolution' That Has Medical Society Up in Arms," *New York Times*, March 14, 1973, 50, www.nytimes.com/1973/03/14/archives/atkins-diet-arevolution-that-has-medical-society-up-in-arms-below.html; Jean Mayer, "A Review of Dr. Atkins' Diet," *Chicago Tribune*, April 19, 1973, S5; Marlene Cimons, "Senate Probes Diet Industry: Dr. Atkins in the Hot Seat," *Los Angeles Times*, April 16, 1973, E1.

57. Shah, "Critics Choke over Dr. Atkins' Diet."

58. Aron, "Nutritionist Hits Fads"; Howard and Treadwell, "Dr. Atkins Says He's Sorry."

59. Jean Mayer, "Diet Revolution: Basically Old Hat," *Washington Post*, April 14, 1973, F1; Jean Mayer, "A Review of Dr. Atkins' Diet," *Chicago Tribune*, April 19, 1973, S5.

60. Shah, "Critics Choke over Dr. Atkins' Diet."

61. Rose Dosti, "More Fad Diets Waiting in Wings," *Los Angeles Times*, May 3, 1973, J5; Shah, "Critics Choke over Dr. Atkins' Diet"; Judith Randal, "Doctor Defends Diet," *Washington Star* (D.C.), April 13, 1973, as cited in *Hearings Before the Select Committee on Nutrition and Human Needs of the United States Senate—Obesity and Fad Diets I*, 93rd Cong. 76 (April 12, 1973), enclosed in Item 3—Articles Pertinent to Hearing Pertaining to Dr. Atkins's "Diet."

62. Shah, "Critics Choke over Dr. Atkins' Diet"; Dosti, "More Fad Diets Waiting in Wings."

63. "Dr. Atkins Is Sued for $7.5-Million," *New York Times*, March 23, 1973, 17, www .nytimes.com/1973/03/23/archives/dr-atking-is-sued-for-75million-diet -revolutionauthor-held-the.html. See also *Gorran v. Atkins Nutritionals, Inc.*, 464 F. Supp.2d 315 (2006), www.leagle.com/decision/2006779464fsupp2d3151749.

64. *Hearings Before the Select Committee on Nutrition and Human Needs of the United States Senate—Obesity and Fad Diets I*, 93rd Cong. (April 12, 1973).

65. Atkins complained to McGovern that he felt he had been unfairly targeted because of his recent success, and his recent tangling with the AMA. It was also a matter of timing, as Atkins became a controversial household name just as the committee investigating dietary fraud first convened. Notably, the tenor with which the committee interrogated diet gurus changed over time, evidenced by the tonal shift in the intervening years between the hearing at which Atkins was scrutinized and the hearing at which Pritikin was highlighted as a potential expert.

66. Cimons, "Senate Probes Diet Industry," E1; Jane E. Brody, "Senate Nutrition Panel to Focus On Perils of Being Overweight," *New York Times*, April 13, 1973, 18.

67. Cimons, "Senate Probes Diet Industry," E1.

68. *Hearings Before the Select Committee on Nutrition and Human Needs of the United States Senate—Obesity and Fad Diets I*, 93rd Cong. (April 12, 1973).

69. This was a regular piece of Atkins's defense in multiple lawsuits.

70. Robert C. Atkins, *Dr. Atkins' New Diet Revolution* (New York: Harper-Collins, 1992), 51.

71. Julie Deardorff, "Skinny but Stinky Thanks to Atkins," *Chicago Tribune*, January 2, 2004, www.chicagotribune.com/news/ct-xpm-2004-05-02-0405020298 -story.html. Bad breath and other bodily odors are an enduring phenomenon with other low-carb diets. See Martha Cliff, "Forget 'Keto Crotch,'—Now 'Keto Breath' Is the Embarrassing Issue Plaguing Women on a Low-Carb Diet," *Sun* (UK) November 1, 2019, www.thesun.co.uk/fabulous/10261513/keto-breath-embarrassing-issue -plaguing-dieters/.

72. There have been more serious concerns regarding the health of ketosis as an extended bodily state, including the suitability of ketones as a fuel for the brain (the body's chief glucose customer), but those are concerns to be developed in future scholarship.

73. Atkins, *Dr. Atkins' New Diet Revolution*, 57; Ball, "Trials of a Famous Fat Doctor."

74. At the hearing, Pawan actually predicated his agreement with the AMA's stance against Atkins on whether the fat mobilizing hormone (FMH) that Atkins credited for burning body fat in the absence of glucose was a true hormone or whether it was merely a fat mobilizing substance (FMS). Tom Zito, "'Diet Revolution' Controversy," *Washington Post*, April 13, 1973, B2, ProQuest.

75. Zito, "'Diet Revolution' Controversy," B2; Shah, "Critics Choke over Dr. Atkins' Diet."

76. Shah, "Critics Choke over Dr. Atkins' Diet."

77. Alex Witchel, "Refighting the Battle of the Bulge: At Lunch with Dr. Robert Atkins," *New York Times*, November 27, 1996, C7, www.nytimes.com/1996/11/27 /garden/refighting-the-battle-of-the-bulge.html.

78. Dosti, "More Fad Diets Waiting in Wings," J5.

79. Ronald M. Deutsch, *The New Nuts among the Berries* (Palo Alto, CA: Bull Publishing, 1977); Jane Skinner, "Nutrition Expert Claims Fad Diets Might Be Damaging," *Palm Beach News*, March 13, 1973, as cited in *Hearings Before the Select Committee on Nutrition and Human Needs of the United States Senate—Obesity and Fad Diets I*, 93rd Cong. 68 (April 12, 1973), enclosed in Item 3—Articles Pertinent to Hearing Pertaining to Dr. Atkins's "Diet"; George Getze, "Food Expert Calls Popular Diet 'Useless'—Perils Cited," *Los Angeles Times*, March 26, 1973, B1.

80. Marilyn Mercer, "The Atkins Diet: Is It Safe?" *McCall's Monthly Newsletter for Women*, April 1973.

81. For examples of prominent followers who had to quit Atkins for this reason, see Lee, "Man Who Took Their Bread Away," ST2.

82. Pierson, "How to S-T-A-Y 10 Lbs. Thinner," 159.

83. Howard and Treadwell, "Dr. Atkins Says He's Sorry."

84. Robert C. Atkins and Shirley Motter Linde, *Dr. Atkins' Superenergy Diet: The Diet Revolution Answer to Fatigue and Depression* (New York: Crown, 1977).

85. US Senate Select Committee on Nutrition and Human Needs, *Dietary Goals for the United States* (Washington, DC: US Government Printing Office, February 1977), also known as the McGovern Report.

86. Shapin highlights the similarity of Atkins's denial of his own guru-ness to the near-identical denials of guru-ness from other gurus like him. Shapin rightly notes that it became somewhat of a trope for gurus like Atkins to deny their status as diet docs. Perhaps in his case, though, Atkins was being truthful. Steven Shapin, "Expertise, Common Sense, and the Atkins Diet," in *Public Science in Liberal Democracy*, eds. Jene Porter and Peter W. B. Phillips, 174–93 (Toronto: University of Toronto Press, 2007).

87. Paul Jacobs, "Diet Book Authors Trade Charges," *Los Angeles Times*, October 15, 1979, B3; Rose Dosti, "Diet Books Offer the Highs and Lows of Proteins and Carbohydrates," *Los Angeles Times*, May 21, 1981, N33; Martha Smiglis, "Pritikin Will Eat No Fat, Atkins Will Eat No Grain—and That Feeds a Fierce Dispute over Diet," *People*, December 3, 1979, https://people.com/archive/pritikin-will-eat-no-fat-atkins -will-eat-no-grain-and-that-feeds-a-fierce-dispute-over-diet-vol-12-no-23/.

88. Nathan Pritikin, interview, *Live at Five*, WNBC-TV, May 27, 1981, broadcast excerpt; Robert Atkins, interview, *Live at Five*, WNBC-TV, May 28, 1981, broadcast excerpt; Nathan Pritikin debates Robert Atkins, *Tomorrow*, WNBC-TV, June 9, 1981, broadcast excerpt; all in box 21, folder "Pritikin-Atkins 'Debate' (Pre-Litigation)," Nathan Pritikin Papers, Library Special Collections, Charles E. Young Research Library, University of California, Los Angeles (hereafter cited as Pritikin Papers).

89. Pritikin kept evidence from the supporters he mentioned and showed it in court. Bernard Rosen to Nathan Pritikin, June 19, 1981; Nell C. Taylor to Tova Leidesdorf, November 10, 1980; both in box 21, folder "*Atkins v. Pritikin* Lawsuit: Legal

Documents," Pritikin Papers. For other accounts of their caustic relationship, see Richard MacManus, *Health Trackers: How Technology Is Helping Us Monitor and Improve Our Health* (Auckland, New Zealand: Rowman & Littlefield, 2015); Susan Yager, *The Hundred Year Diet: America's Voracious Appetite for Losing Weight* (New York: Rodale, 2010); Michael Greger, *Carbophobia: The Scary Truth about America's Low-Carb Craze* (New York: Lantern Books, 2005).

90. Fishman, "The Diet Martyr."

91. Michael Greger claims that Atkins continued trying to sue Pritikin's estate and his "grieving widow," after Pritikin had passed. Greger, *Carbophobia*, 65.

92. Fishman, "The Diet Martyr."

93. Witchel, "Refighting the Battle of the Bulge," C7.

94. "Dr. Robert Atkins and Dr. Dean Ornish: A Chat about Opposing Diet Plans," *CNN: Crossfire*, May 30, 2000, www.cnn.com/community/transcripts/2000/5/30 /atkins.ornish/; Teresa L. Ebert and Mas-ud Zavarzadeh, "In Atkins, Ornish Diets, Class Shapes the Outcomes," *Sun Sentinel* (Florida), September 10, 2000, www.sun -sentinel.com/news/fl-xpm-2000-09-10-0009070851-story.html.

95. USDA Millennium Lecture Series, "Symposium on The Great Nutrition Debate," USDA Center for Nutrition Policy & Promotion, February, 24, 2000, posted online by Gerhardt Steinke, "USDA Great Nutrition Debate," December 13, 2012, YouTube video, 2:55:11, www.youtube.com/watch?v=zJ-2Mo2ON5E; Sean Martin, "Diet Gurus Belly Up to the Debate Table," *WebMD*, February 24, 2000, www.webmd .com/diet/news/20000224/diet-gurus-belly-up-to-the-debate-table#1.

96. Katharine Mieszkowski, "Vegans vs. Atkins," *Salon*, December 9, 2003, www .salon.com/2003/12/08/peta_and_atkins/; Mary Carmichael, "Atkins under Attack," *Newsweek*, February 22, 2004, www.newsweek.com/atkins-under-attack-131403; Rome Neal, "A Warning to Atkins Dieters," *CBS News*, November 19, 2003, www .cbsnews.com/news/a-warning-to-atkins-dieters/; "Group Says Atkins Diet Dangerous," *CNN Health*, November 21, 2003, http://edition.cnn.com/2003/HEALTH/diet .fitness/11/20/diet.heart.reut/.

97. Greger, *Carbophobia*, 65.

98. Robert C. Atkins, *Dr. Atkins' Nutrition Breakthrough: How to Treat Your Medical Condition Without Drugs* (New York: William Morrow, 1981); Robert C. Atkins, *Dr. Atkins' Health Revolution: How Complementary Medicine Can Extend Your Life* (Boston: Houghton Mifflin, 1988).

99. Stein, "The Low-Carb Diet Craze."

100. Ball, "Trials of a Famous Fat Doctor," 174.

101. Robert C.M.D. Atkins, *Dr. Atkins' Nutrition Breakthrough* (New York, Bantam, 1981), 16.

102. Atkins, *Dr. Atkins' New Diet Revolution.*

103. Martin, "Dr. Robert C. Atkins," D9; Julie Dunn, "Restaurant Chains, Too, Watch Their Carbs," *New York Times*, January 4, 2004, BU3, www.nytimes.com /2004/01/04/business/business-restaurant-chains-too-watch-their-carbs.html; Jane E. Allen, "Robert Atkins, 72; His Books Launched High-Protein, Low-Carb 'Diet Revolution,'" *Los Angeles Times*, April 18, 2003, B11, www.latimes.com/archives/la -xpm-2003-apr-18-me-atkins18-story.html; Fishman, "The Diet Martyr."

104. "Who Does What?" *Irish Times*, August 21, 2007, www.irishtimes.com/news /health/who-does-what-1.957066.

105. Jessica Wohl, "Atkins Hires Rob Lowe to Promote Its 'Lifestyle' (It's Not Just a Diet)," *AdAge*, January 3, 2018, https://adage.com/article/cmo-strategy/atkins -hires-rob-lowe-promote-lifestyle-a-diet/311791.

106. Nicola Woolcock and Oliver Poole, "My Lawyers Will Eat You for Breakfast over Atkins Claims, Zeta-Jones Warns," *Telegraph* (London), November 12, 2003, www.telegraph.co.uk/news/worldnews/northamerica/usa/1446508/My-lawyers -will-eat-you-for-breakfast-over-Atkins-claims-Zeta-Jones-warns.html.

107. Ronnie Carr, "Atkins Exposed," *ELLEgirl* Magazine, September–October 2003, 96–97.

108. "Atkins Exposed," 96–97.

109. Robert C. Atkins, *Dr. Atkins Vita-Nutrient Solution: Nature's Answers to Drugs* (New York: Simon and Schuster, 1998); Robert C. Atkins and Sheila Buff, *Dr. Atkins' Age-Defying Diet Revolution* (New York: St. Martin's Press, 2000); Mary C. Vernon and Jacqueline A. Eberstein, *Atkins Diabetes Revolution: The Groundbreaking Approach to Preventing and Controlling Type II Diabetes* (New York: HarperCollins, 2004). The original title of *Atkins Diabetes Revolution* had been *Diobesity*, but was changed after his death; Leith, "Robert Atkins."

110. Gary Taubes, "What If It's All Been a Big Fat Lie?" *New York Times Magazine*, July 7, 2002, www.nytimes.com/2002/07/07/magazine/what-if-it-s-all-been-a -big-fat-lie.html.

111. Fishman, "The Diet Martyr."

112. Michael Fumento, "Big Fat Fake," *Reason*, March 2003, https://reason.com /2003/03/01/big-fat-fake-2/; Gary Taubes, "An Exercise in Vitriol Rather Than Sound Journalism," *Reason*, March 2003, https://reason.com/2003/03/01/an-exercise-in -vitriol-rather/; Michael Fumento, "Gary Taubes Tries to Overwhelm the Reader with Sheer Verbiage," *Reason*, March 2003, https://reason.com/2003/03/01/gary-taubes -tries-to-overwhelm/. Fumento had published a takedown of the Atkins diet in *Reason* the previous year as well: Michael Fumento, "Hold the Lard! The Atkins Diet Still Doesn't Work," *Reason*, December 5, 2002, https://reason.com/2002/12/05/hold -the-lard/.

113. Bonnie Liebman, "The Truth about the Atkins Diet," *Nutrition Action*, November 2002, 3–7.

114. Ellen Ruppel Shell, "It's Not the Carbs, Stupid," *Newsweek*, August 5, 2002, 41.

115. For reports on the scandal, see Camila Domonoske, "50 Years Ago, Sugar Industry Quietly Paid Scientists to Point Blame at Fat," *NPR*, September 13, 2016, www.npr.org/sections/thetwo-way/2016/09/13/493739074/50-years-ago-sugar -industry-quietly-paid-scientists-to-point-blame-at-fat; Anahad O'Connor, "How the Sugar Industry Shifted Blame to Fat," *New York Times*, September 12, 2016, www .nytimes.com/2016/09/13/well/eat/how-the-sugar-industry-shifted-blame-to-fat .html.

116. Gary Taubes, "'Nutrition Heretic' Gary Taubes on the Long Road Back from a Big, Fat Public Shaming," *New York Magazine*, November 23, 2016, https://nymag

.com/vindicated/2016/11/how-a-nutrition-heretic-overcame-a-big-fat-public
-shaming.html; Michael Pollan, *In Defense of Food: An Eater's Manifesto* (London: Penguin, 2009), 49.

117. Stephen Barrett and William T. Jarvis, *The Health Robbers: A Close Look at Quackery in America* (Buffalo, NY: Prometheus, 1993). Quote in section subheading from Nina Burleigh, "The New Healers," *New York Magazine*, April 5, 1999, https:// nymag.com/nymetro/health/features/890/.

118. Burleigh, "The New Healers."

119. Burleigh, "The New Healers."

120. Fishman, "The Diet Martyr."

121. Rogak, *Dr. Robert Atkins*, 95.

122. Rosenfeld, "Going against the Grain," C1.

123. Fredericks was also known for vilifying sugar and overdiagnosing hypogly-cemia. Barrett and Jarvis, *Health Robbers*, 373.

124. Barrett and Jarvis, *Health Robbers*, 376.

125. Ball, "Trials of a Famous Fat Doctor." For dietary supplement history, see Gyorgyi Scrinis, *Nutritionism: The Science and Politics of Dietary Advice* (New York: Columbia University Press, 2013); Catherine Price, *Vitamania: Our Obsessive Quest with Nutritional Perfection* (New York: Penguin, 2015).

126. Smiglis, "Pritikin Will Eat No Fat."

127. Fishman, "The Diet Martyr."

128. Karen Tetlow, "Complementary Design," *Interiors* 153, no. 10 (1994): 70–71.

129. Tetlow, "Complementary Design," 70–71.

130. Stewart, "Thin Memories," C1.

131. Fishman, "The Diet Martyr"; Ramin P. Jaleshgari, "Doctor with a Diet Has a New Message," *New York Times*, April 18, 1999, L125, www.nytimes.com/1999/04 /18/nyregion/on-island-books-of-individualism-doctor-with-a-diet-has-a-new -message.html.

132. Fishman, "The Diet Martyr"; Jaleshgari, "Doctor with a Diet," L125.

133. Ball, "Trials of a Famous Fat Doctor"; Burleigh, "The New Healers"; Fish-man, "The Diet Martyr"; Leith, "Robert Atkins."

134. Burleigh, "The New Healers"; Ball, "Trials of a Famous Fat Doctor."

135. Ball, "Trials of a Famous Fat Doctor," 173.

136. Barrett and Jarvis, *Health Robbers*, 376.

137. Burleigh, "The New Healers"; Barrett and Jarvis, *Health Robbers*, 376.

138. Fishman, "The Diet Martyr."

139. Ball, "Trials of a Famous Fat Doctor," 174.

140. Ball, "Trials of a Famous Fat Doctor," 175.

141. The *Geraldo Show* as quoted in Barrett and Jarvis, *Health Robbers*, 376.

142. USDA Great Nutrition Debate, 2000.

143. Fishman, "The Diet Martyr."

144. Witchel, "Refighting the Battle of the Bulge," C7; Jeanne Lenzer, "Robert Coleman Atkins," *British Medical Journal* 326, no. 7398 (2003): 1090, https://doi.org /10.1136/bmj.326.7398.1090.

145. Atkins, *Nutrition Breakthrough*, 16; Ball, "Trials of a Famous Fat Doctor," 174.

146. For a broader history of sugar substitutes, see Caroline de la Peña, *Empty Pleasures: The Story of Artificial Sweeteners from Saccharin to Splenda* (Chapel Hill: University of North Carolina Press, 2010).

147. W. A. Thomasson, "The Controversy over Saccharin and Health," *Washington Post*, July 1, 1979, www.washingtonpost.com/archive/opinions/1979/07/01/the -controversy-over-saccharin-and-health/94704bca-6ec2-423e-b354-e82f8d6abd5d/. The carcinogenic potential of cyclamates has been challenged, and bans have been reversed in the European Union and around the world. It should be noted that the United States is one of the only nations that still restricts the use of cyclamates on the basis of the Delaney Clause.

148. Howard and Treadwell, "Dr. Atkins Says He's Sorry." Also see Harvey Levenstein, *Paradox of Plenty: A Social History of Eating in Modern America* (Berkeley: University of California Press, 2003), 135–36; Harvey Levenstein, *Appetite for Change: How the Counterculture Took On the Food Industry* (Ithaca, NY: Cornell University Press, 2014), 140.

149. *People v. Atkins*, 76 Misc.2d 661 (1974), www.leagle.com/decision/19747 3776misc2d6611578.

150. *People v. Atkins*.

151. *Ballinger v. Atkins*, 947 F. Supp. 925 (E.D. Va. 1996), https://law.justia.com /cases/federal/district-courts/FSupp/947/925/1453962/.

152. *Ballinger v. Atkins*.

153. Barrett and Jarvis, *Health Robbers*, 412.

154. For a more robust account of the difficulties encountered by clinical ecologists, see Matthew Smith, *Another Person's Poison: A History of Food Allergy* (New York: Columbia University Press, 2015).

155. Barrett and Jarvis, *Health Robbers*, 148.

156. "$900,000 Award in Clinical Ecology Malpractice Case," *NCAHF News* 14, no. 3 (1991), https://quackwatch.org/ncahf/1991-2/5-6/.

157. *Gersten v. Levin*, 150 Misc.2d 594 (1991), www.leagle.com/decision /1991744150misc2d5941639.

158. Robert H. Harris, *Prime Example: The True Story of the Case That Saved Alternative Medicine in New York State* (New York: Morgan James, 2011).

159. Harris, *Prime Example*.

160. Barrett says Atkins's supplements were intended for the treatment of medical conditions, which was illegal, but they were thinly disguised using an obvious code (i.e., Cardiovascular formula was coded as CV). But Atkins managed to skirt the line in part because he considered most chronic diseases to be nutritional deficiencies. Barrett and Jarvis, *Health Robbers*, 376.

161. Burleigh, "The New Healers." The Act has been repeatedly ignored by New York judges, so it is not clear it actually did anything to help CAM practitioners. Barbara L. Atwell, "Mainstreaming Complementary and Alternative Medicine in the Face of Uncertainty," *UMKC Law Review* 72, no. 593 (2004): 593–630.

162. Ball, "Trials of a Famous Fat Doc," 175.

163. Barrett cofounded the National Council against Health Fraud (NCAHF) with William Jarvis in 1983 (an outgrowth of a similar anti-quackery committee he

founded in Allentown, Pennsylvania, in 1969). NCAHF has since become Quackwatch, an organization run by Barrett that publicizes his years of meticulous documentation of cases he believes to be health fraud. He and his regular coauthors, including Herbert and Jarvis, were antagonistic toward and thus deservedly unpopular among alternative healers. In addition to *Health Robbers*, Barrett and Herbert coauthored *Vitamins and 'Health' Foods: The Great American Hustle* (Philadelphia: G. F. Stickley, 1985) and *The Vitamin Pushers: How the "Health Food" Industry Is Selling America a Bill of Goods* (Buffalo, NY: Prometheus, 1994).

164. After four years of investigation, Pepper's committee published a subcommittee report titled "Quackery: A $10 BIllion Scandal," which labeled health fraud the "single most prevalent and damaging of the frauds directed at the elderly." Though diets like Atkins's were specifically excoriated at the hearing, his practices were mild compared to the other procedures cited in the report. At the hearing, Pepper himself said "We found the inventiveness of the quacks to be as unlimited as their callousness and greed. . . . We found promoters who advised arthritics to bury themselves in the earth, sit in an abandoned mine, or stand naked under a 1,000-watt bulb during the full moon. . . . These suffering souls have been wrapped in manure, soaked in mud, injected with snake venom, sprayed with WD-40, bathed in kerosene and made to pay for the privilege of being afflicted that way." Don Colburn, "Quackery," *Washington Post*, June 19, 1985, www.washingtonpost.com/archive/lifestyle/wellness/1985/06/19/quackery/1778d04e-d969-4c78-8eeb-f2df5346e057/.

165. *Atkins v. Guest*, 158 Misc.2d 426 (1993), www.leagle.com/decision/1993584158misc2d4261521; *Atkins v. Guest*, 201 A.D.2d 411 (1994), www.leagle.com/decision/1994612201ad2d4111366.

166. Coy's affidavit was quoted in Kaufman, "Maze of Alternative Medicine," 26.

167. "Doctor's License Restored," *New York Times*, August 18, 1993, B4, www.nytimes.com/1993/08/18/nyregion/doctor-s-license-restored.html.

168. Hampson, "Diet Doc's License Suspended."

169. Fishman, "The Diet Martyr."

170. Ball, "Trials of a Famous Fat Doctor," 176.

171. Ball, "Trials of a Famous Fat Doctor," 176.

172. "Rival Diet Doc Leaks Atkins Death Report," *Smoking Gun*, February 10, 2004, www.thesmokinggun.com/documents/crime/rival-diet-doc-leaks-atkins-death-report.

173. Ball, "Trials of a Famous Fat Doctor."

174. Fishman, "The Diet Martyr."

175. Shah, "Critics Choke over Dr. Atkins' Diet."

176. Theodore Berland, "Best Model for His Own Diet," *Chicago Tribune*, September 22, 1975, B18.

177. Joel Stein, "Paging Dr. Fatkins?" *Time*, February 16, 2004, http://content.time.com/time/magazine/article/0,9171,591316,00.html.

178. "Rival Diet Doc Leaks Atkins Death Report."

179. N. R. Kleinfield, "Just What Killed the Diet Doctor, and What Keeps the Issue Alive?" February 11, 2004, *New York Times*, www.nytimes.com/2004/02/11/nyregion/just-what-killed-the-diet-doctor-and-what-keeps-the-issue-alive.html.

180. Kleinfield, "Just What Killed the Diet Doctor."

181. Jennifer Steinhauer, "Dr. Atkins and the Mayor: The Art of Not Saying Sorry," January 24, 2004, *New York Times*, B3, www.nytimes.com/2004/01/24/nyregion /political-memo-dr-atkins-and-the-mayor-the-art-of-not-saying-sorry.html.

182. John Hockenberry, "Defending Dr. Atkins: Wife of Famous Diet Doctor Fights Critics' Claims," *NBC News*, February 25, 2004, www.nbcnews.com/id/4327741/ns /dateline_nbc/t/defending-dr-atkins/; Edie Magnus, "Florida Man Sues Atkins over Health Problems," *Dateline NBC*, June 6, 2004, www.nbcnews.com/id/5137232/ns /dateline_nbc/t/florida-man-sues-atkins-over-health-problems/.

183. Hockenberry, "Defending Dr. Atkins."

184. Steinhauer, "Dr. Atkins and the Mayor," B3; Winnie Hu, "Bloomberg Offers an Apology to Atkins' Widow," January 25, 2004, *New York Times*, N36, www .nytimes.com/2004/01/25/nyregion/bloomberg-offers-an-apology-to-atkins-s -widow.html.

185. Stein, "Paging Dr. Fatkins?"

186. Hockenberry, "Defending Dr. Atkins."

187. Maxine Frith, "Fighting for a Slice of the Atkins Pie: The Doctors Who Claim to Be His Successor," *Independent* (London), March 22, 2004, www.independent.co .uk/news/world/americas/fighting-for-a-slice-of-the-atkins-pie-the-doctors-who -claim-to-be-his-successor-756860.html.

188. Fred Pascatore, *The Hamptons Diet: Lose Weight Quickly and Safety with the Doctor's Delicious Meal Plans* (Hoboken, NJ: John Wiley & Sons, 2004).

189. Robert C. Atkins, *Atkins for Life: The Complete Controlled Carb Program for Permanent Weight Loss and Good Health* (New York: St. Martin's Press, 2003).

190. See Stuart Trager and Collette Heimowitz, *The All-New Atkins Advantage* (New York: St. Martin's Press, 2007).

191. Fishman, "The Diet Martyr."

Conclusion

1. Eliza Barclay, "Not Your Grandmother's Hospital Food," *NPR: The Salt*, January 23, 2012, www.npr.org/sections/thesalt/2012/01/23/145659005/not-your-grand mothers-hospital-food; Richard Schiffman, "Hospital Food You Can Get Excited About," *New York Times*, September 20, 2018, www.nytimes.com/2018/09/20/well /eat/hospital-food-you-can-get-excited-about.html; "American Hospital Food Is Fast Improving," *Economist*, September 8, 2022, www.economist.com/united -states/2022/09/08/american-hospital-food-is-fast-improving.

2. Gyorgi Scrinis, *Nutritionism: The Science and Politics of Dietary Advice* (New York: Columbia University Press, 2015); Marion Nestle, *Food Politics: How the Food Industry Influences Nutrition and Health* (Berkeley: University of California Press, 2013); Charlotte Biltekoff, *Eating Right in America: The Cultural Politics of Food and Health* (Durham, NC: Duke University Press, 2013); Harvard T. H. Chan School of Public Health, "Healthy Eating Plate and Healthy Eating Pyramid," *Nutrition Source,* January 2015, www.hsph.harvard.edu/nutritionsource/healthy-eating -plate/.

3. Nutrition science is often used as the poster child for scientific uncertainty. Steven Shapin, "Expertise, Common Sense, and the Atkins Diet," in *Public Science in Liberal Democracy*, ed. Jene Porter and Peter W. B. Phillips, 174–93 (Toronto: University of Toronto Press, 2007).

4. Emily Abel, *Sick and Tired: An Intimate History of Fatigue* (Chapel Hill: The University of North Carolina Press, 2021).

5. For a more detailed analysis about public figures who have been heavily scrutinized for their bodies, and especially their medical conditions, see Barron Lerner, *When Illness Goes Public: Celebrity Patients and How We Look at Medicine* (Baltimore: Johns Hopkins University Press, 2006).

6. Eleanor Hoover, "Nathan Pritikin's Diet Book Is Selling Like Hotcakes, a Dish He Sure Hopes You Won't Eat," *People*, August 13, 1979, https://people.com/archive /nathan-pritikins-diet-book-is-selling-like-hotcakes-a-dish-he-sure-hopes-you -wont-eat-vol-12-no-7/.

7. James C. Barks to Nathan Pritikin, August 5, 1980, box 23, folder "Birthday Book Replies III," Nathan Pritikin Papers, Library Special Collections, Charles E. Young Research Library, University of California, Los Angeles (hereafter cited as Pritikin Papers).

8. Dianne Struzzi, "Natural Healer Alvenia Fulton," *Chicago Tribune*, March 20, 1999, 25, www.chicagotribune.com/news/ct-xpm-1999-03-20-9903200076-story .html.

9. Aveline Kushi died, at age seventy-eight, from cancer and used conventional radiation therapy. Douglas Martin, "Aveline Kushi, 78, Advocate of Macrobiotic Diet for Health," *New York Times*, July 23, 2001, B6, www.nytimes.com/2001/07/23 /us/aveline-kushi-78-advocate-of-macrobiotic-diet-for-health.html. The Kushis's daughter Lily also underwent conventional radiation therapy for her stage four cervical cancer.

10. Dick Cavett, "When That Guy Died on My Show," Opinionator, *New York Times*, May 3, 2007, https://opinionator.blogs.nytimes.com/2007/05/03/when-that -guy-died-on-my-show/.

11. Jane Gross, "James F. Fixx Dies Jogging; Author on Running Was 52," *New York Times*, July 22, 1984, 24, www.nytimes.com/1984/07/22/obituaries/james-f -fixx-dies-jogging-author-on-running-was-52.html.

12. "Heart Beat: Ornish, Pritikin Get Medicare Okay for Cardiac Rehab," *Harvard Health Publishing*, December 1, 2010, www.health.harvard.edu/newsletter _article/ornish-pritikin-get-medicare-okay-for-cardiac-rehab. Notably, after Donald Trump's Doral Resorts bought out the Pritikin Longevity Center's former landlord, they forced a room rate change for which they were promptly and successfully sued. Jose Lambiet, "Pritikin Again Wins against Trump National Doral Miami," *Miami Herald*, January 17, 2018, www.miamiherald.com/entertainment/ent -columns-blogs/jose-lambiet/article195228074.html; Martin Vassolo, "Trump Loses Appeal to Doral Golf Resort Tenant in Room-Rate Dispute," *Miami Herald*, August 3, 2018, www.miamiherald.com/news/local/community/miami-dade/doral/article21 6038190.html.

13. Eboni Senai Hawkins, Sam Scipio, and Michael Tekhen Strode, "Episode #1: Fultonia," *Afros & Ceramic Fruit*, WSTS Radio, 2014, 55:00, www.mixcloud.com /wstsradio/afros-ceramic-fruit-episode-1-fultonia/; *Fultonia*, exhibition organized by Propeller Fund at Mana Contemporary, Chicago, October 16, 2014–January 23, 2015, http://propellerfund.org/693/.

14. Marian Burros, "Make That Steak a Bit Smaller, Atkins Advises Today's Dieters," *New York Times*, January 18, 2004, www.nytimes.com/2004/01/18/nyregion /make-that-steak-a-bit-smaller-atkins-advises-today-s-dieters.html.

15. Lizzie Widdicombe, "The End of Food," *New Yorker*, May 5, 2014, www .newyorker.com/magazine/2014/05/12/the-end-of-food. Despite the cannibalistic connotations of its name, Soylent is, in fact, vegan.

16. Soylent was actually founded with the vestiges of the money its three founders had raised for their failed cell tower company. Widdicombe, "The End of Food."

17. The connection between Bitcoin and ZC is a philosophical one. Its proponents argue that just as Bitcoin replaced "fiat" currencies, so should meat replace other "fiat" foods. Jordan Pearson, "Inside the World of the 'Bitcoin Carnivores,'" *Vice*, September 29, 2017, www.vice.com/en_us/article/ne74nw/inside-the-world-of-the -bitcoin-carnivores.

Index

enemas, 22, 34. *See also* colonic cleansing

energy balance theory, 46–47, 149. *See also* calorie, concept of

Erewhon Trading Company, 71, 88, 91, 112, 215n72

Esselstyn, Caldwell, 138

Ethiopian famine, 39–40

ethnobotany, 18

eugenics, 37

Evans County Georgia Heart Study, 26

exercise and fitness trends: daily routines, 109; Dick Gregory's program, 41; fitness cults, 7; fitness trends, 7, 196; 4X supplement for athletic performance, 38–39, 40; group classes, 114; macrobiotic approach, 57, 77; medical advice, standard, 46–47; Pritikin Program, 101, 108–9, 111–22, 127; running and jogging, 7, 100–101, 193, 196

experiential medicine, 171, 174, 176–77

Faces of Death (mondo horror film), 3

Falana, Lola, 23

fasting, 20; Alvenia Moody Fulton's fasting program, 23; Dick Gregory's fasting protests, 38–39; as protest, 16, 22–23, 38–39

fat: Atkins diet, 148, 157–61; avoidance of in Pritikin Program, 107–10; low-fat paradigm, 118, 137–38

fat activism, 46–47

fat-mobilizing hormone (FMH), 159

fat-mobilizing substance (FMS), 159

Fat of the Land (Fumento), 166

FDA (Food and Drug Administration): and diet regulation, 156; and food contaminants, 95; Ohsawa Foundation investigations, 54, 69; and supplement regulation, 145, 173

Federal Trade Commission (FTC), 143

fertilizer. *See* soil health

Fett, Sharla, 18

fibroid tumors, 20

Fishbein, Morris, 15

fitness. *See* exercise and fitness trends

Fixx, Jim, 193

Flack, Roberta, 23

Fleming, Richard, 178

Flockhart, Calista, 165

fluoridation, public water, 93

Food, Drug, and Cosmetic Act (1958), 143. *See also* Delaney Clause (1958)

Food and Drug Administration (FDA). *See* FDA (Food and Drug Administration)

Food Cure Society (Shoku-Yo Kai), 58–59

food faddism, 34, 94–95

food justice/sovereignty, 43

Food Protection Committee, National Research Council, 142

Food Pyramid, 163–164

"food rebels," 32–34, 205–6n87

Food Stamp program, 118

Formula 4X supplement, 38–41, 207n118

Foundation for the Advancement of Innovative Medicine (FAIM), 173

Foxx, Redd, 23

Framingham Heart Study, 26, 134

Fratellone, Patrick, 179, 182

fraud, 15, 36, 94–95, 174–75, 244n164

Fredericks, Carlton, 168

fruitarianism, 22, 195, 202n27

Fry, Stephen, 165

Fuhrman, Joel, 5

Fulton, Alvenia Moody, 11; background and personal health, 17–20, 35, 190; business model, 23–24; Fultonia Health Food and Fasting Center, 21–22, 23, 34–35; impact and legacy, 43–45; influence on Dick Gregory, 22–23; National Health Federation (NHF), 93; nutritional training, 35–36; racial impact on chronic disease, 25–28; soul food, 28–34; white-coded healing practices, 34–38

Fulton, O. M., 19

Fultonia Health Food and Fasting Center, 21–22, 23, 34–35, 193

Pritikin Program: adoption of by hospitals, 117–18; background and overview, 99–105; blandness and unpalatability, 124–26; community, sense of, 131; development of, 105–10; and Dietary Goals for the United States, 118–24; dieters' experiences/cultural limitations, 103, 129–32; in diverse settings, 126–29; guidelines for diet and exercise, 110–13; legacy of, 135–39; letters of testimonial, 130–31, 229n125; Longevity Center, 113–16; Longevity Center, investigation of, 119; medical record-keeping and credibility, 116–18

The Pritikin Program for Diet and Exercise (Pritikin), 111

processed food, 10, 97; avoidance of, 32–33; and beriberi, 66; Stare's support for, 141–42; taste for, 125

Progressive Era, 50

prolotherapy, 170

Protein Power, 150

Pure, White and Deadly (Yudkin), 149

Pure Food and Drug Act (1906), 94–95

Quackwatch, 243–244n163. *See also* anti-quackery

Quaker Oats, 129

racism: anti-Asian, 64–67, 89; impact on chronic disease, 25–28; and macrobiotics, 55; medical racism, 44–45; structural, 26–27; white supremacy and white-normativity, 37–38, 43, 50–51, 101

Radiant Health through Nutrition (Fulton), 18

radiation: as cancer treatment, 77–81; radiation poisoning, recovery from, 72–75, 92

Rastafarian immigrants, 33

Recalled by Life (Sattilaro), 79

Reese, Della, 23

restaurant dining: macrobiotic restaurants, 55, 61, 71; Pritikin approach to, 126–28; soul food restaurants, 28–29, 30–31, 33

Revici, Emanuel, 80

rice: brown rice, role in macrobiotic diet, 70, 212n18; brown vs. white, 57, 65–66; rice cakes, 71; rice diet for kidney disease, 107

Rizzo, Joseph, 172

Roberts, Julia, 165

Robinson, Miles, 143

Rockefeller Foundation, 97

Rodale, Jerome, 48–49, 193

Rodale Press, 49

Rogak, Lisa, 167

royal jelly, 168

Runner's World (magazine), 96

running/jogging culture, 7, 100–101, 193, 196. *See also* exercise and fitness trends

saccharin, 172

salt ratio theory (macrobiotics), 56–58

sanpaku, concept of, 68, 192, 214n60

San Quentin Prison study, 20

Sattilaro, Anthony, 78–80, 81

Sayers, Gale, 23

Schaller, Lorenz K., 74

Schier, Monty, 69

Schweitzer, Albert, 61

science, distrust of, 185–86

Scrinis, Gyorgi, 103

Sears, Barry, 173

sea vegetables/seaweed, 76, 88

Select Committee on Nutrition and Human Needs, 156

714X supplement, 168

Shapin, Steven, 162

shark cartilage, 168

Shell, Ellen Ruppel, 166

Shim, Janet, 29

Shoku-Yo Kai (Food Cure Society), 58–59, 87

Silicon Valley, influence of, 195